PUBLIC HEALTH IN THE 21ST CENTURY

ADVANCES IN DRUG RESISTANCE RESEARCH

PUBLIC HEALTH IN THE 21ST CENTURY

MICHAEL W. POPEJOY - SERIES EDITOR

FLORIDA INTERNATIONAL UNIVERSITY, MIAMI, FLORIDA, USA

Advances in Drug Resistance Research

Christudas Morais (Editor)

2014. ISBN: 978-1-63117-131-4

PUBLIC HEALTH IN THE 21ST CENTURY

ADVANCES IN DRUG RESISTANCE RESEARCH

CHRISTUDAS MORAIS
EDITOR

NOVA BIOMEDICAL

New York

For permission to use material from this book please contact us:
Telephone 631-231-7269; Fax 631-231-8175
Web Site: http://www.novapublishers.com

Additional color graphics may be available in the e-book version of this book.

Library of Congress Cataloging-in-Publication Data

ISBN: 978-1-63117-131-4
LCCN: 2013958458

Published by Nova Science Publishers, Inc. † New York

Contents

Preface

Advances in the understanding of the molecular mechanisms of various diseases have helped the development and implementation of novel therapeutics in clinical practice. Unfortunately patients develop resistance to chemotherapeutics. There are two types of resistance to drug treatment, intrinsic and extrinsic. Intrinsic resistance commonly refers to the innate insensitivity of cells to drug treatment. In contrast, in extrinsic or acquired resistance, the cells are initially sensitive to treatment, but progressively become insensitive. Extrinsic resistance often correlates with time. This book examines the biochemical and molecular mechanisms of innate and extrinsic drug resistance and their clinical relevance. The nine chapters in this book, written by a group of scientists and clinicians, provide an excellent synopsis of the advances in our understanding of drug resistance.

Chapter 1 gives an in-depth view of mechanisms of resistance to cisplatin. In particular, this chapter focuses on the role of deregulated DNA damage repair process, suppressed apoptotic signalling, and clonality as means of developing cisplatin resistance.

Chapter 2 discusses the role of p-glycoprotein and multi-drug resistance molecules, especially the ABC transporters, in drug resistance. It also focuses on the advances made in the field of natural products as effective chemotherapeutics and how they can be used to overcome drug resistance.

Chapter 3 summarizes the different types and origins of fibroblast population that exist within solid tumors, their roles in dictating the response of tumors to therapies and the underlying mechanisms by which the dynamic tumor-fibroblast cell interaction provide a protective niche for tumor cells to escape from cytotoxic effects of chemotherapy.

Chapter 4 gives a comprehensive review of resistance to erythropoiesis stimulating agents (ESA), especially erythropoietin (EPO). EPO is administered to correct anemia in patients with chronic kidney disease. This chapter discusses the causes, epidemiology, clinical sequelae and management of ESA resistance.

Chapters 5 and 6 address the challenges of drug resistance in prostate cancer. Because prostate cancer cells depend on androgen and its receptor for their growth and survival, targeting the androgen signalling has been the major avenue of treatment. However, resistance to therapy continues to be one of the major hurdles for the successful treatment of prostate cancer. These chapters discuss the findings and limitations from ongoing and completed clinical trials, potential mechanisms of therapy resistance, approaches to overcome resistance and future challenges.

Chapters 7-9 cover a number of issues related to drug resistance in renal cell carcinoma. Until the introduction of targeted therapy, immunotherapy used to be the mainstay of treatment for metastatic renal cell carcinoma. Chapter 7 presents an overview of chemotherapy and immunotherapy resistance in metastatic renal cell carcinoma. Despite the initial clinical benefits of targeted therapies, resistance develops after a median of 5–11 months of treatment. Chapter 8 summarizes the current challenges of drug resistance in the effective treatment of metastatic RCC. Chapter 9 specifically focuses on the extrinsic and intrinsic mechanisms of sunitinib resistance in renal cell carcinoma.

It has been a pleasure working with the authors. I am grateful to all the authors for their generosity in sharing their expertise and experience to the scientific community through this book. I am confident this book will be an important contribution to science, and an invaluable tool for researchers who are interested in drug resistance.

Christudas Morais, MSc, MPhil, PhD

In: Advances in Drug Resistance Research
Editor: Christudas Morais
ISBN: 978-1-63117-131-4

Chapter 1

Mechanisms of Cisplatin Resistance: DNA Repair and Cellular Implications

Mark N. Adams [*1,2], ***Nicholas W. Ashton*** [1,2], ***Nicolas Paquet*** [1,2], ***Ken O'Byrne*** [1,2] ***and Derek J. Richard*** [1,2]

[1]Institute of Health and Biomedical Innovation, Queensland University of Technology, Brisbane, Australia

[2]Translational Research Institute, Brisbane, Australia

Abstract

Cisplatin (cis-diamminedichloroplatinum (II)), is a platinum based chemotherapeutic employed in the clinic to treat patients with lung, ovarian, colorectal or head and neck cancers. Cisplatin acts to induce tumor cell death via multiple mechanisms. The best characterized mode of action is through irreversible DNA cross-links which activate DNA damage signals leading to cell death via the intrinsic mitochondrial apoptosis pathway. However, the primary issue with cisplatin is that while patients initially respond favorably, sustained cisplatin therapy often yields chemoresistance resulting in therapeutic failure. In this

[*] Translational Research Institute, 37 Kent Street, Woolloongabba, Queensland, Australia. Email: mn.adams@qut.edu.au.

chapter, we review the DNA damage and repair pathways that contribute to cisplatin resistance. We also examine the cellular implications of cisplatin resistance that may lead to selection of subpopulations of cells within a tumor. In better understanding the mechanisms conferring cisplatin resistance, novel targets may be identified to restore drug sensitivity.

Keywords: Cisplatin resistance, interstrand cross-links, DNA repair, tumor-initiating cell

Introduction

Cisplatin, (cis-diamminedichloroplatinum (II), or CDDP) was first approved for clinical use in 1978 for treatment of testicular and bladder cancers [1]. The observed anti-tumor effects have led to the use of cisplatin as a frontline chemotherapeutic in the treatment regimens for patients with lung, ovarian, colorectal or head and neck cancers [1-3]. While still clinically relevant today, cisplatin has also spawned the platinum-based drug derivatives carboplatin and oxaliplatin. Patients treated with these platinum-based drugs display early therapeutic success with disease regression or a halt in further progression. As with many chemotherapeutic options, adverse events exist for cisplatin with observed kidney, peripheral nerve and inner ear toxicity [4, 5]. Yet the primary issue with cisplatin therapy is that despite initial therapy successes, many patients eventually develop resistant disease [6-8]. Notably, cisplatin refractory disease is also cross-resistant to carboplatin [9]. Given that cisplatin based therapies remain the sole therapeutic option in certain circumstances [10], it is key that the underlying mechanisms potentiating resistance are uncovered.

Mode of Action

As a platinum based compound, cisplatin is inert but is activated through a series of aquation reactions. The aquation process involves the spontaneous substitution of one or both cis-chloro groups with water molecules in the cytoplasm [11, 12]. This process makes aquated cisplatin highly reactive toward intracellular nucleophiles [13]. It is this process that yields the anticancer effects of cisplatin through reactions within the cytoplasm and nucleus. Within the cytoplasm, cisplatin reacts with nucleophiles such as methionine, metallothioneins, reduced glutathione (GSH) and proteins via cysteine residues. In this way, cytoplasmic cisplatin may act like a molecular sponge for reduced species and push a cell towards oxidative stress. Recent evidence that enucleated cytoplasts are responsive to cisplatin further highlights the cytotoxic effects of the cytoplasmic cisplatin module [14, 15]. However, these cytoplasmic reactions may also serve to inactivate cisplatin through antioxidant systems [7].

The best characterized mode of action for cisplatin is via its reactivity with DNA. In the nucleus, aquated cisplatin interacts with high affinity toward nucleophilic N7-sites of purine bases to form interstrand and intrastrand DNA cross-links [16]. However, the cytotoxic effects of nuclear cisplatin are largely caused by the intrastrand DNA cross-links which account for 90% of cisplatin-induced DNA lesions [17, 18]. These lesions distort the DNA structure allowing multiple DNA damage signals to be initiated [19]. One of the initiated signals involves the nucleotide excision repair (NER) complex. This system recognises the distorted DNA and attempts to remove adducts to enable cell survival [20]. Other DNA damage signals involve the mismatch repair (MMR) and base excision repair (BER) systems. Herein, the components of these complexes sense the DNA lesions and commence the signals instructing cell fate [21-23]. Hence, the cell will initially attempt to repair the cisplatin-induced DNA lesion through one of the listed DNA repair mechanisms (see above). However, the cytotoxicity of cisplatin relies on overwhelming incidence of the adducts, as well as the high proliferative rate of the tumor. This leaves the repair of DNA largely unattainable. As a result, cell death will ensue predominantly via the apoptotic cascade.

The key link between DNA damage and apoptosis involves the ataxia telangiectasia mutated (ATM)-and Rad3-related (ATR) kinase and the checkpoint kinase 1 (CHK1). Cisplatin-dependent sequential activation of ATR and CHK1 leads to activation and stabilization of tumor suppressor p53 through phosphorylation at serine 20 [24-27]. p53 is the central mediator of cisplatin-induced apoptosis. In cisplatin-sensitive cells, p53 induces apoptosis via both nuclear and cytoplasmic mechanisms. In the nucleus, p53 transcriptionally up-regulates genes involved in cell cycle arrest and DNA repair [28] as well as multiple pro-apoptotic genes including *NOXA* [29] and *Bax* [30]. These pro-apoptotic factors are involved in initiation of the complex intrinsic mitochondrial apoptosis pathway [31]. Cisplatin induces the p53-mediated localization of both NOXA and Bax to the mitochondria yielding the release of cytochrome *c* which activates caspase-dependent apoptosis [32, 33].

In particular, the balance of cell fate is hinged upon the ratio of Bax with the anti-apoptotic Bcl-2. In cisplatin-sensitive cells, Bcl-2 is lost via proteolysis enabling activation of the apoptosis cascade [34, 35]. Interestingly, cisplatin is also reported to induce apoptosis via mitochondria independent mechanisms, but nonetheless utilizing the caspase 8-caspase 3 pathway via p53 [36, 37].

Mechanisms of Cisplatin Resistance

It is clear that multiple mechanisms are active in sensitizing cells to cisplatin. Alterations to any of these pathways underlie the cisplatin resistant phenotype observed in the clinic. As such, cisplatin resistance can ensue from (i) reduced intracellular cisplatin uptake, (ii) increased efflux of cisplatin from the cell as well as (iii) an enhanced ability of cells to repair cisplatin-induced DNA distortions. Herein, describing the mechanisms relating to cisplatin uptake and drug efflux go largely beyond the scope of this chapter but are adequately reviewed elsewhere [38, 39].

In the following sections we describe three potential mechanisms through which cisplatin resistance may occur, with an especial emphasis on processes downstream of DNA lesion formation. In this sense, we focus on the deregulation of DNA damage repair and suppressed apoptotic signalling as means of developing cisplatin resistance. Also, the role of tumor clonality in cisplatin resistance is discussed.

Deregulation of DNA Damage Repair

As discussed in previous sections, the nucleophilic attack of aquated cisplatin on purine bases can result in the formation of three major lesion types (i) bulky cisplatin adducts on singular purines, (ii) intrastrand cross-links between bases on the same strand and (iii) interstrand cross-links between bases on opposing strands (Figure 1) [40]. In each instance, the cell will initially respond by launching a DNA damage response in an attempt to remove the lesion. This response will vary depending on the nature of the adduct, as well as on the cell cycle phase. For instance, while nucleotide excision repair (NER) is likely the major pathway for removal of cisplatin bulky adducts and intrastrand cross-links outside of S phase of the cell cycle [41], translesion synthesis and/or repair by homologous recombination may represent significant pathways during replication [42]. Furthermore, while intrastrand cross-links may be processed efficiently by translesion repair alone during replication, the overcoming of interstrand cross-links probably involves proteins of the Fanconi anemiahomologous recombination pathway (see below) [43]. While most likely representing minor repair roles, base excision repair and mismatch repair of cisplatin adducts may represent important mechanisms of 'sensing' cisplatin-mediated DNA damage [44].

Here we describe the known DNA repair pathways involved in the recognition and repair of cisplatin adducts, and discuss some of the recognised mechanisms through which resistance may occur.

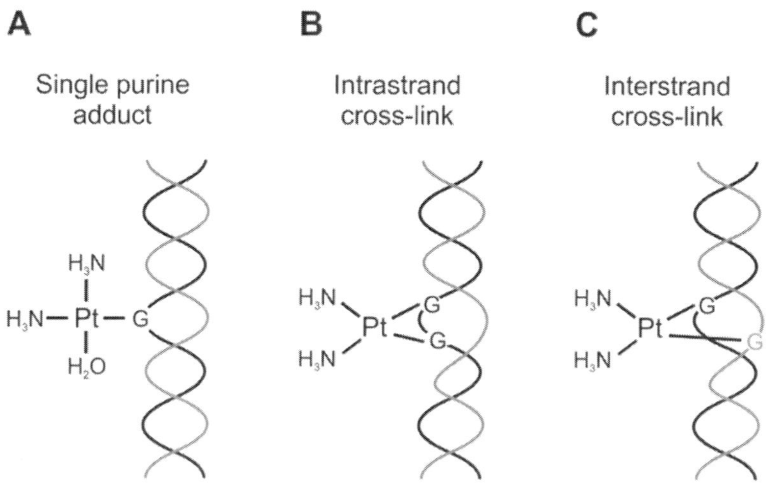

Figure 1. Cisplatin-induced DNA adducts. The predominant DNA adducts caused by cisplatin include (*A*) bulky cisplatin adducts on singular purines, (*B*) intrastrand cross-links between bases on the same strand and (*C*) interstrand cross-links between bases on opposing strands.

Mismatch Repair and Base Excision Repair

Mismatch repair (MMR) is an important cellular pathway in the correction of endogenous polymerase-mediated replication errors [22, 23]. Additionally, MMR may be involved in the repair of small DNA lesions e.g. those caused by alkylating agents [45]. In the earliest instance, base-mismatches are recognized by one of two MutS heterodimers; MutSα (MSH2/MSH6), which binds singular base mismatches or insertions, or MutSβ (MSH2/MSH3), which recognizes larger distortions [46-48]. These complexes are then able to recruit one of three MutL complexes, MutLα (MLH1/PMS2), MutLβ (MLH1/PMS1), or MutLγ (MLH1/MLH3), which, in concert with proliferating cell nuclear antigen (PCNA) and replication factor C (RFC), are able to unwind the helix at the damage site [49, 50]. Exonuclease 1 (EXO1) may then degrade a section of the damaged strand, including the mismatch/lesion, which is replaced by the concerted efforts of DNA polymerase and DNA ligase [51].

Although MMR is not able to repair cisplatin adducts, the MutSβ heterodimer has been documented to interact with cisplatin intrastrand cross-links [52, 53]. Here it is able to recruit MutL complexes, which, being unable to repair the damage, initiate pro-apoptotic signals; this process represents a key aspect of cisplatin-mediated toxicity [54-56]. It is therefore not surprising that these events are often suppressed in cancer cells which are resistant to cisplatin. In particular, the MutS components MSH2, MSH3, and MSH6, as well as MLH1 of the MutL complex, are often under-expressed or mutated in cancer cells displaying platinum resistance [57-61].

The pathway of base excision repair (BER) has also recently been suggested to impact on cisplatin-lesion repair [62]. This pathway primarily functions in the removal of small base damages, primarily as a result of base oxidation or alkylation [21]. DNA adducts are initially recognized by a specific DNA glycosylase, the identity of which depends on the type of base damage [63]. In the case of cisplatin interstrand cross-links, a new model has suggested that adjacent 'extra-helical' bases that have been disrupted by the crosslink may be subject to glycosylase recognition. This is predicted to initiate a pathway of non-productive processing in which the disrupted base is deaminated by the glycosylase, leaving an abasic residue [62]. The phosphodiester backbone is then most likely cleaved by AP endonuclease 1 (APE1), and the residue replaced by DNA polymerase-mediated strand synthesis; the cisplatin cross-link will however remain. While this pathway does not seem to initiate apoptotic signaling akin to that stimulated by MMR, the localization of BER proteins may preclude other DNA repair proteins from binding the site of damage, preventing the proper clearance of the lesion [44]. In this model, and similarly to MMR, BER seems to function in non-reparative cisplatin adduct recognition; unlike MMR however, BER protein localization is likely to suppress apoptosis induction. In agreement, the increased expression of APE1, DNA polymerase β and human 8-oxoguanine DNA glycosylase (hOGG1) has been attributed with cisplatin resistance, presumably through suppression of this signalling [64-66].

Nucleotide Excision Repair

Nucleotide excision repair (NER) represents an important pathway for the repair of a large number of structurally varied DNA adducts [67]. These lesions are seemingly recognized as a result of their disruption to base pairing, and the resulting helical distortion, more so than by their specific chemical nature [68]. In keeping, NER has been found to be the major pathway involved in the removal of cisplatin adducts, and as such, is up-regulated in many platinum-resistant tumors [69, 70].

In the initial stages of NER, damage is recognized by a complex composed of the proteins XPC and hHR23B, which appear to initiate unwinding on either side of the lesion [71]. This is further stimulated by the helicase activity of the TFIIH transcription factor, as well as by XPA and replication protein A (RPA) [72], which help expand the bubble. The exposed adduct may then be excised by the concerted efforts of two major nucleases, XPF-ERCC1, which cleaves the phosphodiester backbone 5` to the lesions, and XPG, which cleaves on the 3` side [73, 74]. These events allow for the removal of an approximately 24-32 nucleotide signal stranded oligomer containing the lesion [75]. This gap may then be replaced by the activities of DNA polymerases δ and ε, which use the intact complementary strand as a template, followed by closing of the phosphate backbone by DNA ligase 1-mediated ligation [76].

While the above seems to reflect the NER response to singular cisplatin adducts and intrastrand cross-links [77-79], the response to interstrand cross-links is apparently more complex. This is most likely due to the damage caused to both strands of the helix, such that neither can function as an appropriate repair template. While a large proportion of cisplatin interstrand cross-links are repaired by translesion repair and homologous recombination during S phase [43, 80, 81], there is compounding evidence that an NER-translesion repair pathway may exist during G1/G0 [82-84]. Following recognition of DNA interstrand cross-links, the NER nucleases are suggested to cleave the phosphodiester backbone on either side of the adduct as per above [85], leaving the 'excised' oligomer covalently bound to the opposing strand through the base crosslink. The cell is then able to bridge the gap by action of a specialized class of DNA polymerases known as translesion polymerases (discussed further below), which are able to insert bases opposite the damage site, although with an increased likelihood of introducing base mismatches when compared to those involved in replication [82, 86, 87]. The remaining 'excised' oligomer, and the section of the opposing strand to which it is bound, is then presumably cleaved and resolved by a second NER excision event [88].

Due to the apparent capacity of the NER system to remove each form of cisplatin adduct, it is not surprising that an upregulation of this pathway is frequently observed as a means of conferring cisplatin resistance. As may be expected, the expression of multiple NER repair proteins has been found to negatively correlate with cisplatin sensitivity, including that of ERCC1 [89-92], XPA [91, 93], and XPC [94]. In the case of XPA, expression levels appear to be regulated by the hypoxia-inducible factor-1α (HIF-1α) [93], an essential transcription factor in the response to hypoxic conditions. Contrasting this, low-level expression of HIF-1α has been correlated with better overall survival in patients with small-cell lung cancer who receive platinum-based chemotherapy, indicating HIF-1 α-mediated NER de-regulation may not be a key mechanism of resistance [95]. In addition, p53-mediated transcriptional regulation of a number of NER proteins also seems to promote resistance to a number of cross-linking agents [96]. For example, acquired cisplatin-resistance in a subset of malignant melanoma cells has recently been attributed to p53-dependent transcriptional up-regulation of XPC [94]. Further, the translational synthesis of XPA, XPC, hHR23B and the RPA subunit RPA32 has also been found to be negatively regulated by eukaryotic initiation factor-3a (eIF3a), the expression of which has been positively correlated with sensitivity to cisplatin [97, 98]. As opposed to deregulated NER protein expression, platinum resistance has also been correlated with gene polymorphic status. Of note, SNPs in *ERCC1* have received recent attention, with a number of studies suggesting an association between some of these variants and cisplatin sensitivity [91, 99-101].

Classical Translesion Repair

Although the NER pathway is able to remove most forms of bulky adduct, in some instances, lesions are able to sustain into S phase. This is especially true of interstrand cross-links, which for this reason, were originally thought only to be processed by homologous recombination. Two possible explanations have been put forward regarding this inefficiency: (i) that interstrand cross-links are not always efficiently recognized when occurring in highly condensed chromatin [43], and (ii) that some of these damage events may be incompletely removed due to their chemical complexity [102].

By any means, the sustainment of bulky DNA adducts into S phase represents a considerable obstacle for the migrating replicative fork, as the processive δ and ε DNA polymerases are not able to insert opposite damaged bases [103]. Additionally, the covalent crosslinking of opposing DNA strands may prevent helicase-mediated unwinding ahead of the fork [104]. In either instance, replication is forced to stall until such time that the adduct is repaired or bypassed.

The pathways of translesion repair and homologous recombination are currently recognized as the major cellular strategies involved in re-starting stalled replicative forks. In the majority of instances, the choice between the two pathways appears largely governed by the mono-ubiquitination of the PCNA sliding clamp, which seems to promote the recruitment of a number of translesion polymerases. The overcoming of interstrand cross-links seems the main exception to this rule (discussed in subsequent sections), where cross-over between the two pathways is apparent [81, 105, 106].

The translesion polymerases largely consist of proteins from the Y-family of polymerases (polη, ι, κ and Rev1), as well as polζ of the B-polymerase family. In response to fork stalling, these polymerases may be recruited to sites of damage, largely as a result of Rad18/Rad6 mediated-mono-ubiquitination of PCNA [107]. PCNA is a central protein in the recruitment and activity of both replicative and translesion polymerases, although its mono-ubiquitination seems to increase its affinity for the later [108]. Although each of the translesion polymerases initially seems to interact with PCNA, 'competition' for bypass of the lesion is resolved by the differing substrate specificities of each enzyme, such that the adduct is overcome by the most appropriate polymerase(s). In the bypass of cisplatin bulky adducts and intrastrand cross-links, the translesion polymerases Polη [109-111], Polζ [112, 113], and Rev1 [114-116] seem to play the most important roles.

Consistent with our discussion on the NER pathway, an upregulation of the translesion synthesis pathway has been associated with cisplatin-resistance. Of particular note, expression of Rev3, the catalytic subunit of Polζ, has been correlated with cisplatin-resistance in head and neck [117] and cervical tumors [118]. Furthermore, suppression of Rev3 in cisplatin-resistant cells in culture [117] and *in vivo* [119] resulted in re-sensitization to platinum therapy, suggesting this as a driving factor of resistance. While increased clearance of cisplatin adducts is likely the major outcome of increased Rev3 expression, the inherent mutagenicity of Polζ translesion replication has also been cited as a potential mechanism of resistance development [120, 121].

In addition to Polζ, a positive correlation between Polη protein expression and platinum resistance has also been observed [122, 123]. Polη represents the major polymerase in the bypass of GpG intrastrand cross-links, where it is able to bypass the lesion in an essentially error-free manner [124]. For this reason, and unlike Polζ, the apparent cisplatin-resistance phenotype afforded by Polη is likely to result purely from increased repair capacity, and not from increased mutagenic rate.

Homologous Recombination at the Replication Fork

As discussed above, cisplatin induces interstrand cross-links which block the DNA replication fork by preventing DNA strand separation. To enable cell survival, restoration of replication by removal and repair of the interstrand cross-link is required. As described in detail below, this process involves interplay between factors involved in homologous recombination double strand break repair as well as members of the Fanconi anemia pathway [43]. Indeed, cells deficient in homologous recombination proteins (such as BRCA1 or BRCA2) or Fanconi anemia proteins, exhibit an increased sensitivity to cisplatin [125].

However, these factors alone are insufficient for DNA repair with other repair pathways, such as base and nucleotide excision repair, or translesion repair, required to complete DNA repair. Despite the contribution of additional pathways, homologous recombination is the primary pathway through which DNA cross-links are removed to allow replication to restart.

Homologous recombination is a series of interrelated pathways that repair DNA double strand breaks in an error free manner by using DNA strand invasion and template directed DNA synthesis. As shown in Figure 2, the initial step of repair requires the processing of the break to generate a 3' overhanging tail of ssDNA that is initially coated and protected by the ssDNA binding protein RPA [126]. Subsequently, BRCA2 (FANCD1) functions to remove and replace RPA with RAD51 to allow formation of the pre-synaptic filament [127].

This RAD51 nucleofilament is involved in the search for and annealing with the homologous template; a process called strand invasion. The newly formed structure is termed a D-loop, where the invading strand is elongated using the invaded duplex DNA as a template [128].

The capture and annealing of the second end of the double strand break is catalyzed by the RAD52 protein and generates a structure called double Holliday junction [129].

This structure of interlaced DNA strands is dissolved in a non cross-over product by a complex formed by the DNA helicase Bloom (BLM) and the topoisomerase TOPOIIIα, ultimately achieving an error- free repair of the DNA break [130].

Repair pathways are activated when replication forks collide with an interstrand cross-link during S phase, blocking the replisome (Figure 3). When one fork encounters such a block, the spontaneous collapsing of the fork generates a one-ended double-strand break.

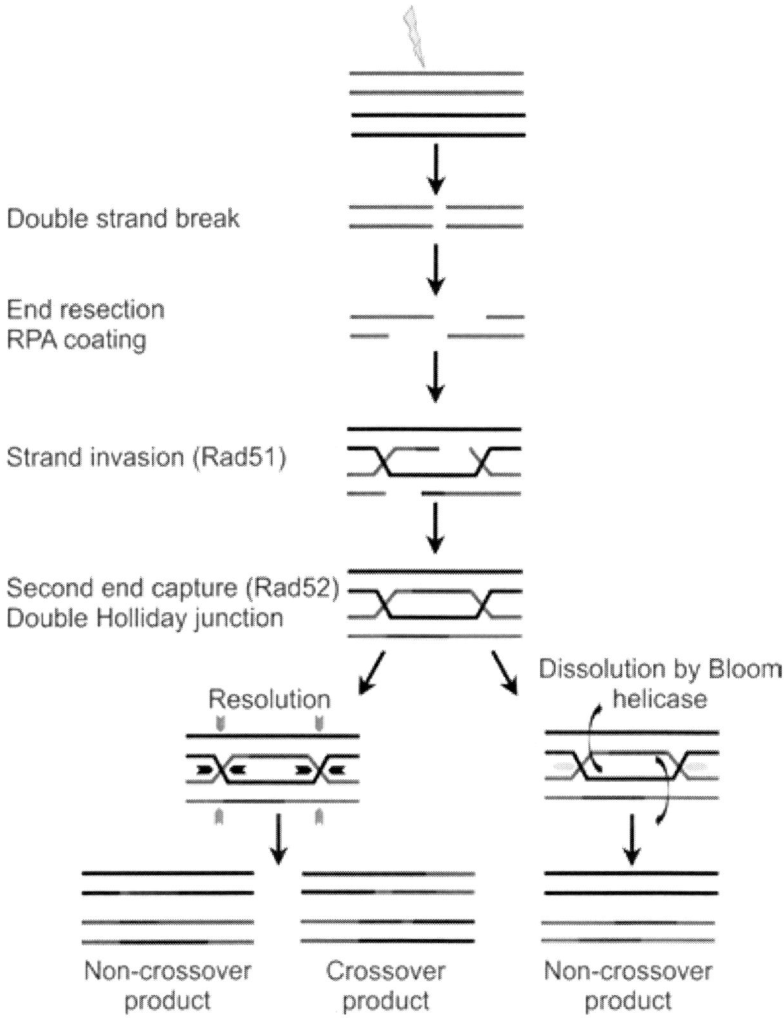

Figure 2. Repair of DNA double strand breaks (DSB) by homologous recombination. Following a DNA double strand break, the DNA is recessed forming a 3' overhang, allowing coating of the ssDNA with RPA. RPA is replaced by Rad51 initiating the search and annealing with a homologous template (strand invasion) to create a D-loop. A double Holliday junction is then formed when the opposite DNA strand from the break anneals to the D-loop strand. The Holliday junction is resolved either creating a chromatid crossover product or non-crossover product.

The repair of the collapsed fork then requires the invasion of the broken strand into the intact double strand of DNA, this pathway is mediated by RAD51, which catalyses the strand invasion, similar to the one use in homologous recombination (see above). The interstrand cross-link is cleaved by the MUS81-EME1 endonuclease complex allowing the bypass of the lesion [131]. The broken leading strand is then extended by translesion synthesis polymerases, completing the homologous recombination. Following this process, replication can then restart.

As shown in Figure 3, such collapses can be avoided by FANCM-mediated fork regression and fork stabilization. Following unhooking of the cross-linked DNA, this stabilized structure allows the leading strand of synthesized DNA to be extended by the translesion synthesis machinery. The one-ended double strand break is then processed and repaired by homologous recombination followed by replication restart. In this setting, the protein FANCM, in complex with FAAP24 and the MHF1/2 histone-fold dimer, recognizes the helix distortion caused by the interstrand cross-link [132]. The specificity of binding for the stalled fork seems to be provided by FAAP24. Although FANCM is a helicase, the protein is not able to catalyze strand separation. Rather, FANCM acts as a dsDNA translocase by remodelling the fork to permit processing and extensive fork regression [133]. At the same time, FANCM/FAAP24 activate an interstrand cross-link specific ATR-CHK1 mediated response, by its ability to generate a ssDNA stretch that is rapidly coated by RPA [134].

Independent of this signalling function, FANCM/FAAP24 recruits the Fanconi anemia core complex to the stalled fork. This complex, which is formed by eight Fanconi anemia proteins (A/B/C/E/F/G/L/M), prevents the fork from collapsing [132, 135]. Together with the activation of the ATR pathway, the recruitment of the Fanconi anemia core complex promotes the monoubiquitination of the FANCD2/I complex, allowing its localization to the chromatin [136].

This modification is catalized by the E3 ligase activity of FANCL and is essential for the scaffolding role of FANCD2, which then binds the DNA repair protein FAN1 [137]. The nuclease FAN1 performs a nucleolytic incision on the 5' side of the lesion. The 3' side is cleaved by the MUS81/EME1 nucleases, finally promoting the unhooking of the cross-link, generating a double strand break and allowing the translesion synthesis polymerases to bypass the lesion. In addition to the recruitment of FAN1, the FANCD2/I complex enables recruitment of the proteins BRCA2 (FANCD1), FANCJ and PALB2 (FANCN) to the site of damage. This process leads to the formation of a RAD51 coated presynaptic filament initiating homologous recombination and replication restart.

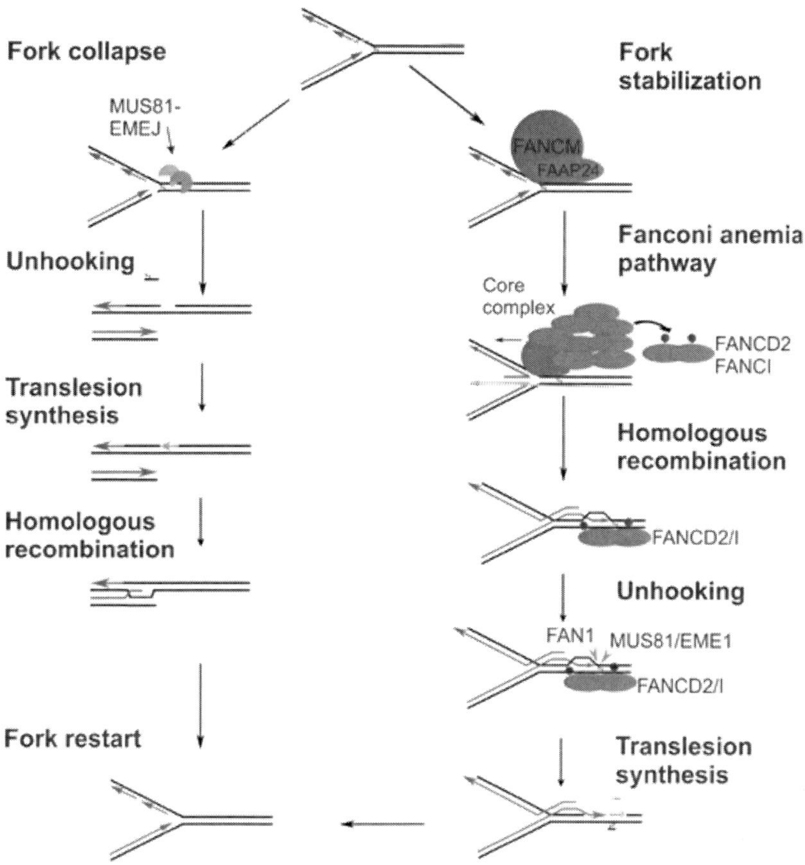

Figure 3. Speculative model of how Fanconi anaemia-associated proteins repair interstrand cross-links during DNA replication. Cisplatin induces an interstrand cross-link preventing progress of the DNA replication fork. Blockade of the replication fork causes either the fork to collapse (left) or the fork to stabilise (right). Replication can only restart after unhooking (removal) of the cross-linked DNA and DNA repair either by homologous recombination (left) or by the Fanconi anemiapathway (right).

An alternative scenario is when two replication forks, arriving from opposite directions, collide at the interstrand cross-link. In this instance, one fork stops 24 nucleotides ahead of the interstrand cross-link while the other fork stops only one nucleotide away from the damage. Each replication fork may be stabilized in a process similar to that of single fork stabilisation. In this way, adduct removal takes place by cutting the leading strand template at either side of the cross-link. A complex series of ligations and elongations of the DNA strands results in the formation of a typical Holliday junction structure. Replication can then restart after resolving the Holliday junction via a complex of multiple factors including BLM helicase, topoisomerase TOPIIIa, RMI1, RMI2 and RPA [138]. Interestingly, although BLM helicase has been shown to have multiple roles in cisplatin removal by the homologous recombination pathway, it has not yet been linked to acquired cisplatin resistance.

Fanconi Anemia and Homologous Recombination Proteins in Cisplatin Resistance

Fanconi anemia is a rare genetic disorder characterized by congenital abnormalities and progressive failure of bone marrow leading to increased susceptibility to haematological cancers [139]. Cells from these patients are highly sensitive to agents inducing interstrand cross-links, resulting in chromosomal aberrations [140]. As such, cisplatin therapy is not able to be used to treat these patients. Our knowledge of the Fanconi anemia and homologous recombination pathways in these patients is aiding out understanding of how these pathways contribute to cisplatin resistance in tumors. For example, hypersensitivity of some ovarian cancer cells to cisplatin is linked with disruption of the Fanconi anemia pathway. In this setting, cells lacking the monoubiquitinated form of FANCD2 are sensitive to cisplatin [141]. This is due to methylation of the FANCF gene lowering its expression. [141]. As part of the Fanconi anemia core complex, FANCF is involved in FANCD2/FANCI ubiquitnation. Interestingly, in cells acquiring cisplatin resistance, FANCF function is restored by endogenous gene demethylation, allowing monoubiquitination of FANCD2 [141]. Sensitivity of other ovarian cancer cells to cisplatin has also been linked with tumors exhibiting *BRCA2* gene mutations [142]. In these cells, prolonged exposure to cisplatin is reported to induced secondary intragenic mutations in *BRCA2* leading to restoration of the reading frame and rescue of gene function, ultimately resulting in cisplatin resistance [142]. A similar mechanism of cisplatin resistance was observed in ovarian cancer cells exhibiting *BRAC1* gene mutations [143]. Secondary mutations in *BRAC1* also yielded cisplatin resistance [143]. Together, these studies highlight the contribution of proteins involved in the Fanconi anemia and homologous recombination pathways to cisplatin resistance.

Suppressed Apoptosis as a Mechanism of Cisplatin Resistance

As discussed above, cisplatin-induced distortion of DNA structure initiates DNA damage signals that link with induction of the apoptotic signal cascade. However, in chemotherapy tolerant cells, failure to induce apoptosis following cisplatin treatment is a documented mechanism conferring drug resistance. A central player in this process is p53. Dysfunction of p53 is a key mechanism of apoptosis evasion with p53 inactivation through gene mutation present in over half of all neoplasms [144-146]. Consistently, in both *in vitro* and *in vivo* settings, cells harboring p53 defects have been linked with poor cisplatin sensitivity [147-149]. In the clinic, ovarian and testicular cancer patients exhibiting expression of wild type p53 are also likely to respond favorably to cisplatin therapy with improved 5-year survival rates compared with patients presenting with mutant p53 [150, 151]. The escape of apoptosis may indeed be context dependent, as there are several reports suggesting that mutant p53 expressing cells remain sensitive to cisplatin [149, 152-154]. Nonetheless, the *in vitro* evidence indicates that in cells expressing mutant p53, the predominant mechanism of cisplatin resistance is via an inability of p53 to initiate the downstream apoptotic cascades [155-159].

Cells expressing wildtype p53 are also capable of developing cisplatin tolerance and resistance. In these instances, mechanisms exist to attenuate p53 function other than by gene mutation. One such example in cisplatin resistant cells is the aberrant overexpression of MDM2, a negative feedback regulator of p53, and potential downregulation of the MDM2 inhibitor, $p14^{ARF}$ [160-163]. In another instance, oncogenic protein phosphatase magnesium-dependent 1 (PPM1D) is reported to confer cisplatin resistance by attenuating both p53 and CHK1 function through dephosphorylation and preventing their stabilization [164]. Mislocalization of p53 may also contribute to cisplatin resistance. For example, cytoplasmic mislocalized p53 is reported to interact with and inhibit caspase-9, allowing evasion of apoptosis [165]. In addition, mutational ablation of p53 nuclear localization signals, leading to cytoplasmic sequestration of p53, is also emerging as a mechanism for conferring cisplatin resistance [166, 167]. In this way, preventing p53 localization to the nucleus enables the manifestation of cisplatin resistance through an inability to transcriptionally upregulate the pro-apoptotic machinery.

Despite the dependence on p53 to decide cell fate, aberrant expression of factors downstream of p53 in the apoptotic cascade is also capable of influencing cisplatin resistance. For example, overexpression of the apoptotic inhibitors survivin and XIAP has been linked with enhancing cisplatin resistance by impacting caspase function [168, 169]. Similarly, overexpression of anti-apoptotic factors Bcl-2, Bcl-X_L and MCL-1 in cisplatin resistant cells is observed *in vitro* and in multiple cancers [170-173]. This is associated with the *in vitro* downregulation of the pro-apoptotic factors BAX and BAK in cisplatin resistance [31, 174, 175]. Together, these reports highlight the complex regulation of the apoptotic cascade involved in yielding cisplatin resistance.

Tumor Clonality in Cisplatin Resistance

In the previous sections, we have reviewed the complex DNA repair mechanisms and signalling pathways contributing to cisplatin tolerance and resistance. In the following sections, we describe the (i) cellular implications of cisplatin resistance within a tumor and (ii) review the current strategies to profile the genomic and epigenetic aspect to cisplatin resistant disease.

The spatial heterogeneity of tumors is a consequence of tumor evolution [176]. Selection pressures enhance survival of cell sub-populations and allow clonal relationships to form within a tumor. Next generation sequencing has exemplified the clonal nature of tumors within a number of primary cancers including breast [177, 178], prostate [179, 180], renal [181] and pancreatic [182, 183] cancers. While clonal relationships develop during tumor evolution as a result of oncogenic mutations [184] or genetic drift, recent evidence suggests that cisplatin also contributes to tumor clonality. For example, *in vitro* and *in vivo* cisplatin treatment of lung cancer cell lines and patient tissue caused an enrichment of 'stem-like' $CD133^+$ cells [185, 186]. Similarly, in tumors collected from ovarian cancer patients, primary platinum treatment enriched for cells expressing the stem-like markers aldehyde dehydrogenase, CD44 and CD133 [187].

An emerging paradigm in chemotherapy is that cells with stem-like characteristics, also termed tumor-initiating cells, are chemotherapeutic resistant [188, 189]. In particular, cisplatin-induced enrichment of these stem-like cells has been reported to confer drug resistance. For instance, Barr et al. showed that cisplatin-induced apoptosis in $CD133^+/CD44^+$ cells enriched from lung cancer cells was markedly reduced versus the bulk population of cells [190]. Moreover, these cells displayed a reduced uptake of cisplatin together with a reduced formation of DNA cross-links [190]. Consistently, in a separate study, $CD133^+$ enriched lung cancer cells with sphere forming characteristics had reduced cisplatin-induced PARP-dependent apoptosis [191]. Most interestingly, implantation of tumor-initiating spheres from H125 lung cancer cells also exhibited a cisplatin resistant phenotype *in vivo* [191]. Similar observations have shown that tumor-initiating cells isolated from other NSCLC cell lines also exhibit a cisplatin refractory phenotype [185, 192, 193].

Moreover, in ovarian cancer, tumor-initiating spheres exhibited cisplatin and paclitaxel resistance as mediated by the stem cell factor receptor c-Kit [194]. Indeed, these reports point to the likelihood that drug resistant tumor clones exhibiting stem-like characteristics contribute to recurrent disease.

How tumor-initiating cells remain refractory to chemotherapy is an active area of research but the mechanisms remain elusive. However, as discussed earlier in this chapter, evidence suggests that tumor-initiating cells also possess the means to evade cisplatin-induced apoptosis and confer drug resistance through the DNA damage repair pathways [195]. For example, a recent report demonstrates that DNA double strand break repair, as assessed by γH2AX foci, is enhanced in cisplatin resistant NSCLC cells enriched for tumor-initiating cell markers CD133^{+}/CD44' and ALDH [190]. Also in NSCLC cells, sphere forming tumor-initiating cells resistant to cisplatin were found to have higher basal levels of γH2AX yet diminished ATM phosphorylation and monoubiquitination of FANCD2 [191]. Pharmacological inhibition of ATM in NSCLC tumor-initiating cells before and during drug treatment also conferred cisplatin resistance [191]. However, further investigations are required to characterise the DNA repair mechanisms that contribute to cisplatin resistance in tumor-initiating cells.

A number of other cell signaling pathways appear to be active during the formation of cisplatin resistant tumor clones. One such pathway is the notch signaling pathway. Classically, notch signaling is particularly prevalent during development but also in stem cells [196, 197]. Activation of the membrane receptor notch by its mammalian ligand, Jagged, induces proteolysis of notch and translocation of the intracellular domain to the nucleus to modulate transcription [198]. Notch expression is associated with cisplatin resistance in a number of tumors including cervical cancer [199], head and neck squamous cell carcinoma (HNSCC) [200] and ovarian cancer [201]. More strikingly, notch signalling also contributes to acquiring cisplatin resistance. Inhibition of notch signalling by pharmacological or knockdown approaches sensitized drug resistant HNSCC cells [200, 202], cervical cancer cells [199], non-small cell lung cancer cells [203] and ovarian cancer cells [204] to cisplatin. Importantly, notch signalling is also a key feature in mediating cisplatin-induced enrichment of CD133^{+} cell subpopulations from lung adenocarcinoma cells [186]. Hence, the notch pathway presents as an interesting therapeutic target in cisplatin resistant cells.

Another pathway of interest in cisplatin resistance is the WNT/β-catenin signalling pathway. The WNTs couple to a complex network of receptors and co-receptors to activate canonical (β-catenin dependent) or non-canonical (β-catenin independent) downstream signaling [205]. These signaling pathways contribute to mammalian development and stem cell proliferation [206]. Recently, the canonical WNT/β-catenin is also suggested to contribute to cisplatin resistance. In drug resistant triple negative breast cancer, WNT signalling via the receptor FZD8 is reported to contribute to *in vivo* tumor-initiating cell enrichment induced by the combinational treatment of cisplatin with TRAIL [207]. Similarly, in chemoresistant ovarian cancer, activation of the WNT/β-catenin signalling pathway by c-Kit confers cisplatin resistance in tumor-initiating cells by upregulating the ABC drug transporter ABCG2 [194]. Notably, both β-catenin and ABCG2 are overexpressed in chemoresistant and recurrent ovarian carcinoma [187, 208]. Further indication that WNT/β-catenin signalling may contribute to drug resistance is the observation that the potent WNT signalling inhibitor Dkk-1 is downregulated in cisplatin resistant glioma cells [209] and head-neck cancer cells [210].

Genomic and Epigenetic Profiling of Cisplatin Resistant Disease

It is clear that cisplatin induces tumor clonality by enriching for drug resistant tumor-initiating cells via several signalling pathways. However, the genetic basis that drives these mechanisms remains unknown. In chemotherapeutic refractory disease, use of genomic profiling has identified mutations and pathways that drive resistance [211, 212]. For example, secondary mutations in KRAS are detected in the blood of colorectal cancer patients undergoing anti-EGFR therapies that confer drug resistance [213, 214]. As discussed earlier in this chapter, secondary mutations on the *BRCA1* and *BRCA2* genes have been discovered in response to cisplatin therapy [142, 143]. However, only a handful of studies have investigated the wider genetic component to cisplatin refractory cancer. In one such study, sequential exome sequencing of circulating tumor DNA from an ovarian cancer patient over a period of 2 years identified an increase in a truncating mutation of the retinoblastoma 1 (RB1) gene [215]. Interestingly, loss of RB1 function is linked with a varied chemotherapeutic response in breast and prostate cancers [216]. In addition, genetic profiling of copy number variants (CNVs) has identified genetic changes in response cisplatin [217]. In particular, 70 cisplatin-associated CNVs were identified (66 as biallelic) of which 87% were deleterious. Of interest, one of the duplicated CNVs predicted the expression of glutathione reductase [217], which is associated with cisplatin sensitivity [218].

In addition to genomic changes in cisplatin resistance, it is also clear that epigenetic changes may contribute to drug resistance. Changes in methylation of CpG islands in cisplatin resistant cells leading to gene downregulation are well documented [219-222]. One example is methylation-dependent downregulation of *MLH1* expression, which is a component of the MMR DNA repair pathway [223]. Cisplatin-induced loss of *MLH1* expression occurs in 25-30% of ovarian cancer patients and is associated with poor patient prognosis [223, 224]. Use of genome-wide DNA methylation profiling is also revealing potential epigenetic drivers of cisplatin resistance. For example, use of demethylating agents and microarray analysis identified several hundered genes downregulated in isogenic cisplatin resistant cancer cells [219]. In this study, bisulfite sequencing also confirmed that 14 genes were hypermethylated in resistant cells but that expression of six of these genes (*SAT*, *C8orf4*, *LAMB3*, *TUBB*, *G0S2*, *MCAM*) were induced following cisplatin treatment in sensitive cells but not resistant cells [219]. More recently, use of isogenic sensitive and resistant ovarian cancer cells has also identified a large array of hypermethylated genes [222]. In this study, of the identified 4092 hypermethylated genes, only 245 genes were silenced while demethylation of 41 of these genes led to cisplatin resensitization [222]. Interestingly, 4 of these 41 genes (*ARMCX2*, *COL1A1*, *MEST*, and *MLH1*) were found to be hypermethylated following acquisition of cisplatin resistance in TICs from IGROV1 ovarian cancer cells [222].

The state of chromatin is also implicated in cisplatin tolerance via histone deacetylases (HDAC). HDACs modify histones enabling chromatin maintenance and transcription. HDAC4 silencing is reported to sensitize drug resistant ovarian cancer cells to cisplatin via a mechanism dependent on STAT1 [225]. Consistently, early use of HDAC inhibitors in drug resistant ovarian cancer cells resensitized cells to cisplatin through an induction of the intrinsic apoptosis pathway independent of p53 [226]. Interestingly, use of HDAC inhibitors has also led to the re-expression of several methylated genes [227, 228], notably *MLH1* in both *in vitro* and *in vivo* settings [229]. Importantly, modified chromatin structure has also been linked with drug resistant TICs. Sharma et al. reported that HDAC inhibitors also yield cisplatin sensitivity in tumor-initiating cells but that chromatin state is altered by the histone demethylase RBP2/KDM5A/Jarid1A in these cells [230].

Together, these studies point to a genetic and epigenetic component to cellular responsiveness to cisplatin. However, further efforts are required to genotype the tumor clones resistant to cisplatin therapy. In particular, monitoring disease before and during cisplatin therapy will elucidate further genetic and epigenetic components as well as pathways leading to chemotherapy refractory disease.

Conclusion

How tumors affect cisplatin resistance is the key issue facing healthcare providers. As discussed in this chapter, there are distinct mechanisms yielding drug resistance through the DNA damage and repair pathways as well as via attenuation of the apoptotic cascade. These signalling pathways are seemingly active within the context of tumor, with subpopulations of cells intrinsically refractory to cisplatin therapy. It is important to note that cisplatin resistance is no doubt multifactorial. Therefore, understanding the multiple mechanisms that are active in cisplatin resistant cells is key to preventing survival of intrinsically resistant cells as well as cells that may gain drug tolerance. In this way, generation of therapeutics and strategies targeting these mechanisms of resistance may restore cisplatin sensitivity and circumvent drug resistance.

References

[1] Prestayko, A.W., et al., (1979). Cisplatin (cis-diamminedichloroplatinum II). *Cancer Treat Rev*. 6, 17-39.

[2] Galanski, M., (2006). Recent developments in the field of anticancer platinum complexes. *Recent Pat Anticancer Drug Discov*. 1, 285-95.

[3] Lebwohl, D. and R. Canetta, (1998). Clinical development of platinum complexes in cancer therapy: an historical perspective and an update. *Eur J Cancer*. 34, 1522-34.

[4] Cvitkovic, E., et al., (1977). Improvement of cis-dichlorodiammineplatinum (NSC 119875): therapeutic index in an animal model. *Cancer*. 39, 1357-61.

[5] Kelland, L., (2007). The resurgence of platinum-based cancer chemotherapy. *Nat. Rev. Cancer*. 7, 573-84.

[6] Giaccone, G., (2000). Clinical perspectives on platinum resistance. *Drugs*. 59 Suppl 4, 9-17; discussion 37-8.

[7] Koberle, B., et al., (2010). Cisplatin resistance: preclinical findings and clinical implications. *Biochim. Biophys. Acta*. 1806, 172-82.

[8] Ozols, R.F., (1991). Ovarian cancer: new clinical approaches. *Cancer Treat. Rev*. 18 Suppl A, 77-83.

[9] Gore, M.E., et al., (1989). Cisplatin/carboplatin cross-resistance in ovarian cancer. *Br. J. Cancer*. 60, 767-9.

[10] Armstrong, D.K., et al., (2006). Intraperitoneal cisplatin and paclitaxel in ovarian cancer. *N. Engl. J. Med*. 354, 34-43.

[11] el-Khateeb, M., et al., (1999). Reactions of cisplatin hydrolytes with methionine, cysteine, and plasma ultrafiltrate studied by a combination of HPLC and NMR techniques. *J. Inorg. Biochem*. 77, 13-21.

[12] Kelland, L.R., (2000). Preclinical perspectives on platinum resistance. *Drugs*. 59 Suppl 4, 1-8; discussion 37-8.

[13] Michalke, B., (2010). Platinum speciation used for elucidating activation or inhibition of Pt-containing anti-cancer drugs. *J. Trace Elem. Med. Biol*. 24, 69-77.

[14] Berndtsson, M., et al., (2007). Acute apoptosis by cisplatin requires induction of reactive oxygen species but is not associated with damage to nuclear DNA. *Int. J. Cancer*. 120, 175-80.

[15] Mandic, A., et al., (2003). Cisplatin induces endoplasmic reticulum stress and nucleus-independent apoptotic signaling. *J. Biol. Chem*. 278, 9100-6.

[16] Eastman, A., (1987). The formation, isolation and characterization of DNA adducts produced by anticancer platinum complexes. *Pharmacol. Ther*. 34, 155-66.

[17] Fraval, H.N. and J.J. Roberts, (1979). Excision repair of cis-diamminedichloroplatinum(II)-induced damage to DNA of Chinese hamster cells. *Cancer Res*. 39, 1793-7.

[18] Kelland, L.R., (1993). New platinum antitumor complexes. *Crit. Rev. Oncol. Hematol*. 15, 191-219.

[19] Bellon, S.F. and S.J. Lippard, (1990). Bending studies of DNA site-specifically modified by cisplatin, trans-diamminedichloroplatinum(II) and cis-[Pt(NH3)2(N3-cytosine)Cl]+. *Biophys. Chem*. 35, 179-88.

[20] Furuta, T., et al., (2002). Transcription-coupled nucleotide excision repair as a determinant of cisplatin sensitivity of human cells. *Cancer Res*. 62, 4899-902.

[21] Dianov, G.L. and U. Hubscher, (2013). Mammalian base excision repair: the forgotten archangel. *Nucleic Acids Res*. 41, 3483-90.

[22] Kunkel, T.A. and D.A. Erie, (2005). DNA mismatch repair. *Annu Rev. Biochem.* 74, 681-710.

[23] Li, G.M., (2008). Mechanisms and functions of DNA mismatch repair. *Cell Res.* 18, 85-98.

[24] Appella, E. and C.W. Anderson, (2001). Post-translational modifications and activation of p53 by genotoxic stresses. *Eur J Biochem.* 268, 2764-72.

[25] Damia, G., et al., (2001). Cisplatinum and taxol induce different patterns of p53 phosphorylation. *Neoplasia.* 3, 10-6.

[26] Shieh, S.Y., et al., (2000). The human homologs of checkpoint kinases Chk1 and Cds1 (Chk2) phosphorylate p53 at multiple DNA damage-inducible sites. *Genes Dev.* 14, 289-300.

[27] Zhao, H. and H. Piwnica-Worms, (2001). ATR-mediated checkpoint pathways regulate phosphorylation and activation of human Chk1. *Mol. Cell Biol.* 21, 4129-39.

[28] Delmastro, D.A., et al., (1997). DNA damage inducible-gene expression following platinum treatment in human ovarian carcinoma cell lines. *Cancer Chemother. Pharmacol.* 39, 245-53.

[29] Oda, E., et al., (2000). Noxa, a BH3-only member of the Bcl-2 family and candidate mediator of p53-induced apoptosis. *Science.* 288, 1053-8.

[30] Hershberger, P.A., et al., (2002). Cisplatin potentiates 1,25-dihydroxyvitamin D3-induced apoptosis in association with increased mitogen-activated protein kinase kinase kinase 1 (MEKK-1) expression. *Mol. Cancer Ther.* 1, 821-9.

[31] Kroemer, G., L. Galluzzi, and C. Brenner, (2007). Mitochondrial membrane permeabilization in cell death. *Physiol. Rev.* 87, 99-163.

[32] Chai, J., et al., (2000). Structural and biochemical basis of apoptotic activation by Smac/DIABLO. *Nature.* 406, 855-62.

[33] Yang, J., et al., (1997). Prevention of apoptosis by Bcl-2: release of cytochrome c from mitochondria blocked. *Science.* 275, 1129-32.

[34] Del Bello, B., et al., (2001). Cleavage of Bcl-2 in oxidant- and cisplatin-induced apoptosis of human melanoma cells. *Oncogene.* 20, 4591-5.

[35] Zhu, J., Y. Yang, and J. Wu, (2007). Bcl-2 cleavages at two adjacent sites by different caspases promote cisplatin-induced apoptosis. *Cell Res.* 17, 441-8.

[36] Micheau, O., et al., (1997). Sensitization of cancer cells treated with cytotoxic drugs to fas-mediated cytotoxicity. *J. Natl. Cancer Inst.* 89, 783-9.

[37] Muller, M., et al., (1998). p53 activates the CD95 (APO-1/Fas) gene in response to DNA damage by anticancer drugs. *J .Exp. Med.* 188, 2033-45.

[38] Galluzzi, L., et al., (2012). Molecular mechanisms of cisplatin resistance. *Oncogene*. 31, 1869-83.

[39] Siddik, Z.H., (2003). Cisplatin: mode of cytotoxic action and molecular basis of resistance. *Oncogene*. 22, 7265-79.

[40] Roos, W.P. and B. Kaina, (2013). DNA damage-induced cell death: from specific DNA lesions to the DNA damage response and apoptosis. *Cancer Lett*. 332, 237-48.

[41] Wang, D., et al., (2003). Nucleotide excision repair from site-specifically platinum-modified nucleosomes. *Biochemistry*. 42, 6747-53.

[42] Wang, D. and S.J. Lippard, (2005). Cellular processing of platinum anticancer drugs. *Nat. Rev. Drug Discov*. 4, 307-20.

[43] Deans, A.J. and S.C. West, (2011). DNA interstrand crosslink repair and cancer. *Nat. Rev. Cancer*. 11, 467-80.

[44] Kothandapani, A., et al., (2013). Epistatic role of base excision repair and mismatch repair pathways in mediating cisplatin cytotoxicity. *Nucleic. Acids Res*. 41, 7332-43.

[45] Fu, D., J.A. Calvo, and L.D. Samson, (2012). Balancing repair and tolerance of DNA damage caused by alkylating agents. *Nat. Rev. Cancer*. 12, 104-20.

[46] Gupta, S., M. Gellert, and W. Yang, (2012). Mechanism of mismatch recognition revealed by human MutSbeta bound to unpaired DNA loops. *Nat. Struct. Mol. Biol*. 19, 72-8.

[47] Qiu, R., et al., (2012). Large conformational changes in MutS during DNA scanning, mismatch recognition and repair signalling. *EMBO J.* 31, 2528-40.

[48] Sharma, A., et al., (2013). Slow Conformational Changes in MutS and DNA Direct Ordered Transitions between Mismatch Search, Recognition and Signaling of DNA Repair. *J. Mol. Biol.*

[49] Kadyrov, F.A., et al., (2006). Endonucleolytic function of MutLalpha in human mismatch repair. *Cell*. 126, 297-308.

[50] Plotz, G., et al., (2003). N-terminus of hMLH1 confers interaction of hMutLalpha and hMutLbeta with hMutSalpha. *Nucleic Acids Res*. 31, 3217-26.

[51] Martin, S.A., C.J. Lord, and A. Ashworth, (2010). Therapeutic targeting of the DNA mismatch repair pathway. *Clin Cancer Res*. 16, 5107-13.

[52] Wu, Q. and K.M. Vasquez, (2008). Human MLH1 protein participates in genomic damage checkpoint signaling in response to DNA interstrand crosslinks, while MSH2 functions in DNA repair. *PLoS Genet.* 4, e1000189.

[53] Zhao, J., et al., (2009). Mismatch repair and nucleotide excision repair proteins cooperate in the recognition of DNA interstrand crosslinks. *Nucleic Acids Res.* 37, 4420-9.

[54] Marinovic-Terzic, I., et al., (2008). Apoptotic function of human PMS2 compromised by the nonsynonymous single-nucleotide polymorphic variant R20Q. *Proc. Natl. Acad. Sci. U S A.* 105, 13993-8.

[55] Vasilyeva, A., et al., (2009). Small molecule induction of MSH2-dependent cell death suggests a vital role of mismatch repair proteins in cell death. *DNA Repair (Amst).* 8, 103-13.

[56] Wu, J., et al., (1999). Mismatch repair processing of carcinogen-DNA adducts triggers apoptosis. *Mol. Cell Biol.* 19, 8292-301.

[57] Clodfelter, J.E., B.G. M, and K. Drotschmann, (2005). MSH2 missense mutations alter cisplatin cytotoxicity and promote cisplatin-induced genome instability. *Nucleic Acids Res.* 33, 3323-30.

[58] Ding, X., et al., (2009). MLH1 expression sensitises ovarian cancer cells to cell death mediated by XIAP inhibition. *Br. J. Cancer.* 101, 269-77.

[59] Takahashi, M., et al., (2011). MSH3 mediates sensitization of colorectal cancer cells to cisplatin, oxaliplatin, and a poly(ADP-ribose) polymerase inhibitor. *J. Biol. Chem.* 286, 12157-65.

[60] Ting, S., et al., (2013). ERCC1, MLH1, MSH2, MSH6, and betaIII-Tubulin: Resistance Proteins Associated With Response and Outcome to Platinum-based Chemotherapy in Malignant Pleural Mesothelioma. *Clin. Lung Cancer.* 14, 558-567 e3.

[61] Park, J.M., et al., (2013). MSH3 mismatch repair protein regulates sensitivity tocytotoxic drugs and a histone deacetylase inhibitor in human colon carcinoma cells. *PLoS One.* 8, e65369.

[62] Kothandapani, A., et al., (2011). Novel role of base excision repair in mediating cisplatin cytotoxicity. *J. Biol. Chem.* 286, 14564-74.

[63] Almeida, K.H. and R.W. Sobol, (2007). A unified view of base excision repair: lesion-dependent protein complexes regulated by post-translational modification. *DNA Repair (Amst).* 6, 695-711.

[64] Bergoglio, V., et al., (2001). Enhanced expression and activity of DNA polymerase beta in human ovarian tumor cells: impact on sensitivity towards antitumor agents. *Oncogene.* 20, 6181-7.

[65] Gao, D., et al., (2013). Effect of hOGG1 Over-Expression on Cisplatin Resistance in Esophageal Squamous Carcinoma Cells. *Cancer Biother Radiopharm*. 28, 433-40.
[66] Wang, D., et al., (2009). APE1 overexpression is associated with cisplatin resistance in non-small cell lung cancer and targeted inhibition of APE1 enhances the activity of cisplatin in A549 cells. *Lung Cancer*. 66, 298-304.
[67] Hoeijmakers, J.H., (2001). Genome maintenance mechanisms for preventing cancer. *Nature*. 411, 366-74.
[68] Wood, R.D., (1999). DNA damage recognition during nucleotide excision repair in mammalian cells. *Biochimie*. 81, 39-44.
[69] Reardon, J.T., et al., (1999). Efficient nucleotide excision repair of cisplatin, oxaliplatin, and Bis-aceto-ammine-dichloro-cyclohexylamine-platinum(IV) (JM216) platinum intrastrand DNA diadducts. *Cancer Res*. 59, 3968-71.
[70] Zamble, D.B., et al., (1996). Repair of cisplatin--DNA adducts by the mammalian excision nuclease. *Biochemistry*. 35, 10004-13.
[71] Sugasawa, K., et al., (1998). Xeroderma pigmentosum group C protein complex is the initiator of global genome nucleotide excision repair. *Mol. Cell*. 2, 223-32.
[72] Ashton, N.W., et al., (2013). Human single-stranded DNA binding proteins are essential for maintaining genomic stability. *BMC Mol. Biol*. 14, 9.
[73] Evans, E., et al., (1997). Mechanism of open complex and dual incision formation by human nucleotide excision repair factors. *EMBO J*. 16, 6559-73.
[74] Mu, D., et al., (1997). Characterization of reaction intermediates of human excision repair nuclease. *J. Biol. Chem*. 272, 28971-9.
[75] Buschta-Hedayat, N., et al., (1999). Recognition of nonhybridizing base pairs during nucleotide excision repair of DNA. *Proc. Natl. Acad. Sci. U S A*. 96, 6090-5.
[76] de Laat, W.L., et al., (1998). DNA-binding polarity of human replication protein A positions nucleases in nucleotide excision repair. *Genes. Dev*. 12, 2598-609.
[77] Kong, S.E. and J.Q. Svejstrup, (2002). Incision of a 1,3-intrastrand d(GpTpG)-cisplatin adduct by nucleotide excision repair proteins from yeast. *DNA Repair (Amst)*. 1, 731-41.

[78] Neher, T.M., et al., (2010). Photo-cross-linking of XPC-Rad23B to cisplatin-damaged DNA reveals contacts with both strands of the DNA duplex and spans the DNA adduct. *Biochemistry*. 49, 669-78.

[79] Smeaton, M.B., et al., (2008). Distortion-dependent unhooking of interstrand cross-links in mammalian cell extracts. *Biochemistry*. 47, 9920-30.

[80] Kumaresan, K.R., et al., (2007). Deficiency in incisions produced by XPF at the site of a DNA interstrand cross-link in Fanconi anemia cells. *Biochemistry*. 46, 14359-68.

[81] Nakanishi, K., et al., (2011). Homology-directed Fanconi anemia pathway cross-link repair is dependent on DNA replication. *Nat. Struct. Mol. Biol*. 18, 500-3.

[82] Enoiu, M., J. Jiricny, and O.D. Scharer, (2012). Repair of cisplatin-induced DNA interstrand crosslinks by a replication-independent pathway involving transcription-coupled repair and translesion synthesis. *Nucleic Acids Res*. 40, 8953-64.

[83] Sarkar, S., et al., (2006). DNA interstrand crosslink repair during G1 involves nucleotide excision repair and DNA polymerase zeta. *EMBO J*. 25, 1285-94.

[84] Zheng, H., et al., (2003). Nucleotide excision repair- and polymerase eta-mediated error-prone removal of mitomycin C interstrand cross-links. *Mol. Cell Biol*. 23, 754-61.

[85] Kumaresan, K.R., B. Hang, and M.W. Lambert, (1995). Human endonucleolytic incision of DNA 3' and 5' to a site-directed psoralen monoadduct and interstrand cross-link. *J. Biol. Chem*. 270, 30709-16.

[86] Shachar, S., et al., (2009). Two-polymerase mechanisms dictate error-free and error-prone translesion DNA synthesis in mammals. *EMBO J*. 28, 383-93.

[87] Waters, L.S., et al., (2009). Eukaryotic translesion polymerases and their roles and regulation in DNA damage tolerance. *Microbiol. Mol. Biol. Rev*. 73, 134-54.

[88] Muniandy, P.A., et al., (2010). DNA interstrand crosslink repair in mammalian cells: step by step. *Crit. Rev. Biochem. Mol. Biol*. 45, 23-49.

[89] Ferry, K.V., T.C. Hamilton, and S.W. Johnson, (2000). Increased nucleotide excision repair in cisplatin-resistant ovarian cancer cells: role of ERCC1-XPF. *Biochem. Pharmacol*. 60, 1305-13.

[90] Huang, J., et al., (2013). A phase II study of biweekly paclitaxel and cisplatin chemotherapy for recurrent or metastatic esophageal squamous

cell carcinoma: ERCC1 expression predicts response to chemotherapy. *Med. Oncol.* 30, 343.

[91] Mendoza, J., et al., (2013). Association between ERCC1 and XPA expression and polymorphisms and the response to cisplatin in testicular germ cell tumours. *Br. J. Cancer.* 109, 68-75.

[92] Usanova, S., et al., (2010). Cisplatin sensitivity of testis tumour cells is due to deficiency in interstrand-crosslink repair and low ERCC1-XPF expression. *Mol. Cancer.* 9, 248.

[93] Liu, Y., et al., (2012). HIF1alpha regulated expression of XPA contributes to cisplatin resistance in lung cancer. *Carcinogenesis.* 33, 1187-92.

[94] Barckhausen, C., et al., (2013). Malignant melanoma cells acquire resistance to DNA interstrand cross-linking chemotherapeutics by p53-triggered upregulation of DDB2/XPC-mediated DNA repair. *Oncogene.*

[95] Lee, G.W., et al., (2012). Hypoxia-inducible factor-1alpha and excision repair cross-complementing 1 in patients with small cell lung cancer who received front-line platinum-based chemotherapy: a retrospective study. *J. Thorac. Oncol.* 7, 528-34.

[96] Christmann, M. and B. Kaina, (2013). Transcriptional regulation of human DNA repair genes following genotoxic stress: trigger mechanisms, inducible responses and genotoxic adaptation. *Nucleic Acids Res.*

[97] Liu, R.Y., et al., (2011). Role of eIF3a in regulating cisplatin sensitivity and in translational control of nucleotide excision repair of nasopharyngeal carcinoma. *Oncogene.* 30, 4814-23.

[98] Yin, J.Y., et al., (2011). Effect of eIF3a on response of lung cancer patients to platinum-based chemotherapy by regulating DNA repair. *Clin. Cancer Res.* 17, 4600-9.

[99] Lee, S.Y., et al., (2013). Polymorphisms in DNA repair and apoptosis-related genes and clinical outcomes of patients with non-small cell lung cancer treated with first-line paclitaxel-cisplatin chemotherapy. *Lung. Cancer.*

[100] Park, S.R., et al., (2011). CYP2A6 and ERCC1 polymorphisms correlate with efficacy of S-1 plus cisplatin in metastatic gastric cancer patients. *Br. J. Cancer.* 104, 1126-34.

[101] Tiseo, M., et al., (2013). ERCC1/BRCA1 expression and gene polymorphisms as prognostic and predictive factors in advanced NSCLC treated with or without cisplatin. *Br. J. Cancer.* 108, 1695-703.

[102] Mu, D., et al., (2000). DNA interstrand cross-links induce futile repair synthesis in mammalian cell extracts. *Mol. Cell Biol.* 20, 2446-54.

[103] Washington, M.T., et al., (2010). Variations on a theme: eukaryotic Y-family DNA polymerases. *Biochim. Biophys. Acta.* 1804, 1113-23.

[104] Nakano, T., et al., (2013). Translocation and stability of replicative DNA helicases upon encountering DNA-protein cross-links. *J. Biol. Chem.* 288, 4649-58.

[105] Knipscheer, P., et al., (2009). The Fanconi anemia pathway promotes replication-dependent DNA interstrand cross-link repair. *Science.* 326, 1698-701.

[106] Raschle, M., et al., (2008). Mechanism of replication-coupled DNA interstrand crosslink repair. *Cell.* 134, 969-80.

[107] Hoege, C., et al., (2002). RAD6-dependent DNA repair is linked to modification of PCNA by ubiquitin and SUMO. *Nature.* 419, 135-41.

[108] Masuda, Y., J. Piao, and K. Kamiya, (2010). DNA replication-coupled PCNA mono-ubiquitination and polymerase switching in a human in vitro system. *J. Mol. Biol.* 396, 487-500.

[109] Albertella, M.R., et al., (2005). A role for polymerase eta in the cellular tolerance to cisplatin-induced damage. *Cancer Res.* 65, 9799-806.

[110] Hicks, J.K., et al., (2010). Differential roles for DNA polymerases eta, zeta, and REV1 in lesion bypass of intrastrand versus interstrand DNA cross-links. *Mol. Cell Biol.* 30, 1217-30.

[111] Vaisman, A., et al., (2000). Efficient translesion replication past oxaliplatin and cisplatin GpG adducts by human DNA polymerase eta. *Biochemistry.* 39, 4575-80.

[112] Sharma, S., et al., (2012). DNA polymerase zeta is a major determinant of resistance to platinum-based chemotherapeutic agents. *Mol. Pharmacol.* 81, 778-87.

[113] Sonoda, E., et al., (2003). Multiple roles of Rev3, the catalytic subunit of polzeta in maintaining genome stability in vertebrates. *EMBO J.* 22, 3188-97.

[114] Lin, X., et al., (2006). Human REV1 modulates the cytotoxicity and mutagenicity of cisplatin in human ovarian carcinoma cells. *Mol. Pharmacol.* 69, 1748-54.

[115] Okuda, T., et al., (2005). Suppression of hREV1 expression reduces the rate at which human ovarian carcinoma cells acquire resistance to cisplatin. *Mol. Pharmacol.* 67, 1852-60.

[116] Wang, Y., et al., (2012). MiR-96 downregulates REV1 and RAD51 to promote cellular sensitivity to cisplatin and PARP inhibition. *Cancer Res.* 72, 4037-46.
[117] Adachi, M., et al., (2008). Hypersensitivity to cisplatin after hRev3 mRNA knockdown in head and neck squamous cell carcinoma cells. *Mol. Med. Rep.* 1, 695-8.
[118] Shi, T.Y., et al., (2013). DNA polymerase zeta as a potential biomarker of chemoradiation resistance and poor prognosis for cervical cancer. *Med. Oncol.* 30, 500.
[119] Doles, J., et al., (2010). Suppression of Rev3, the catalytic subunit of Pol{zeta}, sensitizes drug-resistant lung tumors to chemotherapy. *Proc Natl. Acad. Sci. U S A.* 107, 20786-91.
[120] Lin, X., et al., (2006). DNA polymerase zeta accounts for the reduced cytotoxicity and enhanced mutagenicity of cisplatin in human colon carcinoma cells that have lost DNA mismatch repair. *Clin. Cancer Res.* 12, 563-8.
[121] Wu, F., et al., (2004). DNA polymerase zeta regulates cisplatin cytotoxicity, mutagenicity, and the rate of development of cisplatin resistance. *Cancer Res.* 64, 8029-35.
[122] Ceppi, P., et al., (2009). Polymerase eta mRNA expression predicts survival of non-small cell lung cancer patients treated with platinum-based chemotherapy. *Clin. Cancer Res.* 15, 1039-45.
[123] Teng, K.Y., et al., (2010). DNA polymerase eta protein expression predicts treatment response and survival of metastatic gastric adenocarcinoma patients treated with oxaliplatin-based chemotherapy. *J. Transl Med.* 8, 126.
[124] Ummat, A., et al., (2012). Structural basis for cisplatin DNA damage tolerance by human polymerase eta during cancer chemotherapy. *Nat. Struct. Mol. Biol.* 19, 628-32.
[125] Auerbach, A.D. and P.C. Verlander, (1997). Disorders of DNA replication and repair. *Curr. Opin Pediatr.* 9, 600-16.
[126] Sugiyama, T., E.M. Zaitseva, and S.C. Kowalczykowski, (1997). A single-stranded DNA-binding protein is needed for efficient presynaptic complex formation by the Saccharomyces cerevisiae Rad51 protein. *J. Biol. Chem.* 272, 7940-5.
[127] Jensen, R.B., A. Carreira, and S.C. Kowalczykowski, (2010). Purified human BRCA2 stimulates RAD51-mediated recombination. *Nature.* 467, 678-83.

[128] San Filippo, J., P. Sung, and H. Klein, (2008). Mechanism of eukaryotic homologous recombination. *Annu. Rev. Biochem*. 77, 229-57.

[129] Nimonkar, A.V., R.A. Sica, and S.C. Kowalczykowski, (2009). Rad52 promotes second-end DNA capture in double-stranded break repair to form complement-stabilized joint molecules. *Proc. Natl. Acad. Sci. U S A*. 106, 3077-82.

[130] Plank, J.L., J. Wu, and T.S. Hsieh, (2006). Topoisomerase IIIalpha and Bloom's helicase can resolve a mobile double Holliday junction substrate through convergent branch migration. *Proc. Natl. Acad. Sci. U S A*. 103, 11118-23.

[131] Abraham, J., et al., (2003). Eme1 is involved in DNA damage processing and maintenance of genomic stability in mammalian cells. *EMBO J*. 22, 6137-47.

[132] Ciccia, A., et al., (2007). Identification of FAAP24, a Fanconi anemia core complex protein that interacts with FANCM. *Mol Cell*. 25, 331-43.

[133] Gari, K., et al., (2008). Remodeling of DNA replication structures by the branch point translocase FANCM. *Proc. Natl. Acad. Sci. U S A*. 105, 16107-12.

[134] Collis, S.J., et al., (2008). FANCM and FAAP24 function in ATR-mediated checkpoint signaling independently of the Fanconi anemia core complex. *Mol. Cell*. 32, 313-24.

[135] Kim, J.M., et al., (2008). Cell cycle-dependent chromatin loading of the Fanconi anemia core complex by FANCM/FAAP24. *Blood*. 111, 5215-22.

[136] Liu, T., et al., (2010). FAN1 acts with FANCI-FANCD2 to promote DNA interstrand cross-link repair. *Science*. 329, 693-6.

[137] Meetei, A.R., Z. Yan, and W. Wang, (2004). FANCL replaces BRCA1 as the likely ubiquitin ligase responsible for FANCD2 monoubiquitination. *Cell Cycle*. 3, 179-81.

[138] Singh, T.R., et al., (2008). BLAP18/RMI2, a novel OB-fold-containing protein, is an essential component of the Bloom helicase-double Holliday junction dissolvasome. *Genes. Dev*. 22, 2856-68.

[139] Fanconi, G., (1967). Familial constitutional panmyelocytopathy, Fanconi's anemia (F.A.). I. Clinical aspects. *Semin. Hematol*. 4, 233-40.

[140] Auerbach, A.D., (1988). A test for Fanconi's anemia. *Blood*. 72, 366-7.

[141] Taniguchi, T., et al., (2003). Disruption of the Fanconi anemia-BRCA pathway in cisplatin-sensitive ovarian tumors. *Nat. Med*. 9, 568-74.

[142] Sakai, W., et al., (2008). Secondary mutations as a mechanism of cisplatin resistance in BRCA2-mutated cancers. *Nature*. 451, 1116-20.

[143] Swisher, E.M., et al., (2008). Secondary BRCA1 mutations in BRCA1-mutated ovarian carcinomas with platinum resistance. *Cancer Res.* 68, 2581-6.

[144] Hollstein, M., et al., (1991). p53 mutations in human cancers. *Science.* 253, 49-53.

[145] Soussi, T., (2000). The p53 tumor suppressor gene: from molecular biology to clinical investigation. *Ann. N. Y. Acad. Sci.* 910, 121-37; discussion 137-9.

[146] Vousden, K.H. and D.P. Lane, (2007). p53 in health and disease. *Nat. Rev. Mol. Cell Biol.* 8, 275-83.

[147] Branch, P., et al., (2000). Spontaneous development of drug resistance: mismatch repair and p53 defects in resistance to cisplatin in human tumor cells. *Oncogene.* 19, 3138-45.

[148] Hengstler, J.G., et al., (2001). Metallothionein expression in ovarian cancer in relation to histopathological parameters and molecular markers of prognosis. *Int. J. Cancer.* 95, 121-7.

[149] O'Connor, P.M., et al., (1997). Characterization of the p53 tumor suppressor pathway in cell lines of the National Cancer Institute anticancer drug screen and correlations with the growth-inhibitory potency of 123 anticancer agents. *Cancer Res.* 57, 4285-300.

[150] Feldman, D.R., et al., (2008). Medical treatment of advanced testicular cancer. *JAMA.* 299, 672-84.

[151] Gadducci, A., et al., (2002). Molecular mechanisms of apoptosis and chemosensitivity to platinum and paclitaxel in ovarian cancer: biological data and clinical implications. *Eur. J. Gynaecol. Oncol.* 23, 390-6.

[152] Fan, S., et al., (1995). Disruption of p53 function sensitizes breast cancer MCF-7 cells to cisplatin and pentoxifylline. *Cancer Res.* 55, 1649-54.

[153] Hawkins, D.S., G.W. Demers, and D.A. Galloway, (1996). Inactivation of p53 enhances sensitivity to multiple chemotherapeutic agents. *Cancer Res.* 56, 892-8.

[154] Righetti, S.C., et al., (1996). A comparative study of p53 gene mutations, protein accumulation, and response to cisplatin-based chemotherapy in advanced ovarian carcinoma. *Cancer Res.* 56, 689-93.

[155] Eliopoulos, A.G., et al., (1995). The control of apoptosis and drug resistance in ovarian cancer: influence of p53 and Bcl-2. *Oncogene.* 11, 1217-28.

[156] Fan, S., et al., (1994). p53 gene mutations are associated with decreased sensitivity of human lymphoma cells to DNA damaging agents. *Cancer Res.* 54, 5824-30.

[157] Gallagher, W.M., et al., (1997). Identification of p53 genetic suppressor elements which confer resistance to cisplatin. *Oncogene*. 14, 185-93.

[158] Perego, P., et al., (1996). Association between cisplatin resistance and mutation of p53 gene and reduced bax expression in ovarian carcinoma cell systems. *Cancer Res*. 56, 556-62.

[159] Righetti, S.C., et al., (1999). Emergence of p53 mutant cisplatin-resistant ovarian carcinoma cells following drug exposure: spontaneously mutant selection. *Cell Growth Differ*. 10, 473-8.

[160] Deng, X., et al., (2002). Recombinant adenovirus-mediated p14(ARF) overexpression sensitizes human breast cancer cells to cisplatin. *Biochem Biophys Res Commun*. 296, 792-8.

[161] Mayo, L.D. and D.B. Donner, (2002). The PTEN, Mdm2, p53 tumor suppressor-oncoprotein network. *Trends Biochem. Sci*. 27, 462-7.

[162] Oren, M., et al., (2002). Regulation of p53: intricate loops and delicate balances. *Ann. N. Y. Acad. Sci*. 973, 374-83.

[163] Zhou, B.P. and M.C. Hung, (2002). Novel targets of Akt, p21(Cipl/WAF1), and MDM2. *Semin. Oncol*. 29, 62-70.

[164] Ali, A.Y., M.R. Abedini, and B.K. Tsang, (2012). The oncogenic phosphatase PPM1D confers cisplatin resistance in ovarian carcinoma cells by attenuating checkpoint kinase 1 and p53 activation. *Oncogene*. 31, 2175-86.

[165] Chee, J.L., et al., (2013). Wild-type and mutant p53 mediate cisplatin resistance through interaction and inhibition of active caspase-9. *Cell Cycle*. 12, 278-88.

[166] Komlodi-Pasztor, E., et al., (2009). Impaired p53 binding to importin: a novel mechanism of cytoplasmic sequestration identified in oxaliplatin-resistant cells. *Oncogene*. 28, 3111-20.

[167] Mandic, R., et al., (2005). Reduced cisplatin sensitivity of head and neck squamous cell carcinoma cell lines correlates with mutations affecting the COOH-terminal nuclear localization signal of p53. *Clin. Cancer Res*. 11, 6845-52.

[168] Asselin, E., G.B. Mills, and B.K. Tsang, (2001). XIAP regulates Akt activity and caspase-3-dependent cleavage during cisplatin-induced apoptosis in human ovarian epithelial cancer cells. *Cancer Res*. 61, 1862-8.

[169] Ikeguchi, M., S. Nakamura, and N. Kaibara, (2002). Quantitative analysis of expression levels of bax, bcl-2, and survivin in cancer cells during cisplatin treatment. *Oncol. Rep*. 9, 1121-6.

[170] Erovic, B.M., et al., (2005). Mcl-1, vascular endothelial growth factor-R2, and 14-3-3sigma expression might predict primary response against radiotherapy and chemotherapy in patients with locally advanced squamous cell carcinomas of the head and neck. *Clin. Cancer Res.* 11, 8632-6.

[171] Han, J.Y., et al., (2003). Death receptor 5 and Bcl-2 protein expression as predictors of tumor response to gemcitabine and cisplatin in patients with advanced non-small-cell lung cancer. *Med. Oncol.* 20, 355-62.

[172] Michaud, W.A., et al., (2009). Bcl-2 blocks cisplatin-induced apoptosis and predicts poor outcome following chemoradiation treatment in advanced oropharyngeal squamous cell carcinoma. *Clin. Cancer Res.* 15, 1645-54.

[173] Williams, J., et al., (2005). Expression of Bcl-xL in ovarian carcinoma is associated with chemoresistance and recurrent disease. *Gynecol. Oncol.* 96, 287-95.

[174] Castedo, M., et al., (2006). Apoptosis regulation in tetraploid cancer cells. *EMBO J.* 25, 2584-95.

[175] Tajeddine, N., et al., (2008). Hierarchical involvement of Bak, VDAC1 and Bax in cisplatin-induced cell death. *Oncogene.* 27, 4221-32.

[176] Aparicio, S. and C. Caldas, (2013). The implications of clonal genome evolution for cancer medicine. *N. Engl. J. Med.* 368, 842-51.

[177] Navin, N., et al., (2011). Tumour evolution inferred by single-cell sequencing. *Nature.* 472, 90-4.

[178] Navin, N.E. and J. Hicks, (2010). Tracing the tumor lineage. *Mol. Oncol.* 4, 267-83.

[179] Ruiz, C., et al., (2011). Advancing a clinically relevant perspective of the clonal nature of cancer. *Proc. Natl. Acad. Sci. U S A.* 108, 12054-9.

[180] Grasso, C.S., et al., (2012). The mutational landscape of lethal castration-resistant prostate cancer. *Nature.* 487, 239-43.

[181] Gerlinger, M., et al., (2012). Intratumor heterogeneity and branched evolution revealed by multiregion sequencing. *N. Engl. J. Med.* 366, 883-92.

[182] Campbell, P.J., et al., (2010). The patterns and dynamics of genomic instability in metastatic pancreatic cancer. *Nature.* 467, 1109-13.

[183] Yachida, S., et al., (2010). Distant metastasis occurs late during the genetic evolution of pancreatic cancer. *Nature.* 467, 1114-7.

[184] Sidransky, D., et al., (1992). Clonal expansion of p53 mutant cells is associated with brain tumour progression. *Nature.* 355, 846-7.

[185] Bertolini, G., et al., (2009). Highly tumorigenic lung cancer CD133+ cells display stem-like features and are spared by cisplatin treatment. *Proc. Natl. Acad. Sci. U S A*. 106, 16281-6.

[186] Liu, Y.P., et al., (2013). Cisplatin selects for multidrug-resistant CD133+ cells in lung adenocarcinoma by activating Notch signaling. *Cancer Res*. 73, 406-16.

[187] Steg, A.D., et al., (2012). Stem cell pathways contribute to clinical chemoresistance in ovarian cancer. *Clin. Cancer Res*. 18, 869-81.

[188] Dembinski, J.L. and S. Krauss, (2009). Characterization and functional analysis of a slow cycling stem cell-like subpopulation in pancreas adenocarcinoma. *Clin. Exp. Metastasis*. 26, 611-23.

[189] Li, Y. and J. Laterra, (2012). Cancer stem cells: distinct entities or dynamically regulated phenotypes? *Cancer Res*. 72, 576-80.

[190] Barr, M.P., et al., (2013). Generation and characterisation of cisplatin-resistant non-small cell lung cancer cell lines displaying a stem-like signature. *PLoS One*. 8, e54193.

[191] Lundholm, L., et al., (2013). Resistance to DNA-damaging treatment in non-small cell lung cancer tumor-initiating cells involves reduced DNA-PK/ATM activation and diminished cell cycle arrest. *Cell Death Dis*. 4, e478.

[192] Chen, Y.C., et al., (2008). Oct-4 expression maintained cancer stem-like properties in lung cancer-derived CD133-positive cells. *PLoS One*. 3, e2637.

[193] Eramo, A., et al., (2008). Identification and expansion of the tumorigenic lung cancer stem cell population. *Cell Death Differ*. 15, 504-14.

[194] Chau, W.K., et al., (2013). c-Kit mediates chemoresistance and tumor-initiating capacity of ovarian cancer cells through activation of Wnt/beta-catenin-ATP-binding cassette G2 signaling. *Oncogene*. 32, 2767-81.

[195] Maugeri-Sacca, M., M. Bartucci, and R. De Maria, (2012). DNA damage repair pathways in cancer stem cells. *Mol. Cancer Ther*. 11, 1627-36.

[196] Guruharsha, K.G., M.W. Kankel, and S. Artavanis-Tsakonas, (2012). The Notch signalling system: recent insights into the complexity of a conserved pathway. *Nat. Rev. Genet*. 13, 654-66.

[197] Pannuti, A., et al., (2010). Targeting Notch to target cancer stem cells. *Clin. Cancer Res*. 16, 3141-52.

[198] Bray, S.J., (2006). Notch signalling: a simple pathway becomes complex. *Nat. Rev. Mol. Cell Biol*. 7, 678-89.

[199] Song, L.L., et al., (2008). Notch-1 associates with IKKalpha and regulates IKK activity in cervical cancer cells. *Oncogene*. 27, 5833-44.

[200] Gu, F., et al., (2010). Expression of Stat3 and Notch1 is associated with cisplatin resistance in head and neck squamous cell carcinoma. *Oncol. Rep*. 23, 671-6.

[201] Rahman, M.T., et al., (2012). Notch3 overexpression as potential therapeutic target in advanced stage chemoresistant ovarian cancer. *Am. J. Clin. Pathol*. 138, 535-44.

[202] Lee, S.H., et al., (2013). Epigallocatechin-3-gallate attenuates head and neck cancer stem cell traits through suppression of Notch pathway. *Eur. J. Cancer*.

[203] Ji, X., et al., (2012). Delta-tocotrienol augments cisplatin-induced suppression of non-small cell lung cancer cells via inhibition of the Notch-1 pathway. *Anticancer Res*. 32, 2647-55.

[204] McAuliffe, S.M., et al., (2012). Targeting Notch, a key pathway for ovarian cancer stem cells, sensitizes tumors to platinum therapy. *Proc. Natl. Acad. Sci. U S A*. 109, E2939-48.

[205] Niehrs, C., (2012). The complex world of WNT receptor signalling. *Nat Rev. Mol. Cell Biol*. 13, 767-79.

[206] Wray, J. and C. Hartmann, (2012). WNTing embryonic stem cells. *Trends Cell Biol*. 22, 159-68.

[207] Yin, S., et al., (2013). Tumor-initiating cells and FZD8 play a major role in drug resistance in triple-negative breast cancer. *Mol. Cancer Ther*. 12, 491-8.

[208] Zajchowski, D.A., B.Y. Karlan, and L.K. Shawver, (2012). Treatment-related protein biomarker expression differs between primary and recurrent ovarian carcinomas. *Mol. Cancer Ther*. 11, 492-502.

[209] Shou, J., et al., (2002). Human Dkk-1, a gene encoding a Wnt antagonist, responds to DNA damage and its overexpression sensitizes brain tumor cells to apoptosis following alkylation damage of DNA. *Oncogene*. 21, 878-89.

[210] Gosepath, E.M., et al., (2008). Acquired cisplatin resistance in the head-neck cancer cell line Cal27 is associated with decreased DKK1 expression and can partially be reversed by overexpression of DKK1. *Int. J. Cancer*. 123, 2013-9.

[211] Harismendy, O., et al., (2011). Detection of low prevalence somatic mutations in solid tumors with ultra-deep targeted sequencing. *Genome Biol*. 12, R124.

[212] Heiser, L.M., et al., (2012). Subtype and pathway specific responses to anticancer compounds in breast cancer. *Proc. Natl. Acad. Sci. U S A*. 109, 2724-9.

[213] Diaz, L.A., Jr., et al., (2012). The molecular evolution of acquired resistance to targeted EGFR blockade in colorectal cancers. *Nature*. 486, 537-40.

[214] Misale, S., et al., (2012). Emergence of KRAS mutations and acquired resistance to anti-EGFR therapy in colorectal cancer. *Nature*. 486, 532-6.

[215] Murtaza, M., et al., (2013). Non-invasive analysis of acquired resistance to cancer therapy by sequencing of plasma DNA. *Nature*. 497, 108-12.

[216] Knudsen, E.S. and K.E. Knudsen, (2008). Tailoring to RB: Tumour suppressor status and therapeutic response. *Nat. Rev. Cancer*. 8, 714-24.

[217] Gamazon, E.R., et al., (2011). Copy number polymorphisms and anticancer pharmacogenomics. *Genome Biol*. 12, R46.

[218] Moyer, A.M., et al., (2010). Glutathione pathway genetic polymorphisms and lung cancer survival after platinum-based chemotherapy. *Cancer Epidemiol. Biomarkers Prev*. 19, 811-21.

[219] Chang, X., et al., (2010). Identification of hypermethylated genes associated with cisplatin resistance in human cancers. *Cancer Res*. 70, 2870-9.

[220] Dai, W., et al., (2008). Methylation Linear Discriminant Analysis (MLDA) for identifying differentially methylated CpG islands. *BMC Bioinformatics*. 9, 337.

[221] Teodoridis, J.M., et al., (2005). CpG island methylation of DNA damage response genes in advanced ovarian cancer. *Cancer Res*. 65, 8961-7.

[222] Zeller, C., et al., (2012). Candidate DNA methylation drivers of acquired cisplatin resistance in ovarian cancer identified by methylome and expression profiling. *Oncogene*. 31, 4567-76.

[223] Gifford, G., et al., (2004). The acquisition of hMLH1 methylation in plasma DNA after chemotherapy predicts poor survival for ovarian cancer patients. *Clin. Cancer Res*. 10, 4420-6.

[224] Strathdee, G., et al., (1999). A role for methylation of the hMLH1 promoter in loss of hMLH1 expression and drug resistance in ovarian cancer. *Oncogene*. 18, 2335-41.

[225] Stronach, E.A., et al., (2011). HDAC4-regulated STAT1 activation mediates platinum resistance in ovarian cancer. *Cancer Res*. 71, 4412-22.

[226] Strait, K.A., et al., (2005). Histone deacetylase inhibitors induce G2-checkpoint arrest and apoptosis in cisplatinum-resistant ovarian cancer cells associated with overexpression of the Bcl-2-related protein Bad. *Mol. Cancer Ther.* 4, 603-11.

[227] Cameron, E.E., et al., (1999). Synergy of demethylation and histone deacetylase inhibition in the re-expression of genes silenced in cancer. *Nat. Genet.* 21, 103-7.

[228] Suzuki, H., et al., (2002). A genomic screen for genes upregulated by demethylation and histone deacetylase inhibition in human colorectal cancer. *Nat. Genet.* 31, 141-9.

[229] Steele, N., et al., (2009). Combined inhibition of DNA methylation and histone acetylation enhances gene re-expression and drug sensitivity in vivo. *Br. J. Cancer.* 100, 758-63.

[230] Sharma, S.V., et al., (2010). A chromatin-mediated reversible drug-tolerant state in cancer cell subpopulations. *Cell.* 141, 69-80.

In: Advances in Drug Resistance Research
Editor: Christudas Morais
ISBN: 978-1-63117-131-4

Chapter 2

Multi-Drug Resistance in Cancer and New Approaches for Its Overcoming

Jelena Dinić, Tijana Stanković, Jasna Banković and Milica Pešić*

Institute for Biological Research "Siniša Stanković",
University of Belgrade, Belgrade, Serbia

Abstract

Resistance to chemotherapy is the main obstacle to efficient cancer treatment. The problem of multi-drug resistance (MDR) has been intensively studied for the last three decades. Classically defined as resistance to structurally and/or functionally unrelated drugs, MDR is connected to aggressive, untreatable cancers. There are two types of MDR: inherent (intrinsic) and acquired. Selection pressures within the tumor microenvironment favor the development of intrinsic MDR, while the ordinary dose and schedule chemotherapy practices induce acquired MDR. In recent years, patient-to-patient variability within each type of cancer has arisen as an unsolved problem. Even more, heterogeneous

* Corresponding Author address: Department of Neurobiology, Institute for Biological Research "Siniša Stanković", Despota Stefana 142, 11060 Belgrade, Serbia. Email: vtbvtm@sbb.rs.

populations of cancer cells within one patient must be considered as a cause of chemotherapy impediment.

Several genes and pathways have been found to contribute to the MDR. Tentatively, MDR phenotype could develop from point mutations, gene amplification or other genetic or epigenetic changes that affect biological functions. Therefore, MDR is driven by similar mechanisms as cancerogenesis. This is also supported by the fact that important characteristics of MDR include abnormal tumor vasculature, regions of hypoxia, aerobic glycolysis, and an elevated apoptotic threshold. Understanding these mechanisms and developing agents to target them are important steps in the design of new therapies.

Penetration of drugs into the cancer cell is necessary for their lethal pharmacological effect due to the interaction with intracellular target molecules. Decreased activity of membrane-embedded drug uptake as well as increased activity of efflux pumps reduce the intracellular drug accumulation, thereby preventing drug-target interactions. The discovery of the efflux transporter P-glycoprotein (P-gp) in MDR cancer cells prompted the efforts in overcoming drug resistance by inhibition of P-gp.

The search for nontoxic anti-cancer agents able to overcome MDR has been an imperative in the field of drug design and discovery for many years. Two main approaches in combating the problem of MDR in cancer include (i) development of agents able to preserve cytotoxic activity toward MDR cancer cells; (ii) development of compounds able to restore the cytotoxicity of classic anti-cancer drugs.

In this chapter, we discuss the new findings regarding MDR reversal strategies, the alterations obtained in our artificially developed MDR models and advantages of our different approaches in overcoming MDR.

Keywords: Multi-drug resistance, cancer, P-glycoprotein, natural products, reversal approaches

Introduction

Resistance to anti-cancer drugs is mediated by several mechanisms, which include:

- reduced apoptosis,
- decreased transporter-based drug uptake,
- altered drug metabolism,
- altered site of action,
- increased DNA damage repair,

- increased energy-dependent efflux of free-diffusing hydrophobic anti-cancer agents.

Multi-drug resistance (MDR) is one of the major obstacles to the effective cancer treatment. MDR occurs when cancer cells become progressively insensitive to structurally different drugs. One of the main mechanisms underlying MDR is P-glycoprotein (P-gp) overproduction, an efflux pump encoded by the *mdr1* gene [1,2]. P-gp exports various hydrophobic anti-cancer drugs out of the cell, including anthracyclines, Vinca alkaloids, taxanes, epipodophyllotoxins, imatinib and nilotinib [3]. P-gp overexpression is associated with both intrinsic and acquired drug resistance and has become a major therapeutic target for overcoming MDR. In non-pathological conditions, P-gp is expressed in several tissues such as liver, kidney and gastrointestinal tract, where it has a protective role eliminating potentially harmful substances [4]. Besides P-gp, normal tissues express many other transporters from the same class referred to as ATP Binding Cassette (ABC) transporters. Their function is to export endogenous substrates, like amino acids, bile acids and hormones. Some of them are able to extrude anti-cancer drugs.

ABC transporters use energy from ATP hydrolysis to actively export compounds out of the cell [5]. The ABC transporter super-family is classified into seven subfamilies based on their sequence homology and domain organization. Three efflux pumps: P-gp (MDR1 or ABCB1), multi-drug resistance associated protein 1 (MRP1 or ABCC1) and breast resistance protein (BCRP or ABCG2), have a major impact on cancer chemotherapy [5]. They are responsible for transport of the majority of anti-cancer drugs such as:

- vinca alkaloids,
- anthracyclines,
- mitoxantrone,
- paclitaxel,
- etoposide
- tyrosine kinase inhibitors (gleevec and nilotinib) [6].

Additionally, the physiological role and the localization of efflux pumps in different tissues can greatly influence:

- absorption,
- elimination,

- distribution,
- metabolism,
- toxicity of drugs [7].

Therefore, finding new modalities for inhibition of these transporters is a main stream in re-establishment of drug sensitivity and improvement of the drug effectiveness in cancer therapy [8, 9, 10].

Finding an inhibitor with appropriate specificity, potency and intrinsic toxicity is difficult considering that major ABC drug transporters exhibit significant overlap in substrate specificities and show variability in expression levels and polymorphisms. Additionally, interactions of efflux pump modulators administered with different anti-cancer drugs can cause nonspecific side effects, which make overcoming of MDR extremely difficult.

There are many different approaches for overcoming MDR, which include competitive, noncompetitive and allosteric blocking of the drug binding sites on P-gp, the inhibition of ATP hydrolysis and the modification of membrane lipids [11, 12].

Developing anti-cancer compounds that are not P-gp substrates and consequently not expelled from cancer cells is also considered [13, 14]. There are many molecules with various structures and mechanisms of action which could potentially serve this purpose. These compounds include:

- microtubule stabilizing agents (epothilones and new taxanes),
- microtubule destabilizing agents (cryptophycins and halichondrins),
- inhibitors of topoisomerase I,
- topoisomerase II.

Although some of these drugs have similar structure as P-gp substrates, structural modifications at specific sites allow them to overcome MDR.

In addition to co-administration of inhibitors and cytotoxic substrates of P-gp other approaches for circumventing MDR include:

- P-gp-targeting antibodies,
- *mdr1* gene silencing strategies,
- transcriptional modulators,
- encapsulation of P-gp substrates into liposomes or nanoparticles.

We have studied different treatment modalities for overcoming MDR. To that end, we have developed, characterized and employed MDR cancer cell lines of epithelial origin: non-small cell lung carcinoma (NSCLC), colon carcinoma and glioblastoma.

Herein, we describe our main findings regarding effects of:

- natural compounds – euphodendrophanes (jatrophane diterpenoides) with high anti-P-gp activity,
- tipifarnib (farnesyl transferase/Ras inhibitor) that acts also as P-gp inhibitor,
- sulfinosine (purine nucleoside analog) that decreases P-gp expression,
- NK-2 host defense antimicrobial peptide that possesses unique selectivity towards P-gp overexpressing cells.

Considering that finding a selective, potent and relatively non-toxic compound, which inhibits ABC transporters and restores drug sensitivity in MDR cancer cells, is a major challenge in cancer treatment, the aim of this chapter is to shed new light on this problem and to contribute in its resolving.

Role of Natural Products in Overcoming MDR

History of ABC Transporters Inhibition

Three generations of compounds have been developed to modulate the activity of ABC transporters. First-generation of MDR1 inhibitors are compounds that are developed to treat other conditions: verapamil (a calcium channel blocker used as an antihypertensive), quinine (as an antimalarial) and cyclosporine A (as an immunosuppressant). Although these modulators inhibited P-gp-dependent drug efflux *in vitro*[15], they had low binding affinity and numerous adverse side effects such as dose-limiting toxicity andcardiac toxicity in the case of verapamil [16, 17].

In the development of second-generation of MDR1 inhibitors, efforts were focused on increasing the specificity for P-gp, while decreasing toxicities. Valspodar (PSC-833), a derivative of cyclosporine A, is representative of second-generation P-gp inhibitors. It showed higher potency and no immunosuppressive side effects in comparison with cyclosporine A and other first-generation inhibitors [18]. In addition, enhanced therapeutic effect of certain drugs in patients with acute myeloid leukemia was observed [19]. However, its further development was discontinued since in several Phase III clinical trials it did not improve patients' outcome and was associated with higher toxicity [20, 21].

It was shown that PSC-833 and other inhibitors exert their toxicity by inhibiting cytochrome P450 3A (CYP3A) function and decreasing CYP3A-mediated drug metabolism [22]. Another second-generation inhibitor Biricodar (VX-710) was shown to be potent modulator of both P-gp and MRP1-mediated MDR *in vitro*[23, 24]. However, in clinical trials it showed substantial level of toxicity [25, 26].

Therefore, the next, third, generation of inhibitors were designed to be more potent without interfering with pharmacokinetics of other anticancer drugs that cause undesired side effects. Tariquidar (an anthranilamide, XR9576), Elacridar (an acridone caroxamide), Zosuquidar (LY335979, quinolone derivative), CBT-1 (quinolone derivative) and Laniquidar (a piperidine) are representatives of this group of inhibitors. Generally, third-generation of P-gp inhibitors are less toxic, do not interfere with pharmacokinetics of anti-cancer drugs and have better outcomes in clinical trials than first- and second generation of inhibitors [27-30].

Inhibitors of other ABC transporters were also identified. The leukotriene LTD4 receptor antagonist MK571 was reported to specifically modulate MRP1 associated resistance [31]. Moreover, several compounds were identified to target multiple ABC transporters. Elacridar, a dual P-gp and BCRP inhibitor was reported to increase the bioavailability of topotecan[32], while biricodar has been identified as an inhibitor of both P-gp and MRP1 [24].

Since none of the available ABC transporter inhibitors is successful enough to fully restore sensitivity of MDR cells to chemotherapeutics there is constant search for the novel compounds that would be more specific and more potent inhibitors than the present ones [33].

Natural Sources Modulators: Fourth Generation Inhibitors

ABC transporter modulators or inhibitors, which arise from natural products, represent fourth generation inhibitors. Screening for new natural product modulators attracts a lot of attention in recent years, as they possess the potential to be more efficient than many of the modulators from earlier generations and with generally lower toxicity. Source material for biologically active compounds is very diverse and includes plants, fungi and marine organisms. The main goal is finding candidates from natural extracts, which strongly modulate the function or the expression of drug transporters. After purification, characterization and subsequent structure-activity relationship studies, many of the lead compounds undergo modifications to optimize their potency. As an example, fumitremorgin C, a toxin isolated from a fungus, is shown to be an effective ABCG2 inhibitor but exhibits high neurotoxicity [34]. For this reason, the toxin was modified into a less toxic analog with higher potency and specificity Ko143, making it more appropriate for clinical trials [35].

Curcumin

In recent years, curcumin has become one of the most investigated modulators isolated from natural products. It exhibits inhibitory effect on various ABC drug transporters and possesses many favorable biological actions such as anti-inflammatory [36], anti-viral [37] and anti-cancer [38]. Curcuminoids purified from *Curcuma longa* turmeric powder are mainly comprised of curcumin (curcumin I), demethoxycurcumin (curcumin II) and bisdemothoxycurcumin (curcumin III) [39]. Curcumin was shown to directly inhibit the functions of P-gp, MRP1and BCRP [40-42] and restore drug sensitivity in MDR cancer cells. It was also found to be active against MDR tumors in mice [42]. It wasshown to suppress NF-κB activation induced by TNF, phorbor esters and hydrogen peroxide through suppression of IκB degradation [43, 44]. Curcumin also inhibits the TPA-induced expression of cyclooxygenase-2 by suppressing NF-κB activation [45]. Curcumin also affects the Wnt signaling pathway, ß-catenin-induced c-Myc expression, the amount of nuclear ß-catenin and TCF-4 proteins [46, 47]. A serine/threonine kinase, the mammalian target of rapamycin (mTOR), acts downstream of thephosphatidylinositol 3-kinase (PI3K)/Akt (protein kinase B) and regulates the cell growth and survival [48]. Curcumin inhibits mTOR signaling in cancer cells through a protein phosphatase-dependent dephosphorylation mechanism [49, 50]. Curcumin has an inhibitory effect on P-gp function in KB-C2 cells and in addition to chemosensitizing potency, shows chemopreventive properties [51].

One of the main problems in clinical administration of curcumin is its very low level in plasma and tissues because of its lipophilic and insoluble nature.

Curcumin is also very rapidly metabolized requiring the administration of very high doses in order to reach biological effectiveness. However, even in high doses curcumin is well-tolerated and provided significant improvement in cancer patients with low drug-curcumin interactions [52]. Curcumin treatment can also improve the outcome in patients with rheumatoid arthritis [53], chronic anterior uveitis [54], inflammatory bowel disease [55], psoriasis[56] and in patients with advanced pancreatic cancer [57]. Various approaches have been proposed to improve the system delivery of curcumin, such as nanoparticles [58, 59], liposome encapsulated curcumin [60], curcumin phospholipid complex and structural analogues [61] and the curcumin-piperine combination. Piperine blocks the metabolism of curcumin and has the potential to increase the bioavailability of orally given curcumin in humans [62].

Flavonoids

Flavonoids are a well-studied group of natural product modulators, which include flavonols, flavones, isoflavones, flavanols, flavanolols, flavanones and chalcones. Their biological actions include anti-cancer, anti-mitotic and anti-viral properties [63-65]. They also exhibit kinase inhibiting [66], radical scavenging, metal ion chelating [67] and modulation activity against major ABC drug transporters [68, 69]. By modulating the function of ABC transporters, they modify drug absorption, penetration and elimination. Depending on the substrate of interest, flavonoids can both stimulate and inhibit the function of ABC transporters. The ability of flavonoids to inhibit P-gp-, MRP1- and BCRP-mediated drug efflux and restore drug sensitivity in MDR cancer cells has been extensively studied [68,69]. Flavonoids competitively bind to substrate-binding sites of ABC transporters [68, 69] and some of them can also affect ATP binding or hydrolysis at the nucleotide binding domains, or alter the surface expression level of ABC transporters [70].

Marine Products

In the past several decades a variety of new biologically active compounds have been isolated from marine sources, such as sponge, algae, coral and ascidian [71, 72] and many of them are considered to be cytotoxic against tumor cells [71]. In addition, marine compounds able to reverse MDR include: agosterol A, ecteinascidin 743, sipholane triterpenoids, bryostatin 1 and welwintolidones.

Agosterol A, a polyhydroxylated sterol acetate isolated from the marine sponge, was identified as the most active compound by bioassay-guided separation. It showed growth inhibition of colchicine treated MDR cancer cell line KB-C2 and showed no cytotoxicity against parental KB-3-1 cells at the same concentration [73]. The Agosterol A also completely reversed the resistance to vincristine, colchicine, doxorubicin and etoposide in KB-C2 and KB-CV60 cells [73] and inhibited drug efflux through P-gp and MRP1 [74].

Ecteinascidins are tetrahydroisoquinolone alkaloids isolated from the Caribbean tunicate *Ecteinascidia turbinate*[75]. Ecteinascidin 743 binds to the minor groove of DNA, bending the DNA helix towards the major groove [76] and interferes with cellular transcription-coupled nucleotide excision repair to induce cell death and cytotoxicity [77].Results obtained on KB-8-5 and KB-C2 MDR cells showed that a nontoxic concentration of Ecteinascidin 743 partially reversed the resistance to both doxorubicin and vincristine [78]. Best results with ecteinascidin 743 were obtained in breast, ovarian and mesenchymal tumors in phase I trials and in refractory soft tissue sarcoma, breast and ovarian cancer in phase II trials [79]. In 2007, ecteinascidin 743 (trabectedin, brand name Yondelis; PharmaMar) was approved in the European Union for advanced soft tissue sarcoma [80].

Triterpenoids, isolated from the Red Sea sponge *Callyspongia siphonella*, consist of four different skeletons: sipholane, siphonellane, neviotane and dahabane [81, 82]. Sipholane triterpenoids include sipholenol A, sipholenone E, sipholenol L and siphonellinol D. Sipholenol A has been shown to reverse P-gp-mediated MDR in cancer cells by directly inhibiting P-gp function [83].Sipholenol A increased the cytotoxicity of colchicine, vinblastine and paclitaxel in KB-C2 and KB-V1 cells but did not affect the sensitivity of vincristine and mitoxantrone. Sipholenone E, sipholenol L and siphonellinol D were also found to inhibit the function of P-gp and enhanced the cytotoxicity of several P-gp substrate in KB-C2 cells [80], but had no effect in MRP1-, MRP7- and BCRP-overexpressing cells.

Bryostatin 1 is a macrocyclic lactone isolated from the marine bryozoan *Bugula neritina* which activates protein kinase C (PKC) [84], induces the translocation of PKC from the cytosol to the membrane [85] and enhances the activity of P-gp by a PKC-mediated phosphorylation [86].

Welwitindolinones are alkaloids isolated from the blue-green alga *Hapalosiphon welwitschii*, which have the ability to reverse P-gp MDR [87].

N-Methylwelwitindolinone C increased the cytotoxicity of actinomycin D and daunomycin in SK-VLB-1 cells and the cytotoxicity of vinblastine, taxol, actinomycin D, colchicine and daunomycin in the drug-resistant breast carcinoma MCF-7/ADR cells.

MDR and Other Natural Compounds

P-gp is abundant in the apical membranes of intestinal epithelium, renal proximal tubular epithelium and the blood-brain barrier [5, 88] where it plays important roles in the absorption, distribution and elimination of many drugs, determining their efficacy and toxicity. Inhibition of P-gp activity can be an important factor in modifying the bioavailability and tissue distribution of P-glycoprotein substrates. Drug absorption, disposition and elimination can also be affected by different foods [89].

Many natural compounds obtained from herbs, food and dietary supplements exhibit much lower toxicity to the human body than medical drugs. In fact, a number of natural products including quercetin, (-)-epigallocatechin gallate, curcumin, capsaicin and [6]-gingerol, are promising anti-cancer drug efflux pump inhibitors [90,19, 51].

Consumption of tea *(Camellia sinensis)* has been linked to reduced risk of a variety of tumors including the skin, oral cavity, esophagus, stomach, intestine, lung, liver, pancreas, mammary gland, urinary bladder and prostate [5]. (-)-Epigallocatechin gallate (EGCG), the active tea compound with the cancer preventive effects, has been reported to have inhibitory effect on NF-κB pathway in JB6 mouse epidermal cells [91] and human epidermal keratinocytes [92]. The inhibition of heterocyclic amine 2-amino-1-methyl-6-phenylimidazo [4,5-b]pyridine (PhIP)-induced formation of intestinal polyps bytea constituentswas reported in Apcminmouse [93]. EGCG also inhibited ß-catenin/TCF (T – cell factor)reporter activity in human embryonic kidney cells HEK293 [183] and Wnt/ß-catenin signaling in human invasive breast cancer cells [94]. EGCG and other tea catechins have inhibitory effects on P-gp in human MDR epidermal carcinoma cell line KB-C2 cells, which overexpresses this membrane transporter [95-97].

Capsaicin, extracted from hot and red chili pepper *(Capsicum annuum)*, exhibits chemopreventive properties and suppresses carcinogenesis of the skin, colon, lung, tongue and prostate [43]. Capsaicin inhibits TNF-induced NF-κB activation in human myeloid ML-1a cells by blocking the degradation of IκB and nuclear translocation of NF-κB [98] and also inhibits the TPA (*12-O-*

tetradecanoylphorbol-13-acetate)-induced activation of NF-κB in mouse skin [99]. [6]-Gingerol, a phenol isolated from ginger *(Zingiber officinale)*, inhibits the proliferation of cancer cells including prostate, gastric and breast [43]. [6]-gingerol inhibits the activation of NF-κB and down-regulates ß-catenin-depenent cyclin D1 levels inducing apoptosis in cancer cells [100, 101]. Capsaicin and [6]-gingerol can also inhibit human P-gp, increasing the cytotoxicity of vinblastine and partially reversing MDR [51].

Phenolic diterpenes and triterpenes extracted from *Rosmarinus officinalis* are shown to possess strong anti-oxidative, anti-inflammatory, anti-microbial and anti-cancer properties [102-105]. Anti-oxidative activity of rosemary extracts is mainly derived from carnosic acid and carnosol [102]. Rosemary also yields substantial quantities of the polyphenolic antioxidant rosmarinic acid. Rosemary derived compounds such as carnosic acid, carnosol, rosmarinic acid and ursolic acid also act as potential chemopreventive agents. Carnosol reduces metalloproteinase-9 activity through inhibition of NF-κB, restricting the invasion of B16/F10 mouse melanoma cells [105]. Carnosol blocks the phosphorylation and degradation of IκB as well as nuclear translocation of NF-κB [106] and prevents ß-catenin/APC (Adenomatous polyposis coli)-associated intestinal carcinogenesis[107]. Carnosic acid, carnosol and ursolic acid are inhibitory to P-gp function in human MDR KB-C2 cells [108]. Carnosic acid chemosensitized KB-C2 cells to vinblastine, reversing P-gp-mediated MDR by increasing the intracellular accumulation of anti-cancer drug [108].

The ingestion of citrus fruit has been reported to be beneficial for the reduction of certain types of human cancer. A variety of compounds isolated from citrus such as monoterpenes, limonoids, flavonoids and coumarins were shown to possess anti-cancer activity [109]. Auraptene (7-geranyloxycoumarin) and nobiletin (5,6,7,8,3',4'-hexamethoxyflavone), have shown potential as chemopreventive agents. Coumarin auraptene inhibited 4-nitroquinoline 1-oxide-induced oral carcinogenesis in rats and suppressed the growth of human prostate carcinoma cells [110-112]. In addition, it showed suppression of TPA- and LPS (lipopolysaccharide)- induced inflammatory responses [113]. Nobiletin inhibited the production of NO and O2 in leukocytes and showed strong inhibitory effects on the growth of human prostate carcinoma cells, TPA-induced skin inflammation and oxidative stress in mice [114]. Auraptene or nobiletin were also shown to stimulate the basal ATPase activity of P-gp and further enhance the verapamil-stimulated ATPase activity of P-gp [115] suggesting that they could be substrates for P-gp competitively interacting at its drug binding site.

Plant sterols are essential structural components of membranes in plant cells. In addition to their activity as efficient modulators of plasma low-density lipoprotein (LDL) cholesterols in humans [116], their protective role in colon, breast and prostate cancer has been reported [117].

Plant sterol guggulsterone from the guggul tree (*Commiphora mukul*) suppresses TNF-induced phosphorylation, degradation of IκB and translocation of NF-κB to the nucleus [118]. Guggulsterone also promotes apoptosis in human lung carcinoma cells by inhibiting the activation of NF-κB and expression of anti-apoptotic gene products. Moreover, guggulsterone increased the cellular accumulation of daunorubicin in P-gp overexpressing KB-C2 cells [119].

A variety of other natural products have been reported to possess cancer preventive properties [5] and exhibit inhibitory effect on human P-gp, including:

- resveratrol (a phytoalexin isolated from grapes - *Vitis vinifera*),
- sesamin (a lignan found only in sesame - *Sesamum indicum*),
- seeds and matairesinol from soybean - *Glycine max*,
- glycyrrhetinic acid and glabridin from licorice - *Glycyrrhiza glabra*,
- extract and ginsenosides from the root of *Panax ginseng* [51, 120, 19].

There is also a number of natural products with inhibitory effects on MRP1 transport pump. Quercetin, EGCG and curcumin are all reported to interact with human MRP1 [121-123]. Citrus phytochemical nobiletin inhibits the function of MRP1 [115] as well as guggulsterone and glycyrrhetinic acid [119, 120]. Glycyrrhetinic acid has a chemosensitizing effect, reversing P-gp and MRP1-mediated MDR by increasing the intracellular accumulation of anti-cancer drugs [120].

Emerging Techniques for Overcoming MDR

Silencing of MDR1 Gene

New RNA interference (RNAi) technology was employed in overcoming MDR (Figure 1). This technology exploits short interfering RNAs (siRNAs) that are synthetic analogs of RNAi. Many authors reported promising results regarding suppression of P-gp expression by this method. For example, Stierle and collaborators reached maximum of 50% of P-gp mRNA suppression using 5nM siRNA delivered by OligofectamineTM in MCF7 resistant cells [124]. Compared to the conventional P-gp inhibitors, siRNAs tend to have reduced toxicity toward non-target tissues and higher specificity for desired gene targets [125, 126]. Most of the studies focused on MDR reversal by siRNA methodology use *in vitro* systems while there are only several publications on animal models. Notably, 80% P-gp down-regulation was observed in Balb/c nude mice bearing NCI-H460 xenograft tumors upon StealthTM RNAi delivery. It ultimately resulted in reduction of tumor size after 13 days of vinorelbine treatment [127]. However, there are several obstacles for successful siRNA delivery and subsequent P-gp knockdown. Initially, anionic siRNA has to cross the plasma membrane and therefore choice of adequate carrier with high affinity to siRNA is crucial step. Furthermore, P-gp protein has long half-life, while siRNA is rapidly degraded and therefore needs chemical modification to increase its half-life and activity [128]. Although siRNAs are sequence specific they can cause undesired silencing of genes other than targeted one; probably due to similarities in mRNA sequences [129]. Another aspect that can limit therapeutic effect of siRNA in *in vivo* systems is the activation of the innate immune system due to siRNA recognition in the endosomes [130]. Delivery of other molecules such as micro-RNAs (miRNAs), hammerhead ribozymes and antisense oligonucleotides (ASO) may be efficient in overcoming MDR through sequence-specific down-regulation of P-gp. Zhu et al. showed that specific miRNA delivered by OligofectamineTM decreased P-gp levels by 40% and increased sensitivity to vinblastine in the human ovarian cancer cell line, A2780, and its MDR counterpart, A2780DX5 [131]. Similarly, hammerhead ribozymes against P-gp mRNA were able to increase sensitivity to doxorubicin and etoposide in a human colon cancer cell line (HCT-8DDP) [51]. Administration of ASOs by liposomal delivery system could also increase accumulation of doxorubicin in drug-resistant MCF-7 cells by reducing P-gp expression [132].

Inhibition of Nuclear Receptors

Another promising approach in solving MDR problem is its prevention rather than reversal that can be achieved by down-regulation of drug-mediated *mdr1* overexpression. The transcription of *mdr1* gene is regulated by many factors including nuclear receptors such as pregnane X receptor (PXR) [133]. This xenobiotic receptor was shown to bind and activate promoter of *mdr1* gene in response to applied drugs [133]. The association between the activity of PXR and drug resistance, as well as successful down-regulation of PXR that increase effectiveness of anti-cancer drugs was reported in several cancer types such as osteosarcoma, prostate, colon and endometrial cancer[134-137]. Hence, recentefforts are directedtoward search/development of PXR antagonists and inhibitors that would prevent drug-mediated activation of PXR and subsequent overexpression of P-gp (Figure 1).

Nanotechnology

Application of nanotechnology is widely studied in cancer treatment. Use of nanoparticles for site-specific release of chemotherapeutic agents has several advantages over conventional therapies including overcoming MDR. Regarding main obstacles in chemotherapy, nanoparticles are developed to inhibit or bypass efflux pumps on the membrane or to enhance endocytosis in MDR tumors (Figure 1).It increases drug uptake and protects drugs from P-gp recognition.

Various nanoparticles-based drug-delivery systems were developed so far:

- liposomal nanoparticle,
- solid lipid nanoparticle,
- gold nanoparticle,
- nanodiamond,
- magnetic nanovector,
- carbon nanotube,
- quantum dot nanocarrier,
- polymeric nanoparticle,
- dendrimer nanoparticle,
- virus-mediated nanocarrier [138, 139].

Doxorubicin-loaded nanoparticles were shown to be efficient in overcoming MDR in breast and ovarian cancer cells [140, 141] while paclitaxel delivered by various nanoparticles was effective in resistant colon and breast cancer cells [142, 143]. Doxorubicin conjugated gold nanoparticles were shown to increase intracellular uptake and drug citotoxicity in MDR hepatocellular and breast carcinoma cell lines [144, 22]. Nanotechnology offers the possibility to deliver simultaneously multiple compounds, such as anti-cancer agents and P-gp inhibitors, into MDR tumor cells. Similarly, successful delivery of conventional therapeutic doxorubicin along with P-gp siRNA was achieved using mesoporous silica nanoparticles, as well as RGD (Arg–Gly–Asp)-modified liposomes, in drug resistant tumors [145, 146].

Collateral Sensitivity

Collateral sensitivity (CS) is phenomenon referred to as drug hypersensitivity of resistant cancer cells compared to the non-resistant parental cells [147]. Namely, developing resistance towards one agent is accompanied by the development of hypersensitivity towards another compound. The existence of such phenomenon allows us to search for substances that selectively modulate MDR (Figure 1). Verapamil, as a classical P-gp inhibitor, was shown to induce CS in P-gp expressing cells [148]. Its S-isomer can also be efficient CS inducing agent in MRP1-transfected cells [149]. Xanthones were also found to be potent MRP1-selective CS agents with less cardiotoxic side effects compared to verapamil [150]. Glucose analog 2-Deoxy-D-glucose (2-DG) was reported to induce CS in resistant breast MCF7/ADR and cervical adenocarcinoma KB-V1 cells compared to their sensitive counterparts [151, 152]. The flavonoid desmosdumotin B and its derivatives have been shown to selectively eliminate the P-gp-expressing cell lines KB-VIN and Hep3B-VIN [153, 154]. NSC73306 is an isatin-β-thiosemicarbazone that was also reported to elicit CS towards numerous P-gp-expressing cells lines [155, 156]. The iron chelator di-2-pyridkylketone-4,4,-dimethyl-3-thiosemicarbazone (Dp44mT) exerted CS towards the P-gp-expressing human adenocarcinoma cell line KB-V1, while lacking CS towards the MRP1-expressing MCF7-VP16 breast cancer cell line [157]. Moreover, it has been demonstrated that several P-gp expressing human adenocarcinoma cell lines (KB-A1, KB-8-5, KB-8-5-11 and KB-V1) as well as the breast cancer cell line MCF-7/ VP-16 expressing MRP1 are collaterally sensitive to tiopronin [158].

Tyrosine Kinase Inhibitors

Although tyrosine kinase inhibitors (TKIs) in many cases were proven to be successful anti-cancer agents, MDR can also greatly affect their efficacy in cancer treatment. There is complex association between TKIs and MDR [3]. Namely, ABC transporters are involved in resistance to TKIs, while on the contrary some TKIs can inhibit ABC transporter-mediated drug efflux and therefore contribute to solving problem of resistance to conventional chemotherapeutics [159]. Most of the TKIs (imatinib, nilotinib, dasatinib, gefitinib, danusertib) are substrates for BCRP pump [160-164]. Additionally, both P-gp and MRP1 can also confer resistance to imatinib [165-167], while resistance to nilotinib can also be P-gp mediated [168]. Moreover, MRP2 can contribute to resistance to TKIs as was shown for sorafenib [169]. Several studies have shown that imatinib can reverse resistance to classical chemotherapeutic drugs in cells overexpressing P-gp, as well as BCRP [170, 171]. Although nilotinib is substrate for P-gp and BCRP it was reported that nilotinib increases intracellular accumulation of paclitaxel in cell lines overexpressing P-gp and mitoxantronein cells transfected with BCRP [172]. Another TKI, erlotinib, was also shown to reverse P-gp and BCRP-mediated MDR in cancer cells by directly inhibiting the drug efflux function of these transporters [173]. Gefitinib, as an analogue of erlotinib, has been reported to reverse BCRP-mediated resistance to topotecan and mitoxantrone in resistant cells by inhibiting the function of BCRP [174]. It was also capable of modulating resistance to paclitaxel and docetaxel by direct interaction with P-gp in lung and breast cancer cells overexpressing this ABC transporter [175]. However, sorafenib restored sensitivity to conventional anticancer compounds in MDR hepatocellular carcinoma cells probably through downregulation of either gene or P-gp protein expression. It was also shown that this TKI works effectively in combination with doxorubicin or gemcitabin in resistant hepatocellular carcinoma [176].

Targeting Resistance to Apoptosis

An important feature of MDR is resistance to apoptosis, which prevents action of various cytotoxic drugs. Therefore, developing strategies for inducing apoptosis is essential for overcoming MDR in cancer cells (Figure 1). P53, a tumorsuppressor molecule, is commonly altered in human cancers [177, 178] and is also associated with acquisition of MDR, since wild-type p53 represses *mdr1* expression. Adenovirus-mediated *p53* gene (Ad-p53) transfection was shown to enhance doxorubicin cytotoxicity and reverse doxorubicin resistance in human breast cancer cells [179]. Moreover, nutlin-3, a non-genotoxic MDM2 inhibitor that activates p53 pathway, inhibits P-gp and

MRP1 and sensitizes chemoresistant neuroblastoma and rhabdomyosarcoma cell lines to vincristine [180]. Compounds that interfere with mitochondrial apoptotic machinery, such as obatoclax, were shown to restore sensitivity to several anticancer drugs [181]. Inhibitors of NF-kB, transcription factor that suppresses the apoptotic potential of chemotherapeutic agents, were also shown to sensitize cells to anticancer drugs [182]. PI3K induce apoptosis through Akt-mediated inhibition of pro-apoptotic Bad and therefore its inhibitors show potential for overcoming apoptotic resistance in MDR cells [183, 184]. Direct Akt down-regulation using specific siRNA also increases cell sensitivity towards various chemotherapeutic drugs [94]. Additionally, transfection of wild-type PTEN, a negative regulator of PI3K/Akt signaling pathway that is frequently inactivated in human cancers [177, 185], reverse drug resistance in K562/ADM leukemic cells [186].

MDR cells often have decreased level of ceramide, second messenger that induces immune response and apoptosis. *In vitro* and *in vivo* studies showed that combination treatments with ceramide and paclitaxel, delivered by nanocarrier system, were effective in overcoming MDR [187, 188]. Moreover, silencing of overexpressed glucosylceramide synthase, enzyme that converts ceramide into inactive form, successfully down-regulates P-gp and resensitizes MDR breast cancer cells to anti-cancer drugs [189].

Physical Techniques

MDR can also be successfully overcome using different physical approaches in combination with conventional therapies. Namely, work on MDR cervical carcinoma cells showed that hyperthermia sensitized cells to doxorubicin delivered by liposomes [190]. Similarly, application of ultrasound in combination with nanoparticles loaded with doxorubicin increased the efficacy of the drug in both MDR and drug sensitive cells [191, 192].

Immunotherapy

Administration of immunotherapy with the aim to treat successfully MDR-expressing cancer cells has been studied extensively. In the beginning of immunotherapy investigations, cytokines were used to treat MDR cancer cells. Early studies showed that TNF-alpha, interferon-gamma and IL-2 reduced *mdr1* expression in various human cancer cell lines and sensitized cells to subsequent treatment with vincristine and doxorubicin (Figure 1) [193].

In one approach, an IL-2/granzyme A fusion protein was used to deliver granzyme A, an immune protein inducing caspase-independent apoptosis, to IL-2 receptor-expressing cells and increased their sensitivity to doxorubicin (Figure 1) [194].

Alkylphospholipids

Alkylphospholipids (ALPs), such as edelfosine, miltefosine, perifosine, erucylphosphocholine and erufosine, represent a relatively new class of synthetic compounds that act on cell membranes, selectively target proliferating cancer cells, inducing growth arrest and apoptosis. Moreover, they are potent sensitizers of conventional chemo- and radiotherapy. Specifically, miltefosine showed synergistic effect with paclitaxel in resistant glioblastoma cells [195]. Similarly, perifosine enhanced response of mouse neuroblastoma model system to etoposid through the Akt inhibition [196]. Simultaneous inhibition of ErbB signaling by gefitinib and inhibition of Akt by perifosine was recently shown to overcome tamoxifen resistance in breast carcinoma cells (Figure 1) [197].

MDR *In Vitro* Models

We have developed several MDR cancer cell lines in order to study different approaches for overcoming MDR. Resistant colon cancer and glioma cell lines, DLD1-TxR and U87-TxR, respectively, were selected after continuous exposure of their sensitive counterparts (DLD1 and U87) to stepwise increasing concentrations of paclitaxel [198]. Resistant NSCLC cell line, NCI-H460/R, was obtained from its sensitive parental cells (NCI-H460) using the same approach but with doxorubicin as selective agent [199]. The obtained cells exhibit classical MDR phenotype with cross-resistance to several anti-cancer agents (Table 1). DLD1- TxR showed significant cross-resistance to vinblastine, epirubicin, doxorubicin and etoposide, and slight cross-resistance to cisplatin. U87-TxR has considerable cross-resistance only to vinblastine and slight cross-resistance to epirubicin, doxorubicin, etoposide and cisplatin [199]. NCI-H460/R cells were characterized by marked cross-resistance to paclitaxel, moderate cross-resistance to vinblastine, etoposide and epirubicin [199].

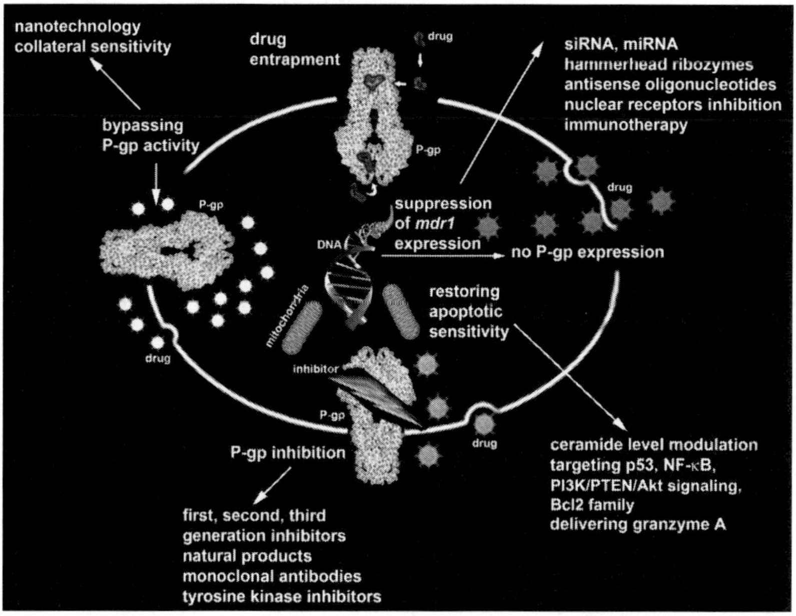

Figure 1. Different approaches for overcoming MDR. Main strategies for circumventing MDR are P-gp inhibition, suppression of *mdr1* expression, bypassing P-gp activity and restoring apoptotic sensitivity. P-gp inhibition can be achieved using either first, second, third generation of inhibitors, natural products as fourth generation of inhibitors, monoclonal antibodies or tyrosine kinase inhibitors. Several approaches can be exploited to suppress *mdr1* expression such as targeted silencing by siRNA, miRNA, hammerhead rybozomes or antisense oliginucleotides, inhibition of nuclear receptors such as PXR as well as use of immunotherapy. Nanotechnology achievements and collateral sensitivity could be used to bypass P-gp activity. Finally, modulation of ceramide level, delivering granzyme A or targeting p53, NF-κB, Bcl-2 family or PTEN/PI3K/Akt pathway could be utilized to restore apoptotic sensitivity and therefore overcome MDR.

Our Approaches for Overcoming MDR

Resistant phenotype in all three newly established cancer cell lines is mainly a consequence of significant increase in expression of *mdr1* gene and its product P-gp (Table 1) [198-203]. It is followed by significant drop in the intracellular accumulation of P-gp substrates (Rho 123 and DOX) in resistant compared to sensitive cell lines [198, 199, 201, 204]. The composition of plasma membrane is altered in NCI-H460/R and DLD1-TxR cells. They possess more phosphatidylserine on the surface of membrane than their parental cells [205].

Furthermore, the induction of MDR decreased the *mrp1* expression in DLD1-TxR and U87-TxR [198], while it was not significantly changed in NCI-H460/R cells [199, 204]. NCI-H460/R is additionally characterized by decreased *topo IIa* mRNA level due to continuous doxorubicin application and development of doxorubicin resistance [199, 201].

Glutathione detoxification system was not affected by the acquisition of MDR in DLD1-TxR cell line. However, in U87-TxR cells, the level of *gst-π* gene expression was decreased by 43% and it was accompanied with significant depletion of GSH concentration compared to U87 cells (Table 1) [199]. On the contrary, in NCI-H460/R cells expression of *gst-π* is significantly increased compared to its sensitive counterpart [200]. However, these two cell lines did not differ in the level of reduced glutathione [201].

Further characterization of the resistant cell lines revealed a disturbance of cell cycle kinetics (Table 1). Flow-cytometric analysis showed significant decrease in the percentage of cells in G1 and S phases and increase in cell death in subG0 in DLD1-TxR cell line. The changes in cell cycle distribution in U87-TxR and NCI-H460/R compared to their parental cells are due to decrease in G1 phase and increase in S and G2/M phase [198, 201].

Genotypic analyses revealed that acquisition of MDR caused selection of mutations in *p53* tumor suppressor gene in NCI-H460/R cell line and the loss of the region containing this gene in U87-TxR cells (Table 1) [200, 203]. DLD1-TxR cell line was derived from the sensitive cells that already carried mutation in *p53*[206]. Moreover, *PTEN* gene was affected by the induction of MDR, specifically in DLD1-TxR cells where it suffered the loss of heterozygousity (Table 1). NCI-H460/R cells stayed genetically unchanged in the case of *PTEN*, while U87-TxR is *PTEN* null since its sensitive counterpart already had such aberration (Table 1) [206, 207].

Cytogenetic analyses revealed gross chromosomal alterations in all three resistant cancer cell lines compared to their parental cells (Table 1). The NCI-H460/R cells possess several numerical and structural aberrations compared to their sensitive cells including gains of chromosomes, 13, 17 and 19 and losses of 4p, 5q, 6q and chromosomes Y, 9, 10, 12, 21 and 22 with the decrease in overall number of chromosomes. The DLD1-TxR cells obtained another set of chromosomal aberrations such as loss of chromosome Y, del(4)(q35) and del(6)(q23.3q25.1).

Table 1. Major changes developed after MDR induction in NCI-H460/R, DLD1-TxR and U87-TxR cells

	NCI-H460	NCI-H460/R	DLD1	DLD1-TxR	U87	U87-TxR
IC50 (PTX)	35 nM	2500 nM	40 nM	1800 nM	90 nM	1200 nM
IC50 (DOX)	40 nM	2000 nM	30 nM	4000 nM	300 nM	1000 nM
mdr1 mRNA	basal expression	15 fold increase	existing expression	4 fold increase	no expression	induced expression
p53 status	wild type	mutated	mutated	mutated	wild type	LOH
PTEN alterations	expressed	expressed	expressed	LOH	null	null
GSH concentration		unchanged		unchanged		significantly decreased
cell cycle disturbance		G1 phase↓ S phase↑ G2/M phase↑		G1 phase↓ S phase↓		G1 phase↓ S phase↑ G2/M phase↑
chromosomal alterations		numerical: chromosome number decrease structural: loss of 6q and Y		structural: Y, del(4)(q35) del(6)(q23.3q25.1)	aneuploidy 67–76 chromosomes	numerical: one ploidy reduction 45–50 chromosomes

U87-TxR mostly retained characteristic clonal structural rearrangements of their sensitive counterpart, but the karyotype of most cells (~90 %) was byproduct of one level ploidy reduction, with the reduction in mitotic chromosome number from 67–76 in U87 to 45–50 in U87-TxR [203].

Euphodendrophanes (Jatrophane Diterpenoids)

Euphorbiaceae are known since ancient times as plants that cure cancer and as such, they have been described in the literature of antique Greeks and Romans. Recent studies have recognized macrocyclic jatrophane diterpenoids from Euphorbia species as new leading inhibitors of P-gp [208, 209].

Spurge plants (*Euphorbia dendroides*) from Sardinia and Montenegro are plentiful source of jatrophane diterpenoids [210-212]. Apart from the moderate difference in stereochemistry and polarity between jatrophanes from two geographical sources, they all possess high anti-P-gp activity.

We have tested jatrophane diterpenoids (euphodendrophanes) for their anti-P-gp activity on three different human MDR cancer cell lines developed in our laboratory [198, 199]. P-gp functional assay with Rhodamine 123 was employed. The potential of the tested compounds to inhibit P-gp was measured by flow-cytometry as an increase in accumulation of Rhodamine 123 and expressed through fluorescence activity ratio (FAR). We have observed that investigated jatrophanes significantly differ in the degree of inhibition of the efflux activity of P-gp in NCI-H460/R and DLD1-TxR cells, while they exert similar activity against P-gp in U87-TxR cells.

According to the FAR values, we have classified jatrophanes as moderate ($2 < FAR < 10$), strong ($10 < FAR < 20$) and very strong P-gp inhibitors ($FAR > 20$) [110]. In addition, we have tested the cell growth inhibitory effect of jatrophanes by Sulforhodamine B viability assay. The IC50 values (the concentration of jatrophanes necessary to inhibit the cell growth by 50% compared to untreated control) were further correlated next to FAR values (Figure 2). Pearson test revealed strong negative correlation between anti-P-gp activity (FAR) and IC50 values in NCI-H460/R and DLD1-TxR cells expressed by **r** index (-0.7333 and -0.7314, respectively). Obviously, jatrophanes with higher anti-P-gp activity (higher FAR values) are better cell growth inhibitors (lesser IC50 values). No correlation (**r** index close to zero) was found in U87-TxR where all tested jatrophanes showed the same moderate anti-P-gp activity ($2 < FAR < 10$) (Figure 2).

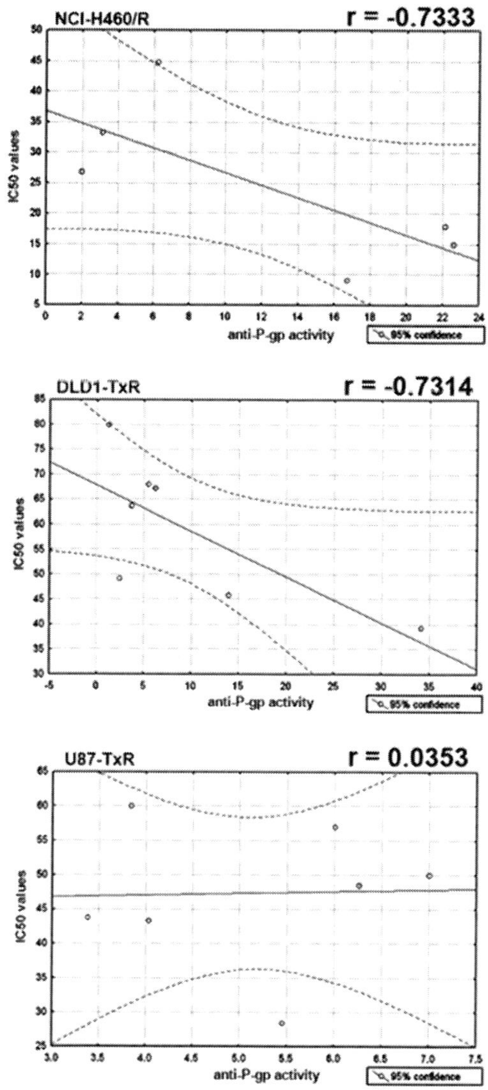

Figure 2. Relation between anti-cancer and anti-P-gp activities of euphodendrophanes. Euphodendrophanes' anti-cancer activity expressed by IC50 value was correlated with euphodendropanes' anti-P-gp activity expressed by FAR index in three MDR cancer cell lines (NCI-H460/R, DLD1-TxR and U87-TxR). Pearson correlation was employed. If r index is between 0 and 1, the correlation is considered as positive. If r index is between -1 and 0, the correlation is considered as negative.

Some of the investigated euphodendrophanes were found to be more powerful inhibitors of P-gp than R + verapamil and tariquidar (the second and third generation of P-gp modulators) [212]. The highest increase in the accumulation of Rhodamine123 and complete blockade of P-gp pump were observed in colorectal MDR cells (DLD1-TxR). Structure–activity relationship showed no obvious difference in the activity of jatrophanes with 6,17 exo- and those with 5,6 endo double bond [212]. Our jatrophanes possess homogeneous skeleton with main differences in the substitution pattern on medium sized ring. Their activity is strongly affected by the OBz group at the positions C-8 and C-9 for jatrophanes with exo- and endo double bond, respectively [212].

Considering high anti-P-gp activity, euphodendrophanes can be used as valuable tools for drug development and the improvement of chemotherapy in MDR cancers. However, the effective reversion of MDR requires both, the inhibition of transport proteins, such as P-gp and modulation of other mechanisms of resistance.

The effectiveness of anti-cancer agents is often limited by appearance of MDR. However, we observed that the existence of MDR phenotype in non-small cell lung carcinoma do not influence the effect of most tested euphodendrophanes (Table 2). They showed similar effect on MDR cancer cell line (NCI-H460/R) and its sensitive counterpart (NCI-H460). The lack of cross-resistance to euphodendrophanes implies that these compounds are not transported by P-gp pump.

Table 2. Growth inhibition potential of jatrophanes in sensitive and MDR NSCLC cell lines (NCI-H460 and NCI-H460/R)

jatrophanes	NCI-H460		NCI-H460/R	
	IC30[a)]	IC50[b)]	IC30	IC50
Euph A	31.0	46.6	26.6	44.8
Euph B	6.1	16.2	3.9	17.2
Euph H	2.4	6.0	5.5	15.0
Euph I	17.3	39.6	16.8	33.3
Euph K	2.3	4.7	6.6	18.0
Euph L	2.8	6.4	3.3	9.1
Euph Q	2.2	11.2	8.7	26.8
Euph R	3.5	10.0	6.4	17.0

[a)] Concentration necessary to inhibit 30% of cell growth in μM.
[b)] Concentration necessary to inhibit 50% of cell growth in μM.

Moreover, our jatrophanes significantly reduced the level of *mdr1* expression (codes for P-gp) in sensitive cells, suggesting that they could not induce the development of resistance. In contrast, paclitaxel (PTX), which is a P-gp substrate, increased the *mdr1* expression in sensitive (NCI-H460) cells [204].

In addition, we have found that our jatrophanes were non-toxic to normal cells in the range of concentrations necessary to inhibit the growth of cancer cells [204].

Importantly, we have found that jatrophanes are able to enhance the growth inhibition of PTX and reverse PTX resistance [204]. Further, we were searching for the mechanism, other than P-gp inhibition, by which jatrophane compounds exert their synergistic effects with PTX.

Considering PTX's ability to promote cell cycle arrest at G2/M phase by microtubule polymerization and stabilization of mitotic spindle, we examined whether the disturbance of cell cycle kinetics contributed to the observed synergism. Other authors found that some jatrophanes exhibit microtubule-interacting activity similar to PTX, but without inducing cell cycle arrest in G2/M phase [213]. We confirmed the stimulation of purified tubulin assembly *in vitro* by our jatrophanes within the range of concentrations that effectively inhibit cell growth [204].

The results showed that euphodendrophane alone as well as PTX in lower concentration (40 nM) increase the portion of cells in G2/M phase. However, the cell cycle arrest at G2/M phase was more pronounced in combination with a euphodendrophane (Figure 3).

Although the exact mechanism of jatrophanes-mediated cell cycle disturbance needs to be clarified, the synergism between euphodendrophanes and PTX is partly due to their mutual effect on microtubule assembly.

Next, our results showed that jatrophane type compounds could exert their anti-cancer effect through inhibition of vascular endothelial growth factor (VEGF) secretion. This effect was also more pronounced in combination with PTX.

Besides anti-P-gp activity, we have observed the synergistic effect of euphodendrophanes and PTX, induction of G2/M arrest and even anti-angiogenic activity [204].

In view of the wide distribution and availability of *Euphorbia* plants and relatively easy isolation of jatrophanes, further examinations of new cancer treatment and prevention approaches with jatrophanes should be promising.

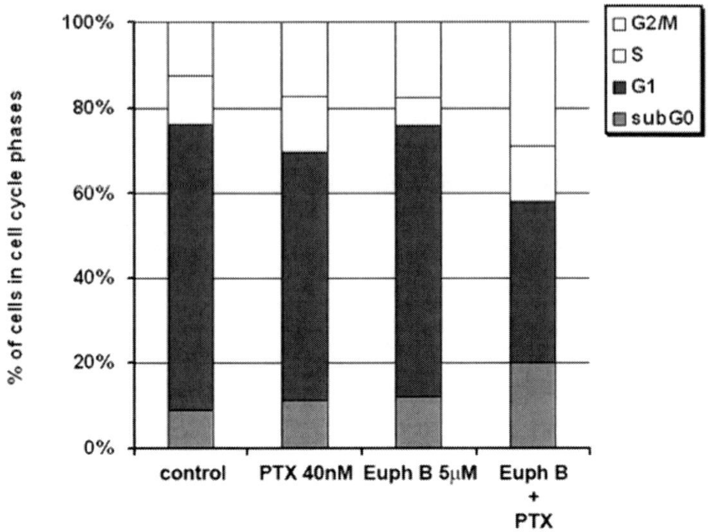

Figure 3. Combinations of Euph B with PTX induce disturbance of cell cycle kinetics. Synchronized NCI-H460/R cells were incubated for 72 h in complete medium. Single treatment of PTX, Euph B and their combination were applied for 72 h. Cell cycle analysis was performed by FACScalibur flow cytometry, using Mod-FIT software.

Tipifarnib (Farnesyl Transferase/Ras Inhibitor)

Besides P-gp inhibitors (jatrophane diterpenoids), we have evaluated the potential for overcoming drug resistance with signaling pathway inhibitors (Akt inhibitor—GSK690693 and Ras inhibitor—Tipifarnib) using our MDR *in vitro* models.

It is known that increased activity of PI3K/Akt and Ras/MEK/ERK signaling pathways can lead to drug resistance considering their positive role in extended cell survival [214]. In addition, activation of PI3K/Akt and Ras/MEK/ERK pathways can modulate the expression of *mdr1* gene [215].

Tipifarnib demonstrated strong growth inhibitory effect making no difference between sensitive and resistant cell lines. However, the presence of MDR phenotype in NCI-H460/R and DLD1-TxR changed the inhibitory potential of Akt inhibitor—GSK690693. The relative resistance to GSK690693 in DLD1-TxR cells was in accordance with the inactivation of PTEN tumor suppressor in this cell line [203]. Since there was no LOH in PTEN tumor suppressor in NCI-H460/R cells, we assumed that the resistance to GSK690693 was driven by mutated *p53* observed earlier [200]. GSK690693 showed moderate inhibitory effect against both glioma cell lines (U87 and U87-TxR).

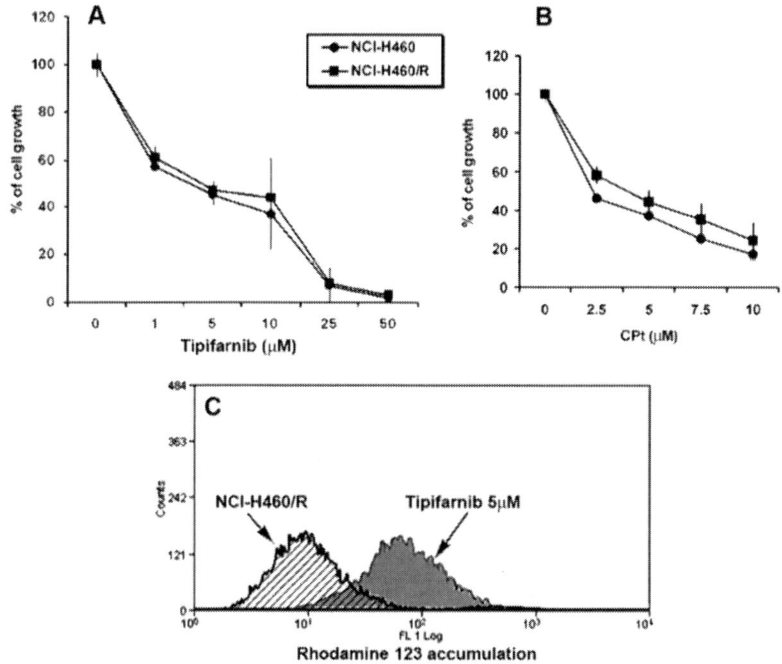

Figure 4. Cell growth inhibition and anti-P-gp activity of tipifarnib. Cell growth inhibition of NCI-H460 and NCI-H460/R induced by tipifarnib (A) and cisplatin (B). The results were assessed by sulforhodamine B (SRB) assay. All values represent average ± SD obtained from five independent experiments, n = 5. Flow cytometric profiles of Rhodamine 123 accumulation in NCI-H460/R cells untreated and treated with 5 μM tipifarnib (C). Two independent experiments were performed (a minimum of 10,000 events were collected for each experimental sample).

Considering that inhibitors of the PI3K/Akt and Ras/MEK/ERK pathways are being rapidly evaluated in preclinical models and in clinical studies in order to restore therapeutic sensitivity to classic anti-cancer drugs [216, 217], we decided to study the effects of simultaneous combination of Akt/Ras inhibitors and PTX. The obtained results pointed to the potential of both Akt and Ras inhibitors to enhance PTX activity [203]. However, Ras inhibitor-Tipifarnib caused significantly higher improvement of PTX effect (declination of IC50 for PTX) compared to Akt inhibitor-GSK690693. We confirmed that anti-P-gp effect of Tipifarnib further contributes to its effectiveness in re-establishment of sensitivity to PTX. Actually, Tipifarnib significantly increased Rhodamine 123 accumulation in all tested MDR cancer cell lines [203].

In addition, we have compared the capacity of Tipifarnib and cisplatin (CPt) to inhibit the growth of the sensitive NSCLC cell line (NCI-H460) and its resistant counterpart (NCI-H460/R) (Figure 4A,B). Inhibitory profiles of both compounds were not affected by the presence of MDR phenotype. It is known that CPt is not a substrate for P-gp [218] and this effect was expected. In contrast to CPt, Tipifarnib showed significant anti-P-gp activity in NCI-H460/R cells (Figure 4C). Therefore, Tipifarnib may pass the P-gp barrier in MDR cancer cells, exert its specific effect and even more inhibit the P-gp activity. By this means, Tipifarnib possesses significant potential for MDR reversal and its application in MDR cancers should be considered.

Sulfinosine (Purine Nucleoside Analog)

Sulfinosine or SF ([R,S]-2-amino-9-b-D-ribofuranosylpurine-6-sulfinamide) is the oxidized form of 6-thioguanosine [219]. It is a quite unexplored anti-cancer agent in comparison to other thiopurines (6-thioguanine and 6-mercaptopurine). SF inhibits cancer cell growth, at least partially, by the incorporation of its phosphorylated derivative into DNA. The metabolic conversion of SF to corresponding nucleotide-monophosphate derivative is more complex than that of other thiopurines [220]. Since SF utilizes different metabolic pathways for its intracellular activation, SF treatment does not induce resistance in cancer cells.

The metabolism of SF involves the cells' glutathione (GSH) system. SF readily adducts to sulfhydryl compounds (GSH and cysteine). By suppressing the glutathione detoxification system and elevating the concentration of reactive oxygen species (ROS), SF may induce the death of cancer cells [220].

In addition, SF showed considerable anti-angiogenic activities through inhibition of VEGF secretion and expression [221]. It was shown that some purine analogs closely related to SF showed considerable anti-angiogenic activities [222, 223].

In view of its considerable efficacy in cancer treatment and moderate toxicity to normal cells [16], SF is suitable for combining with other chemotherapeutic agents. SF acts synergistically with 8-Cl-cAMP, doxorubicin, curcumin and verapamil [224, 200, 202].

We have shown that all mentioned anticancer effects of SF could be useful for the reversion of resistance to chemotherapeutics [221].

Cellular redox environment is a delicate balance between the levels of reactive oxygen species (i.e., superoxide and hydrogen peroxide) and the antioxidant system that scavenges them (i.e., glutathione/glutathione peroxidase and tioredoxin/peroxiredoxin pathways) [225]. Considering that ROS can be generated from exogenous sources (e.g. ionizing radiation, chemicals), we examined whether SF changes the ROS concentration in MDR cancer cells.

SF increased the level of ROS, depleted intracellular GSH and inhibited the expression of key enzymes involved in GSH synthesis and cell detoxification [221].We also found that SF inhibits P-gp expression and its function. This anti-P-gp as well as anti-VEGF effects of SF were mediated through the decrease of HIF-1α expression. It was shown that besides VEGF, HIF-1α could regulate the expression of P-gp [226].By modulating cellular redox status through GSH depletion, SF changes the expression pattern of HIF-1α which down-regulates *mdr1* gene (Figure 5). However, in our studies [198] we observed that classic cytostatic agent PTX up-regulates mdr1 expression although it also depletes cellular GSH (Figure 5).

Namely, the induction of MDR by PTX in U87-TxR cell line caused significant depletion of *gst-π* gene expression and GSH concentration. The levels of *mrp1* mRNA that codes for another membrane transporter that could be involved in MDR development was lower than in their sensitive counterparts [198]. These results are consistent with another study revealing that acquisition of PTX resistance caused decrease in mrp1 and gst-π gene expression [227].

PTX, a diterpene natural product [228], is an antimitotic drug that binds specifically to the β-tubulin subunit in polymerized microtubules. As a consequence, dynamics of mitotic spindle is suppressed, leading to cell cycle arrest at G2/M phase and eventually cell death by apoptosis [229] or slippage back into the G1-phase of the cell cycle without cell division [230]. PTX also affects the process of tumor-angiogenesis through inhibition of matrix metaloproteinases production [231] and VEGF secretion [232].

Despite its high antineoplastic activity, PTX's effectiveness is often limited by the appearance of MDR. In an attempt to define cellular processes, which influence drug efficacy, different mechanisms involved in resistance to PTX were examined so far [233]. However, the main mechanism which prevents the action of PTX is over-expression of P-gp.

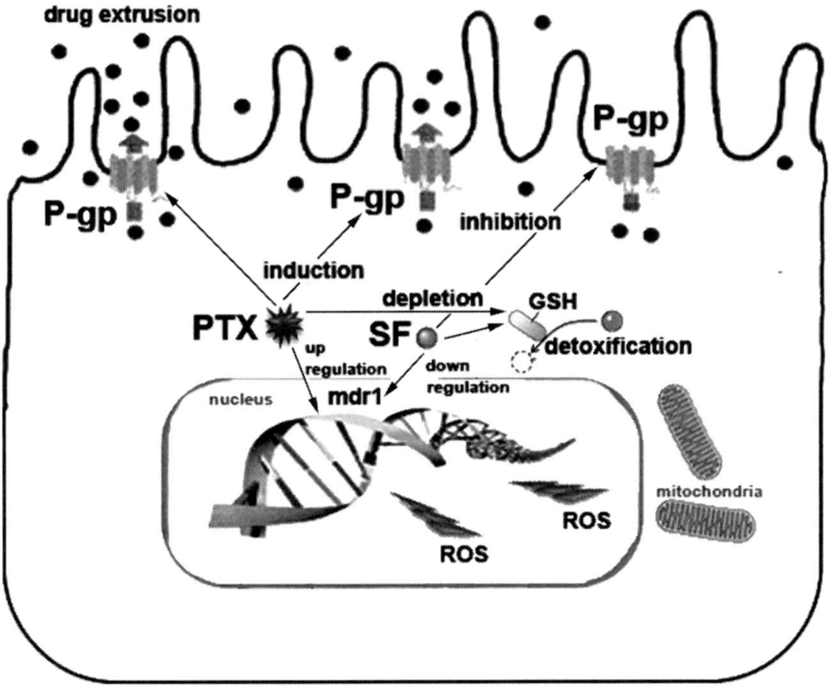

Figure 5. The effects of paclitaxel (PTX) and purine nucleoside analog - sulfinosine (SF) on *mdr1* expression and intracellular redox status. Both PTX and SF generate reactive oxygene species (ROS) and deplete glutathione (GSH). However, their effects on *mdr1* gene expression are distinct. PTX up-regulates *mdr1* and consequently induces P-gp expression, while SF down-regulates *mdr1* and P-gp expression.

NK-2 (Antimicrobial Host Defense Peptide)

Antimicrobial peptides (AMPs), also referred to as innate immunity peptides, possess a unique mechanism of cancer cell killing that involves membrane lysis [234]. They are gene-encoded peptides, which normally provide a first line of defense against invading microbes on epithelial tissues. Interaction of AMPs with target cell membranes eventually leads to the disturbance or destruction of membrane potential and its barrier function [235]. It has been shown that some cancer cells are killed by certain AMPs, whereas normal cells, such as blood lymphocytes, endothelial cells and fibroblasts were not affected [236-238]. This differential sensitivity is driven by electrostatic interactions with the negatively charged lipids of the bacterial membranes [239].

Negatively charged phosphatidylserine (PS), a constituent of the inner layer of human cytoplasmic membranes, can be translocated to the outer leaflet during the loss of membrane asymmetry [240]. Surface exposed PS then serves as a marker for the clearance of pathological or aged erythrocytes and apoptotic cells from the bloodstream by monocytes and macrophages [241-243].

Though it is not well recognized, it has been shown that various cancer cells have elevated surface levels of negatively charged phospholipids, i.e., PS [244-247]. It has been suggested that surface-exposed PS makes these cells susceptible to the cationic, membranolytic peptides [246]. There are evidences that P-gp expressed on plasma membrane of many cells (normal and pathologically changed) and involved as drug-efflux transporter in the development of multi-drug resistance (MDR) in cancer [248], also transports endogenous PS [249]. The increase of negatively charged PS on the surface of MDR cells, due to P-gp activity, could make these cells more vulnerable to AMPs than other cancer cells that possess less P-gp molecules.

The tight association of both P-gp and its substrates with the plasma membrane suggests that P-gp function could be influenced by the composition of the lipid bilayer. Changes in the levels of phospholipids, gangliosides, cholesterol and fatty acids have been reported in P-gp overexpressing cell lines compared to drug sensitive cells. [250-252]. Agents that alter the membrane lipid composition of the resistant cell lines such as cholesterol [251, 253] or ganglioside [254] levels or change the state of the membrane fluidity [255], can modify the extent of drug resistance, providing indirect evidence that P-gp function is highly sensitive to the lipid environment. It was reported that after delipidation, P-gp loses its ATPase activity although the ATP binding sites are not in contact with lipids [256]. This lipid stabilization of the membrane-spanning regions of P-gp is essential for the catalytic activity of the nucleotide binding domains or that the structural and functional integrity of the nucleotide binding domains depends on the presence of phospholipids.

However, P-gp activity appears to be sensitive to the nature of the surrounding lipids since the stimulation of the ATPase activity in response to verapamil differed in proteoliposomes composed of phosphatidylcholine, dimyristoyl-phosphatidylcholine, or dipalmitoylphosphatidylcholine [257, 258]. Reports showed that P-gp is located in lipid raft microdomains, together with several other membrane proteins, which are involved in cell signaling [259-261]. Lipid rafts are plasma membrane microdomains consisted mainly of cholesterol and spingholipids, which possess saturated acyl chains resulting in tight packing of the lipids and little lateral movement in the region. In addition to the presence of signaling molecules, the structure and formation of raft microdomains has been linked to presence of actin filaments and phosphatidylinositol 4,5-bisphosphate, a lipid that links the plasma membrane to the cytoskeleton [262-266]. It was demonstrated that in LS-174-T human colon carcinoma cells, a significant fraction of P-gp resides in rafts and is associated with the cytoskeleton either directly or through microdomains indicating that this localization may influence its transporter function [267].

P-gp was reported to have a higher affinity for its substrates when the surrounding lipids are in the gel-like phase rather than in liquid-crystalline phase [238]. It was also shown that cholesterol sensitizes P-gp to modulators such as verapamil and progesterone and enhances its basal ATPase activity [268], which could be assigned to a cholesterol-dependent conformation of P-gp. The close association of P-gp with lipid raft microdomains suggests that they could provide an optimal lipid microenvironment for P-gp activity which could be strongly influenced by their direct interaction or modulation of physical properties of the surrounding membrane.

We have tested the hypothesis regarding the anti-cancer effects of peptide NK-2. It is an internal fragment of porcine NK-lysin consisting of 27 amino acid residues with an overall positive net charge, which adopts an amphipathic, α-helical secondary structure upon membrane interaction [269].

We found that NK-2 selectivity towards MDR cancer cells correlates to differences in the membrane phospholipid composition between P-gp negative (or low- expressing cells) and P-gp high-expressing cells [205]. This is supported by the fact that among a variety of substrates, P-gp also transports endogenous PS, the trans-location of which to the outer leaflet of cell membrane contributes to the net negative charge of the cell membrane [249]. Other authors suggested that one of the P-gp functions is to catalyze ATP-dependent proton extrusion [1, 270]. Therefore, P-gp expressing cells exhibit cytoplasmatic alkalinization and extracellular acidification, which could also be the reason for the attraction of cationic peptides. In fact, findings directly relating cytosolic alkalinization with abnormalities in membrane depolarization in P-gp-positive MDR cancer cells have been published [271]. The energetic alterations of cell membrane depolarization, low transmembrane potential, decrease in extracellular pH, as well as perturbations in cellular ion transport are considered as characteristics of MDR cancer cells [272]. At the same time, these characteristics are favorable for the action of cationic peptides, such as NK-2.

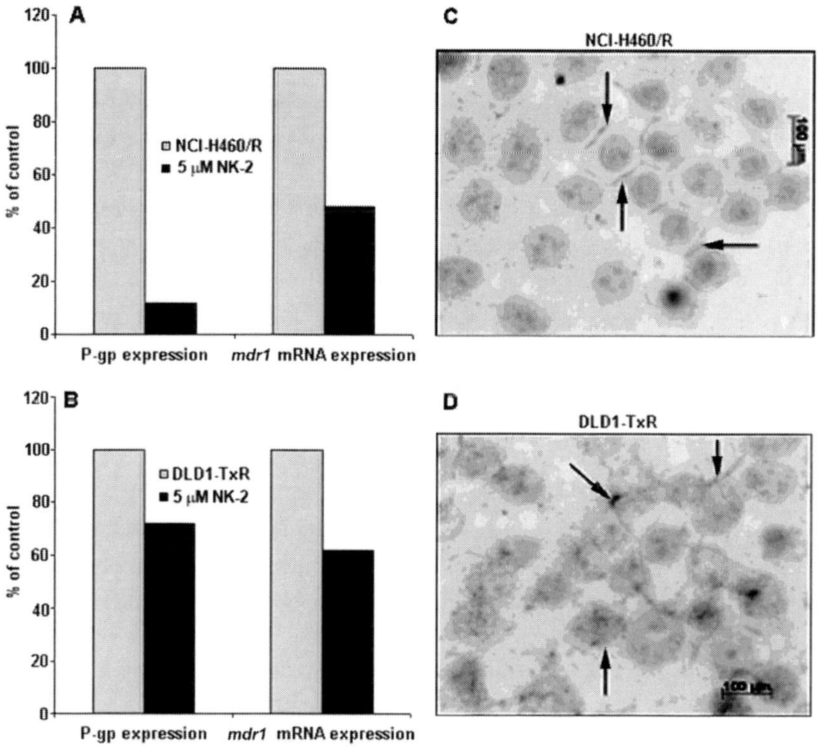

Figure 6. NK-2 decreases P-gp expression in MDR cancer cells and co-localizes with P-gp. P-gp and *mdr1* mRNA expression in untreated MDR cancer cells, as well as in MDR cancer cells treated with 5 μM NK-2 and left to recover for 72 h (A, B). P-gp expression was assessed by flow-cytometry, while *mdr1* mRNA was analyzed by RT-PCR. Merge of red (Rh-NK-2), green (anti-P-gp) and blue (DAPI) fluorescence (arrows point to co-localized P-gp and Rh-NK-2 on cell membrane directly after Rh-NK-2 application) (C, D). Scale bar = 100 μm.

Further, we have examined the interaction of NK-2 with P-gp in MDR cancer cells. We found that P-gp and *mdr1* mRNA expression was significantly lower in MDR cancer cells recovered after NK-2 treatment (Figure 6A, B). In addition, the population of MDR cancer cells that survived NK-2 treatment was more susceptible to doxorubicin [205]. Considering NK-2-specific action on cell membrane lysis accompanied with massive cell death, we did not believe that NK-2 has direct impact on P-gp expression. Rather, we assumed that NK-2 kills more readily the MDR cancer cells with higher P-gp expression and thus higher PS exposure, and that the remained population of

MDR cancer cells possesses less P-gp. It is likely that an enhanced PS content of the outer leaflet of the cell membrane triggers NK-2 binding and membrane permeabilization.

Finally, by using fluorescently-labeled NK-2, we have further confirmed its affinity for P-gp high-expressing cells as well as its co-localization with the P-gp (Figure 6C, D).

In contrast to the classical MDR modulators, NK-2 could exploit P-gp overexpression as the most relevant MDR mechanism and sensitize MDR cancers by selective killing of the P-gp high-expressing cell population. Hence, NK-2 pretreatment could enable further application of classical chemotherapeutics.

Conclusion

Major problem in cancer chemotherapy is development of MDR against variety of drugs. Many MDR inhibitors have been identified, but problems in clinical practice still exist. Continuous discovery of new non-toxic MDR inhibitors, which lack pharmacokinetic interactions with anti-cancer drugs, is needed. In addition, new approaches for overcoming MDR are in focus such as multifunctional nanocarriers and RNAi therapy. Despite all efforts, there is no final conclusion about clinical utility of new therapeutic modalities.

Constant need for improvement of reversal techniques in cancer therapy encouraged us to conduct studies on MDR cancer cells with different compounds that could directly inhibit P-gp, suppress its expression or selectively kill P-gp overexpressing cells. Hoping that our approaches will contribute to understanding of MDR and ways to circumvent this problem, herein we describe the main findings.

Our MDR cancer cell lines developed after continuous exposure to doxorubicin or paclitaxel are cell-type specific with considerable differences in chromosomal instability and tumor suppressors' gene settings, but the similar resistant phenotype due to elevated P-gp expression in all of them. We have used them as *in vitro* models for preclinical testing of different compounds in the search for new efficient MDR inhibitors.

We have shown that euphodendrophanes, isolated from *Euphorbia dendroides*, are non-toxic and potent MDR modulators with new anti-cancer features. Their growth inhibitory potential is connected with their ability to inhibit P-gp, while the synergistic effect with paclitaxel is caused also by G2/M arrest. Considering the wide distribution and availability of their source plants, we suggest further examinations of these compounds in cancer treatment approaches and prevention.

Our study of Ras inhibitor-tipifarnib showed its high potency in improving the paclitaxel efficacy confirming that inhibition of mitogene activated protein kinase (MAPK) pro-survival pathway is rational in combination with paclitaxel. In addition, tipifarnib inhibits P-gp activity, which was confirmed with the increase in P-gp substrate (Rhodamine 123) accumulation. These features elicit treatment with tipifarnib as useful strategy for re-establishment of drug sensitivity.

We have shown that sulfinosine, a poorly studied purine nucleoside analog, possesses anti-cancer effects in MDR cells. Sulfinosine depletes glutathione and reverts MDR through inhibition of P-gp expression and activity. The mechanisms beyond these effects are modification of redox status and HIF-1α regulation. Given together, our results rationalize the use of sulfinosine alone or in combination with conventional anti-cancer agents.

We have provided strong evidences for the interaction between a cationic and amphipathic anti-cancer peptide NK-2 and P-gp. NK-2 preferentially bounds to P-gp high-expressing cancer cells, eliminates them from cell population leading to P-gp expression decrease in cells recovered after NK-2 treatment. By this unique mechanism, NK-2 may sensitize MDR cancers.

References

[1] Roepe, P.D., Wei, L.Y., Cruz, J., Carlson, D., 1993. Lower electrical membrane potential and altered pHi homeostasis in multidrug-resistant (MDR) cells: further characterization of a series of MDR cell lines expressing different levels of P-glycoprotein. *Biochemistry*, 32, 11042–11056.

[2] Gros, P., Croop, J., Housman, D., 1986. Mammalian multidrug resistance gene: complete cDNA sequence indicates strong homology to bacterial transport proteins. *Cell*,47, 371-380.

[3] Pesic, M., Bankovic, J., Tanic, N., 2013. Targeted Anti-Cancer Therapy, Acquiring and Overcoming Multi-Drug Resistance. Atta-ur-Rahman & M. Iqbal Choudhary (Eds.) Bentham Science Publishers. *Frontiers in Anti-Cancer Drug Discovery*, 2(11)

[4] Faber, K.N., Muller, M., Jansen, P.L., 2003. Drug transport proteins in the liver. *Adv. Drug Deliv. Rev.*, 55, 107-124.

[5] Szakács a, G., Paterson, J.K., Ludwig, J.A., Booth-Genthe, C., Gottesman, M.M., 2006. Targeting multidrug resistance in cancer. *Nat. Rev. Drug Discov.*, 5, 219-234.

[6] Shukla, S., Wu, C.P., Ambudkar, S.V., 2008. Development of inhibitors of ATP-binding cassette drug transporters: present status and challenges. *Expert. Opin. Drug Metab. Toxicol.*, 4,205-223.

[7] Szakács b, G., Váradi, A., Ozvegy-Laczka, C., Sarkadi, B., 2008. The role of ABC transporters in drug absorption, distribution, metabolism, excretion and toxicity (ADME-Tox). *Drug Discov. Today*, 13,379-393.

[8] Penson, R.T., Oliva, E., Skates, S.J., Glyptis, T., Fuller, AF. Jr., Goodman, A., Seiden, M.V., 2004. Expression of multidrug resistance-1 protein inversely correlates with paclitaxel response and survival in ovarian cancer patients: a study in serial samples. Gynecol. Oncol., 93, 98-106.

[9] Steinbach, D., Sell, W., Voigt, A., Hermann, J., Zintl, F., Sauerbrey, A., 2002. BCRP gene expression is associated with a poor response to remission induction therapy in childhood acute myeloid leukemia. *Leukemia*, 16, 1443-1447.

[10] van den Heuvel-Eibrink, M.M., Wiemer, E.A., Prins, A., Meijerink, J.P., Vossebeld, P.J., van der Holt, B., Pieters, R., Sonneveld, P., 2002. Increased expression of the breast cancer resistance protein (BCRP) in relapsed or refractory acute myeloid leukemia (AML). *Leukemia,* 16,833-839.

[11] Yang, K., Wu, J., Li, X., 2008. Recent advances in the research of P-glycoprotein inhibitors. *Biosci. Trends*, 2, 137-146.

[12] Aoki, S., Yoshioka, Y., Miyamoto, Y., Higuchi, K., Setiawan, A., Murakami, N., Chen, Z.S., Sumizawa, T., Akiyama, S., Kobayashi, M., 1998. Agosterol A, a novel polyhydroxylated sterol acetate reversing multidrug resistance from a marine sponge of Spongia sp. *Tetrahedron Lett.*, 39, 6303–6306.

[13] Nobili, S., Landini, I., Mazzei, T., Mini, E., 2012. Overcoming tumor multidrug resistance using drugs able to evade P-glycoprotein or to exploit its expression. *Med. Res. Rev.*, 32,1220-1262.

[14] Cortes, J., Baselga, J., 2007. Targeting the microtubules in breast cancer beyond taxanes: the epothilones. *Oncologist*, 12,271-280.

[15] Tsuruo, T., Iida, H., Tsukagoshi, S., Sakurai, Y., 1981. Overcoming of vincristine resistance in P388 leukemia in vivo and in vitro through enhanced cytotoxicity of vincristine and vinblastine by verapamil.*Cancer Res.*, 41, 1967-1972.

[16] Daenen, S., van der Holt, B., Verhoef, G.E., Löwenberg, B., Wijermans, P.W., Huijgens, P.C., van Marwijk Kooy, R., Schouten, H.C., Kramer, M.H., Ferrant, A., van den Berg, E., Steijaert, M.M., Verdonck, L.F., Sonneveld, P., 2004. Addition of cyclosporin A to the combination of mitoxantrone and etoposide to overcome resistance to chemotherapy in refractory or relapsing acute myeloid leukaemia: a randomised phase II trial from HOVON, the Dutch-Belgian Haemato-Oncology Working Group for adults.*Leuk. Res.,* 28, 1057-1067.

[17] Ozols, R.F., Cunnion, R.E., Klecker, RW. Jr., Hamilton, T.C., Ostchega, Y., Parrillo, J.E., Young, R.C., 1987. Verapamil and adriamycin in the treatment of drug-resistant ovarian cancer patients. *J. Clin. Oncol.*, 5, 641-647.

[18] Boesch, D., Gavériaux, C., Jachez, B., Pourtier-Manzanedo, A., Bollinger, P., Loor, F., 1991. In vivo circumvention of P-glycoprotein-mediated multidrug resistance of tumor cells with SDZ PSC 833. *Cancer Res.*, 51, 4226-4233.

[19] Kitagawa, S., Takahashi, T., Nabekura, T., Tachikawa, E., Hasegawa, H., 2007. Inhibitory effects of ginsenosides and their hydrolyzed metabolites on daunorubicin transport in KB-C2 cells. *Biol. Pharm. Bull.,* 30, 1979-1981.

[20] Friedenberg, W.R., Rue, M., Blood, E.A., Dalton, W.S., Shustik, C., Larson, R.A., Sonneveld, P., Greipp, P.R., 2006. Phase III study of PSC-833 (valspodar) in combination with vincristine, doxorubicin, and dexamethasone (valspodar/VAD) versus VAD alone in patients with recurring or refractory multiple myeloma (E1A95): a trial of the Eastern Cooperative Oncology Group. *Cancer*, 106, 830-838.

[21] Baer, M.R., George, S.L., Dodge, R.K., O'Loughlin, K.L., Minderman, H., Caligiuri, M.A., Anastasi, J., Powell, B.L., Kolitz, J.E., Schiffer, C.A., Bloomfield, C.D., Larson, R.A., 2002. Phase 3 study of the multidrug resistance modulator PSC-833 in previously untreated patients 60 years of age and older with acute myeloid leukemia: Cancer and Leukemia Group B Study 9720. *Blood*, 100, 1224-1232.

[22] Wang, F., Wang, Y-C., Dou, S., Xiong, M-H., Sun, T-M., Wang, J., 2011. Doxorubicin-tethered responsive gold nanoparticles facilitate intracellular drug delivery for overcoming multidrug resistance in cancer cells. *ACS Nano*, 5, 3679–3692.

[23] Germann, U.A., Ford, P.J., Shlyakhter, D., Mason, V.S., Harding, M.W., 1997. Chemosensitization and drug accumulation effects of VX-710, verapamil, cyclosporin A, MS-209 and GF120918 in multidrug resistant

HL60/ADR cells expressing the multidrug resistance-associated protein MRP. *Anticancer Drugs.*, 8, 141-155.

[24] Germann, U.A., Shlyakhter, D., Mason, V.S., Zelle, R.E., Duffy, J.P., Galullo, V., Armistead, D.M., Saunders, J.O., Boger, J., Harding, M.W., 1997. Cellular and biochemical characterization of VX-710 as a chemosensitizer: reversal of P-glycoprotein-mediated multidrug resistance in vitro. *Anticancer Drugs.*, 8, 125-140.

[25] Seiden, M.V., Swenerton, K.D., Matulonis, U., Campos, S., Rose, P., Batist, G., Ette, E., Garg, V., Fuller, A., Harding, M.W., Charpentier, D., 2002. A phase II study of the MDR inhibitor biricodar (INCEL, VX-710) and paclitaxel in women with advanced ovarian cancer refractory to paclitaxel therapy. *Gynecol. Oncol.*, 86, 302-310.

[26] Gandhi, L., Harding, M.W., Neubauer, M., Langer, C.J., Moore, M., Ross, H.J., Johnson, B.E., Lynch, T.J., 2007. A phase II study of the safety and efficacy of the multidrug resistance inhibitor VX-710 combined with doxorubicin and vincristine in patients with recurrent small cell lung cancer. *Cancer*, 109, 924-932.

[27] Abraham, J., Edgerly, M., Wilson, R., Chen, C., Rutt, A., Bakke, S., Robey, R., Dwyer, A., Goldspiel, B., Balis, F., Van Tellingen, O., Bates, S.E., Fojo, T., 2009. A phase I study of the P-glycoprotein antagonist tariquidar in combination with vinorelbine. *Clin. Cancer Res.*, 15, 3574-3582.

[28] Fracasso, P.M., Goldstein, L.J., de Alwis, D.P., Rader, J.S., Arquette, M.A., Goodner, S.A., Wright, L.P., Fears, C.L., Gazak, R.J., Andre, V.A., Burgess, M.F., Slapak, C.A., Schellens, J.H., 2004. Phase I study of docetaxel in combination with the P-glycoprotein inhibitor, zosuquidar, in resistant malignancies. *Clin. Cancer Res.*, 10, 7220-7228.

[29] Lancet, J.E., Baer, M.R., Duran, G.E., List, A.F., Fielding, R., Marcelletti, J.F., Multani, P.S., Sikic, B.I., 2009. A phase I trial of continuous infusion of the multidrug resistance inhibitor zosuquidar with daunorubicin and cytarabine in acute myeloid leukemia. *Leuk. Res.*, 33, 1055-1061.

[30] Stewart, A., Steiner, J., Mellows, G., Laguda, B., Norris, D., Bevan, P., 2000. Phase I trial of XR9576 in healthy volunteers demonstrates modulation of P-glycoprotein in CD56+ lymphocytes after oral and intravenous administration. *Clin. Cancer Res.*, 6, 4186-4191.

[31] Gekeler, V., Ise, W., Sanders, K.H., Ulrich, W.R., Beck, J., 1995. The leukotriene LTD4 receptor antagonist MK571 specifically modulates

MRP associated multidrug resistance. *Biochem. Biophys. Res. Commun.*, 208, 345-352.

[32] Kruijtzer, C.M., Beijnen, J.H., Rosing, H., ten Bokkel Huinink, W.W., Schot, M., Jewell, R.C., Paul, E.M., Schellens, J.H., 2002. Increased oral bioavailability of topotecan in combination with the breast cancer resistance protein and P-glycoprotein inhibitor GF120918. *J. Clin. Oncol.*, 20, 2943-2950.

[33] Xu, Y., Zhi, F., Xu, G., Tang, X., Lu, S., Wu, J., Hu, Y., 2012. Overcoming multidrug-resistance in vitro and in vivo using the novel P-glycoprotein inhibitor 1416. *Biosci. Rep.*, 32, 559-566.

[34] Rabindran, S.K., Ross, D.D., Doyle, L.A., Yang, W., Greenberger, L.M., 2000. Fumitremorgin C reverses multidrug resistance in cells transfected with the breast cancer resistance protein. *Cancer Res.*, 60, 47-50.

[35] Allen, J.D., van Loevezijn, A., Lakhai, J.M., van der Valk, M., van Tellingen, O., Reid, G., Schellens, J.H., Koomen, G.J., Schinkel, A.H., 2002. Potent and specific inhibition of the breast cancer resistance protein multidrug transporter in vitro and in mouse intestine by a novel analogue of fumitremorgin C. *Mol. Cancer Ther.*, 1, 417-425.

[36] Bisht, K., Wagner, K.H., Bulmer, A.C., 2010. Curcumin, resveratrol and flavonoids as anti-inflammatory, cyto- and DNA-protective dietary compounds. *Toxicology*, 278,88-100.

[37] Shishodia, S., Singh, T., Chaturvedi, M.M., 2007. Modulation of transcription factors by curcumin. *Adv. Exp. Med. Biol.*, 595,127-148.

[38] Aggarwal, B.B., Kumar, A., Bharti, A.C., 2003. Anticancer potential of curcumin: preclinical and clinical studies. *Anticancer Res.*, 23, 363-398.

[39] Chearwae, W., Anuchapreeda, S., Nandigama, K., Ambudkar, S.V., Limtrakul, P., 2004. Biochemical mechanism of modulation of human P-glycoprotein (ABCB1) by curcumin I, II, and III purified from Turmeric powder. *Biochem. Pharmacol.*, 68, 2043-52.

[40] Limtrakul, P., Chearwae, W., Shukla, S., Phisalphong, C., Ambudkar, S.V., 2007. Modulation of function of three ABC drug transporters, P-glycoprotein (ABCB1), mitoxantrone resistance protein (ABCG2) and multidrug resistance protein 1 (ABCC1) by tetrahydrocurcumin, a major metabolite of curcumin. *Mol. Cell Biochem.*, 296,85-95.

[41] Chearwae, W., Wu, C.P., Chu, H.Y., Lee, T.R., Ambudkar, S.V., Limtrakul, P., 2006. Curcuminoids purified from turmeric powder modulate the function of human multidrug resistance protein 1 (ABCC1). *Cancer Chemother. Pharmacol.*, 57,376-88.

[42] Chearwae, W., Shukla, S., Limtrakul, P., Ambudkar, S.V., 2006. Modulation of the function of the multidrug resistance-linked ATP-binding cassette transporter ABCG2 by the cancer chemopreventive agent curcumin. *Mol. Cancer Ther.*, 5, 1995-2006.

[43] Aggarwal, B.B., Van Kuiken, M.E., Iyer, L.H., Harikumar, K.B., Sung, B., 2009. Molecular targets of nutraceuticals derived from dietary spices: potential role in suppression of inflammation and tumorigenesis. *Exp. Biol. Med.* (Maywood), 234, 825-49.

[44] Singh, S., Aggarwal, B.B., 1995. Activation of transcription factor NF-kappa B is suppressed by curcumin (diferuloylmethane) [corrected]. *J. Biol. Chem.*, 270, 24995-25000.

[45] Chun, K.S., Keum, Y.S., Han, S.S., Song, Y.S., Kim, S.H., Surh, Y.J., 2003. Curcumin inhibits phorbol ester-induced expression of cyclooxygenase-2 in mouse skin through suppression of extracellular signal-regulated kinase activity and NF-kappaB activation. *Carcinogenesis*, 24,1515-1524.

[46] Park, C.H., Hahm, E.R., Park, S., Kim, H.K., Yang, C.H., 2005. The inhibitory mechanism of curcumin and its derivative against beta-catenin/Tcf signaling. *FEBS Lett.*, 579,2965-2971.

[47] Jaiswal, A.S., Marlow, B.P., Gupta, N., Narayan, S. Beta-catenin-mediated transactivation and cell-cell adhesion pathways are important in curcumin (diferuylmethane)-induced growth arrest and apoptosis in colon cancer cells. *Oncogene*, 21,8414-27.

[48] Guertin, D.A., Sabatini, D.M., 2007. Defining the role of mTOR in cancer. *Cancer Cell*, 12, 9-22.

[49] Beevers, C.S., Li, F., Liu, L., Huang, S., 2006.Curcumin inhibits the mammalian target of rapamycin-mediated signaling pathways in cancer cells. *Int. J. Cancer*, 119, 757-764.

[50] Yu, S., Shen, G., Khor, T.O., Kim, J.H., Kong, A.N., 2008. Curcumin inhibits Akt/mammalian target of rapamycin signaling through protein phosphatase-dependent mechanism. *Mol. Cancer Ther.*, 7, 2609-2620.

[51] Nabekura, T., Kamiyama, S., Kitagawa, S., 2005. Effects of dietary chemopreventive phytochemicals on P-glycoprotein function. *Biochem. Biophys. Res. Commun.*, 327,866-870.

[52] Cheng, A.L., Hsu, C.H., Lin, J.K., Hsu, M.M., Ho, Y.F., Shen, T.S., Ko, J.Y., Lin, J.T., Lin, B.R., Ming-Shiang, W., Yu, H.S., Jee, S.H., Chen, G.S., Chen, T.M., Chen, C.A., Lai, M.K., Pu, Y.S., Pan, M.H., Wang, Y.J., Tsai CC, Hsieh CY., 2001. Phase I clinical trial of curcumin, a

chemopreventive agent, in patients with high-risk or pre-malignant lesions. *Anticancer Res.*, 21, 2895-2900.

[53] Deodhar, S.D., Sethi, R., Srimal, R.C., 1980. Preliminary study on antirheumatic activity of curcumin (diferuloyl methane). *Indian. J. Med. Res.*, 71, 632-634.

[54] Lal, B., et al., *Efficacy of curcumin in the management of chronic anterior uveitis.* Phytother Res, 1999. 13(4): p. 318-22.

[55] Hsu, C.H., Cheng A.L., 2007. Clinical studies with curcumin. *Adv. Exp. Med. Biol.*, 595, 471-480.

[56] Heng, M.C., Song, M.K., Harker, J., Heng, M.K., 2000. Drug-induced suppression of phosphorylase kinase activity correlates with resolution of psoriasis as assessed by clinical, histological and immunohistochemical parameters.*Br. J. Dermatol.*, 143, 937-949.

[57] Dhillon, N., Aggarwal, B.B., Newman, R.A., Wolff, R.A., Kunnumakkara, A.B., Abbruzzese, J.L., Ng, C.S., Badmaev, V., Kurzrock, R., 2008. Phase II trial of curcumin in patients with advanced pancreatic cancer. *Clin. Cancer Res.*, 14, 4491-4499.

[58] Bisht, S., Feldmann, G., Soni, S., Ravi, R., Karikar, C., Maitra, A., Maitra, A., 2007. Polymeric nanoparticle-encapsulated curcumin ("nanocurcumin"): a novel strategy for human cancer therapy. *J. Nanobiotechnology*, 5, 3.

[59] Shaikh, J., Ankola, D.D., Beniwal, V., Singh, D., Kumar, M.N., 2009. Nanoparticle encapsulation improves oral bioavailability of curcumin by at least 9-fold when compared to curcumin administered with piperine as absorption enhancer.*Eur. J. Pharm. Sci.*, 37, 223-230.

[60] Li, L., Braiteh, F.S., Kurzrock, R., 2005. Liposome-encapsulated curcumin: in vitro and in vivo effects on proliferation, apoptosis, signaling, and angiogenesis. *Cancer*, 104, 1322-1331.

[61] Mosley, C.A., D.C. Liotta, and J.P. Snyder, *Highly active anticancer curcumin analogues.* Adv Exp Med Biol, 2007. 595: p. 77-103.

[62] Shoba, G., Joy, D., Joseph, T., Majeed, M., Rajendran, R., 1998. Srinivas PS.Influence of piperine on the pharmacokinetics of curcumin in animals and human volunteers. *Planta Med.*, 64,353-356.

[63] Wang, H.K., Xia, Y., Yang, Z.Y., Natschke, S.L., Lee, K.H., 1998. Recent advances in the discovery and development of flavonoids and their analogues as antitumor and anti-HIV agents. *Adv. Exp. Med. Biol.*, 439,191-225.

[64] Choi, S.U., Ryu, S.Y., Yoon, S.K., Jung, N.P., Park, S.H., Kim, K.H., Choi, E.J., Lee, C.O., 1999. Effects of flavonoids on the growth and cell cycle of cancer cells. *Anticancer Res.*, 19, 5229-5233.

[65] Selway, J.W., 1986. Antiviral activity of flavones and flavans. *Prog. Clin. Biol. Res.*, 213,521-36.

[66] Cushman, M., Zhu, H., Geahlen, R.L., Kraker, A.J., 1994. Synthesis and biochemical evaluation of a series of aminoflavones as potential inhibitors of protein-tyrosine kinases p56lck, EGFr, and p60v-src. *J. Med. Chem.*, 37, 3353-3362.

[67] Cotelle, N., Bernier, J.L., Hénichart, J.P., Catteau, J.P., Gaydou, E., Wallet, J.C., 1992. Scavenger and antioxidant properties of ten synthetic flavones. *Free Radic. Biol. Med.*, 13,211-219.

[68] Leslie, E.M., Mao, Q,, Oleschuk, C.J., Deeley, R.G., Cole, S.P., 2001. Modulation of multidrug resistance protein 1 (MRP1/ABCC1) transport and atpase activities by interaction with dietary flavonoids. *Mol. Pharmacol.*, 59, 1171-1180.

[69] Wu, C.P., Calcagno, A.M., Hladky, S.B., Ambudkar, S.V., Barrand, M.A., 2005. Modulatory effects of plant phenols on human multidrug-resistance proteins 1, 4 and 5 (ABCC1, 4 and 5). *FEBS J.*, 272, 4725-4740.

[70] Zhou, S., Lim, L.Y., Chowbay, B., 2004. Herbal modulation of P-glycoprotein. *Drug Metab. Rev.*, 36, 57-104.

[71] Haefner, B., 2003. Drugs from the deep: marine natural products as drug candidates. *Drug Discov. Today*, 8, 536-544.

[72] Hu, G.P., Yuan, J., Sun, L., She, Z.G., Wu, J.H., Lan, X.J., Zhu, X., Lin, Y.C., Chen, S.P., 2011. Statistical research on marine natural products based on data obtained between 1985 and 2008. *Mar. Drugs*, 9, 514-525.

[73] Aoki, S., Chen, Z.S., Higasiyama, K., Setiawan, A., Akiyama, S., Kobayashi, M., 2001. Reversing effect of agosterol A, a spongean sterol acetate, on multidrug resistance in human carcinoma cells. *Jpn. J. Cancer Res.*, 92, 886-895.

[74] Chen, Z.S., Aoki, S., Komatsu, M., Ueda, K., Sumizawa, T., Furukawa, T., Okumura, H., Ren, X.Q., Belinsky, M.G., Lee, K., Kruh, G.D., Kobayashi, M., Akiyama, S., 2001. Reversal of drug resistance mediated by multidrug resistance protein (MRP) 1 by dual effects of agosterol A on MRP1 function. *Int. J. Cancer*, 93,107-113.

[75] Rinehart, K.L., 2000. Antitumor compounds from tunicates. *Med. Res. Rev.*, 20, 1-27.

[76] Zewail-Foote, M., Hurley, L.H., 1999. Ecteinascidin 743: a minor groove alkylator that bends DNA toward the major groove. *J. Med. Chem.*, 42, 2493-2497.

[77] Nebl, T., Pestonjamasp, K.N., Leszyk, J.D., Crowley, J.L., Oh, S.W., Luna, E.J., 2002. Proteomic analysis of a detergent-resistant membrane skeleton from neutrophil plasma membranes. *J. Biol. Chem.*, 277, 43399-43409.

[78] Kanzaki, A., Takebayashi, Y., Ren, X.Q., Miyashita, H., Mori, S., Akiyama, S., Pommier, Y., 2002. Overcoming multidrug drug resistance in P-glycoprotein/MDR1-overexpressing cell lines by ecteinascidin 743. *Mol. Cancer Ther.*, **1,** 1327-1334.

[79] Amador, M.L., Jimeno, J., Paz-Ares, L., Cortes-Funes, H., Hidalgo, M., 2003. Progress in the development and acquisition of anticancer agents from marine sources. *Ann. Oncol.*, 14,1607-1615.

[80] Abraham, I., El Sayed, K., Chen, Z.S., Guo, H., 2012. Current status on marine products with reversal effect on cancer multidrug resistance. *Mar. Drugs.*, 10,2312-2321.

[81] Jain, S., Laphookhieo, S., Shi, Z., Fu, L.W., Akiyama, S., Chen, Z.S., Youssef, D.T., van Soest, R.W., El Sayed, K.A., 2007. Reversal of P-glycoprotein-mediated multidrug resistance by sipholane triterpenoids. *J. Nat. Prod.*, 70,928-931.

[82] Jain, S., Abraham, I., Carvalho, P., Kuang, Y.H., Shaala, L.A., Youssef, D.T., Avery, M.A., Chen, Z.S., El Sayed, K.A., 2009. Sipholane triterpenoids: chemistry, reversal of ABCB1/P-glycoprotein-mediated multidrug resistance, and pharmacophore modeling. *J. Nat. Prod.*, 72,1291-1298.

[83] Shi, Z., Peng, X.X., Kim, I.W., Shukla, S., Si, Q.S., Robey, R.W., Bates, S.E., Shen, T., Ashby, C.R.Jr., Fu, L.W., Ambudkar, S.V., Chen, Z.S., 2007. Erlotinib (Tarceva, OSI-774) antagonizes ATP-binding cassette subfamily B member 1 and ATP-binding cassette subfamily G member 2-mediated drug resistance. *Cancer Res.*, 67, 11012-11020.

[84] Kraft, A.S., Smith, J.B., Berkow, R.L., 1986. Bryostatin, an activator of the calcium phospholipid-dependent protein kinase, blocks phorbol ester-induced differentiation of human promyelocytic leukemia cells HL-60. *Proc. Natl. Acad. Sci. U S A*,. 83, 1334-1338.

[85] Isakov, N., Galron, D., Mustelin, T., Pettit, G.R., Altman, A., 1993.Inhibition of phorbol ester-induced T cell proliferation by bryostatin is associated with rapid degradation of protein kinase C. *J. Immunol.*, 150,1195-1204.

[86] Chambers, T.C., McAvoy, E.M., Jacobs, J.W., Eilon, G., 1990. Protein kinase C phosphorylates P-glycoprotein in multidrug resistant human KB carcinoma cells. *J. Biol. Chem.*, 265, 7679-7686.

[87] Smith, C.D., Zilfou, J.T., Stratmann, K., Patterson, G.M., Moore, R.E., 1995. Welwitindolinone analogues that reverse P-glycoprotein-mediated multiple drug resistance. *Mol. Pharmacol.*, 47, 241-247.

[88] Eckford, P.D., Sharom, F.J., 2009. ABC efflux pump-based resistance to chemotherapy drugs. *Chem. Rev.*, 109, 2989-3011.

[89] Dahan, A., Altman, H., 2004. Food-drug interaction: grapefruit juice augments drug bioavailability--mechanism, extent and relevance. *Eur. J. Clin. Nutr.*, 58, 1-9.

[90] Conseil, G., Baubichon-Cortay, H., Dayan, G., Jault, J.M., Barron, D., Di Pietro, A., 1998.Flavonoids: a class of modulators with bifunctional interactions at vicinal ATP- and steroid-binding sites on mouse P-glycoprotein. *Proc. Natl. Acad. Sci. U S A*, 95, 9831-9836.

[91] Nomura, M., Ma, W., Chen, N., Bode, A.M., Dong, Z., 2000. Inhibition of 12-O-tetradecanoylphorbol-13-acetate-induced NF-kappaB activation by tea polyphenols, (-)-epigallocatechin gallate and theaflavins. *Carcinogenesis*, 21, 1885-1890.

[92] Afaq, F., Adhami, V.M., Ahmad, N., Mukhtar, H., 2003. Inhibition of ultraviolet B-mediated activation of nuclear factor kappaB in normal human epidermal keratinocytes by green tea Constituent (-)-epigallocatechin-3-gallate. *Oncogene*, 22, 1035-1044.

[93] Orner, G.A., Dashwood, W.M., Blum, C.A., Díaz, G.D., Li, Q., Al-Fageeh, M., Tebbutt, N., Heath, J.K., Ernst, M., Dashwood, R.H., 2002. Response of Apc(min) and A33 (delta N beta-cat) mutant mice to treatment with tea, sulindac, and 2-amino-1-methyl-6-phenylimidazo[4,5-b]pyridine (PhIP). *Mutat. Res.*, 506-507, 121-127.

[94] Kim, J., Zhang, X., Rieger-Christ, K.M., Summerhayes, I.C., Wazer, D.E., Paulson, K.E., Yee, A.S., 2006. Suppression of Wnt signaling by the green tea compound (-)-epigallocatechin 3-gallate (EGCG) in invasive breast cancer cells. Requirement of the transcriptional repressor HBP1. *J. Biol. Chem.*, 281,10865-10875.

[95] Kitagawa, S., Nabekura, T., Kamiyama, S., 2004. Inhibition of P-glycoprotein function by tea catechins in KB-C2 cells. *J. Pharm. Pharmacol.*, 56, 1001-1005.

[96] Roninson, I.B., Chin, J.E., Choi, K.G., Gros, P., Housman, D.E., Fojo, A., Shen, D.W., Gottesman, M.M., Pastan, I., 1986. Isolation of human

mdr DNA sequences amplified in multidrug-resistant KB carcinoma cells. *Proc. Natl. Acad. Sci. U S A*, 83, 4538-4542.

[97] Akiyama, S., Fojo, A., Hanover, J.A., Pastan, I., Gottesman, M.M., 1985. Isolation and genetic characterization of human KB cell lines resistant to multiple drugs. *Somat. Cell Mol. Genet.*, 11, 117-126.

[98] Singh, S., Natarajan, K., Aggarwal, B.B., 1996. Capsaicin (8-methyl-N-vanillyl-6-nonenamide) is a potent inhibitor of nuclear transcription factor-kappa B activation by diverse agents. *J. Immunol.*, 157, 4412-4420.

[99] Han, S.S., Keum, Y.S., Seo, H.J., Chun, K.S., Lee, S.S., Surh, Y.J., 2001. Capsaicin suppresses phorbol ester-induced activation of NF-kappaB/Rel and AP-1 transcription factors in mouse epidermis. *Cancer Lett.*, 164, 119-126.

[100] Kim, S.O., Chun, K.S., Kundu, J.K., Surh, Y.J., 2004. Inhibitory effects of [6]-gingerol on PMA-induced COX-2 expression and activation of NF-kappaB and p38 MAPK in mouse skin. *Biofactors*, 21, 27-31.

[101] Lee, S.H., Cekanova, M., Baek, S.J., 2008. Multiple mechanisms are involved in 6-gingerol-induced cell growth arrest and apoptosis in human colorectal cancer cells. *Mol. Carcinog.*, 47, 197-208.

[102] Wellwood, C.R., Cole, R.A., 2004. Relevance of carnosic acid concentrations to the selection of rosemary, Rosmarinus officinalis (L.), accessions for optimization of antioxidant yield. *J. Agric. Food. Chem.*, 52, 6101-6107.

[103] Yu b, M.H., Choi, J.H., Chae, I.G., Im, H.G., Yang, S.A., More, K., Lee, I.S., Lee, J., 2013. Suppression of LPS-induced inflammatory activities by Rosmarinus officinalis L. *Food Chem*., 136, 1047-1054.

[104] Huang, M.T., Ho, C.T., Wang, Z.Y., Ferraro, T., Lou, Y.R., Stauber, K., Ma, W., Georgiadis, C., Laskin, J.D., and Conney, A.H., 1994. Inhibition of skin tumorigenesis by rosemary and its constituents carnosol and ursolic acid. *Cancer Res.,* 54, 701-708.

[105] Huang, S.C., Ho, C.T., Lin-Shiau, S.Y., Lin, J.K., 2005. Carnosol inhibits the invasion of B16/F10 mouse melanoma cells by suppressing metalloproteinase-9 through down-regulating nuclear factor-kappa B and c-Jun. *Biochem. Pharmacol.,* 69, 221-232.

[106] Lo, A.H., Liang, Y.C., Lin-Shiau, S.Y., Ho, C.T., Lin, J.K., 2002. Carnosol, an antioxidant in rosemary, suppresses inducible nitric oxide synthase through down-regulating nuclear factor-kappaB in mouse macrophages. *Carcinogenesis,23*, 983-991.

[107] Moran, A.E., Carothers, A.M., Weyant, M.J., Redston, M., Bertagnolli, M.M., 2005. Carnosol inhibits beta-catenin tyrosine phosphorylation and prevents adenoma formation in the C57BL/6J/Min/+ (Min/+) mouse. *Cancer Res.,* 65, 1097-1104.

[108] Nabekura, T., Yamaki, T., Hiroi, T., Ueno, K., Kitagawa, S., 2010. Inhibition of anticancer drug efflux transporter P-glycoprotein by rosemary phytochemicals, *Pharmacol. Res.,* 61, 259-263.

[109] Ju-Ichi, M., 2005. [Chemical study of citrus plants in the search for cancer chemopreventive agents]. *Yakugaku Zasshi,* 125, 231-254.

[110] Tanaka a, T., Kawabata, K., Kakumoto, M., Makita, H., Hara, A., Mori, H., Satoh, K., Murakami, A., Kuki, W., Takahashi, Y., Yonei, H., Koshimizu, K., Ohigashi, H., 1997. Citrus auraptene inhibits chemically induced colonic aberrant crypt foci in male F344 rats. *Carcinogenesis,* 18, 2155-2161.

[111] Tanaka b, T., Kawabata, K., Kakumoto, M., Matsunaga, K., Mori, H., Murakami, A., Kuki, W., Takahashi, Y., Yonei, H., Satoh, K., Hara, A., Maeda, M., Ota, T., Odashima, S., Koshimizu, K., Ohigashi, H., 1998. Chemoprevention of 4-nitroquinoline 1-oxide-induced oral carcinogenesis by citrus auraptene in rats, *Carcinogenesis,* 19, 425-431.

[112] Tang, M., Ogawa, K., Asamoto, M., Hokaiwado, N., Seeni, A., Suzuki, S., Takahashi, S., Tanaka, T., Ichikawa, K., Shirai, T., 2007. Protective effects of citrus nobiletin and auraptene in transgenic rats developing adenocarcinoma of the prostate (TRAP) and human prostate carcinoma cells. *Cancer Sci.,* 98, 471-477.

[113] Murakami, A., Nakamura, Y., Tanaka, T., Kawabata, K., Takahashi, D., Koshimizu, K., Ohigashi, H., 2000. Suppression by citrus auraptene of phorbol ester-and endotoxin-induced inflammatory responses: role of attenuation of leukocyte activation. *Carcinogenesis,* 21, 1843-1850.

[114] Murakami, A., Nakamura, Y., Torikai, K., Tanaka, T., Koshiba, T., Koshimizu, K., Kuwahara, S., Takahashi, Y., Ogawa, K., Yano, M., Tokuda, H., Nishino, H., Mimaki, Y., Sashida, Y., Kitanaka, S., Ohigashi, H., 2000. Inhibitory effect of citrus nobiletin on phorbol ester-induced skin inflammation, oxidative stress, and tumor promotion in mice. *Cancer Res.,* 60, 5059-5066.

[115] Nabekura, T., Yamaki, T., Kitagawa, S., 2008. Effects of chemopreventive citrus phytochemicals on human P-glycoprotein and multidrug resistance protein 1. *Eur. J. Pharmacol.,* 600, 45-49.

[116] Katan, M.B., Grundy, S.M., Jones, P., Law, M., Miettinen, T., Paoletti, R., 2003. Efficacy and safety of plant stanols and sterols in the management of blood cholesterol levels. *Mayo Clin. Proc.,* 78, 965-978.

[117] Awad, A.B., Fink, C.S., 2000. Phytosterols as anticancer dietary components: evidence and mechanism of action. *J. Nutr.,* 130, 2127-2130.

[118] Shishodia, S., Aggarwal, B.B. 2004. Guggulsterone inhibits NF-kappaB and IkappaBalpha kinase activation, suppresses expression of anti-apoptotic gene products, and enhances apoptosis. *J Biol. Chem* 279, 47148-47158.

[119] Nabekura, T., Yamaki, T., Ueno, K., Kitagawa, S., 2008. Effects of plant sterols on human multidrug transporters ABCB1 and ABCC1. *Biochem. Biophys. Res. Commun.,* 369, 363-368.

[120] Nabekura, T., Yamaki, T., Ueno, K., Kitagawa, S., 2008. Inhibition of P-glycoprotein and multidrug resistance protein 1 by dietary phytochemicals. *Cancer. Chemother. Pharmacol.,* 62, 867-873.

[121] Wortelboer, H.M., Usta, M., van Zanden, J.J., van Bladeren, P.J., Rietjens, I.M., Cnubben, N.H., 2005. Inhibition of multidrug resistance proteins MRP1 and MRP2 by a series of alpha,beta-unsaturated carbonyl compounds. *Biochem. Pharmacol.,* 69, 1879-1890.

[122] Hong, J., Lambert, J.D., Lee, S.H., Sinko, P.J., Yang, C. S., 2003. Involvement of multidrug resistance-associated proteins in regulating cellular levels of (-)-epigallocatechin-3-gallate and its methyl metabolites. *Biochem. Biophys. Res. Commun.,* 310, 222-227.

[123] Newman, D.J., Cragg, G.M., 2004. Marine natural products and related compounds in clinical and advanced preclinical trials. *J. Nat. Prod.*, 67, 1216-1238.

[124] Stierlé, V., Laigle, A., Jollès, B., 2005.Modulation of MDR1 gene expression in multidrug resistant MCF7 cells by low concentrations of small interfering RNAs.*Biochem. Pharmacol.*, 70, 1424-1430.

[125] Luo, Q., Kang, Q., Song, W.X., Luu, H.H., Luo, X., An, N., Luo, J., Deng, Z.L., Jiang, W., Yin, H., Chen, J., Sharff, K.A., Tang, N., Bennett, E., Haydon, R.C., He, T.C., 2007. Selection and validation of optimal siRNA target sites for RNAi-mediated gene silencing. *Gene,* 395, 160-169.

[126] Fuchs, U., Borkhardt, A., 2007. The application of siRNA technology to cancer biology discovery. *Adv. Cancer Res.*, 96, 75-102.

[127] Xiao, H., Wu, Z., Shen, H., Luo, A.L., Yang, Y.F., Li, X.B., Zhu, D.Y., 2008. In vivo reversal of P-glycoprotein-mediated multidrug resistance

by efficient delivery of stealth RNAi. *Basic Clin. Pharmacol. Toxicol.*, 103, 342-348.

[128] Allerson, C.R., Sioufi, N., Jarres, R., Prakash, T.P., Naik, N., Berdeja, A., Wanders, L., Griffey, R.H., Swayze, E.E., Bhat, B., 2005. Fully 2'-modified oligonucleotide duplexes with improved in vitro potency and stability compared to unmodified small interfering RNA. *J. Med. Chem.*, 48, 901-904.

[129] Bartz, J.A.L., Schelter, S.R., Schelter, J., Kobayashi, S.V., Burchard, J., Mao, M., Li, B., Cavet, G., Linsley, P.S., 2003. Expression profiling reveals off-target gene regulation by RNAi. *Nat. Biotechnol.*, 21, 635–637.

[130] Diebold, S.S., Kaisho, T., Hemmi, H., Akira, S., Reis e Sousa, C., 2004. Innate antiviral responses by means of TLR7-mediated recognition of single-stranded RNA. *Science*, 303,1529-1531.

[131] Zhu, H., Wu, H., Liu, X., Evans, B.R., Medina, D.J., Liu, C.G., Yang, J.M., 2008. Role of MicroRNA miR-27a and miR-451 in the regulation of MDR1/P-glycoprotein expression in human cancer cells.*Biochem. Pharmacol.*, 76, 582-588.

[132] Pakunlu, R.I., Wang, Y., Saad, M., Khandare, J.J., Starovoytov, V., Minko, T., 2006. In vitro and in vivo intracellular liposomal delivery of antisense oligonucleotides and anticancer drug. *J. Control. Release.*, 114, 153-162.

[133] Cerveny, L., Svecova, L., Anzenbacherova, E., Vrzal, R., Staud, F., Dvorak, Z., Ulrichova, J., Anzenbacher, P., Pavek, P., 2007. Valproic acid induces CYP3A4 and MDR1 gene expression by activation of constitutive androstane receptor and pregnane X receptor pathways. *Drug Metab. Dispos.*, 35, 1032-1041.

[134] Mensah-Osman, E.J., Thomas, D.G., Tabb, M.M., Larios, J.M., Hughes, D.P., Giordano, T.J., Lizyness, M.L., Rae, J.M., Blumberg, B., Hollenberg, P.F., Baker, L.H., 2007. Expression levels and activation of a PXR variant are directly related to drug resistance in osteosarcoma cell lines. *Cancer*, 109, 957-965.

[135] Chen, Y., Tang, Y., Wang, M.T., Zeng, S., Nie, D., 2007. Human pregnane X receptor and resistance to chemotherapy in prostate cancer. *Cancer Res.*, 67, 10361-10367.

[136] Raynal, C., Pascussi, J.M., Leguelinel, G., Breuker, C., Kantar, J., Lallemant, B., Poujol, S., Bonnans, C., Joubert, D., Hollande, F., Lumbroso, S., Brouillet, J.P., Evrard, A., 2010. Pregnane X Receptor (PXR) expression in colorectal cancer cells restricts irinotecan

chemosensitivity through enhanced SN-38 glucuronidation. *Mol. Cancer*, 9:46.

[137] Masuyama, H., Hiramatsu, Y., Kodama, J., Kudo, T., 2003. Expression and potential roles of pregnane X receptor in endometrial cancer. *J. Clin. Endocrinol. Metab.*88, 4446-4454.

[138] Cho, K., Wang, X., Nie, S., Chen, Z., Shin, D.M., 2008. Therapeutic Nanoparticles for Drug Delivery in Cancer. *Clin. Cancer Res.*, 14, 1310–1316.

[139] McBain, S.C., Yiu, H.H.P., Dobson, J., 2008. Magnetic nanoparticles for gene and drug delivery. *Int. J. Nanomedicine.*, 3, 169–180.

[140] Kang, K.W., Chun, M.K., Kim, O., Subedi, R.K., Ahn, S.G., Yoon, J.H., Choi, H.K., 2010. Doxorubicin-loaded solid lipid nanoparticles to overcome multidrug resistance in cancer therapy. *Nanomedicine.*, 6, 210–213.

[141] Chen, A.M., Zhang, M., Wei, D., Stueber, D., Taratula, O., Minko, T., He, H., 2009.Co-delivery of doxorubicin and Bcl-2 siRNA by mesoporous silica nanoparticles enhances the efficacy of chemotherapy in multidrug-resistant cancer cells. *Small*, 5, 2673–2677.

[142] Koziara, J.M., Whisman, T.R., Tseng, M.T., Mumper, R.J., 2006. In-vivo efficacy of novel paclitaxel nanoparticles in paclitaxel-resistant human colorectal tumors. *J. Control Release.*, 112, 312–319.

[143] Zhang, Y., Tang, L., Sun, L., Bao, J., Song, C., Huang, L., Liu, K., Tian, Y., Tian, G., Li, Z., Sun, H., Mei, L., 2010. A novel paclitaxel-loaded poly (epsilon-caprolactone)/Poloxamer 188 blend nanoparticle overcoming multidrug resistance for cancer treatment. *Acta. Biomater.*, 6, 2045–2052.

[144] Gu, Y-J., Cheng, J., Man, CW-Y., Wong, W-T., Cheng, S.H., 2011. Gold-doxorubicin nanoconjugates for overcoming multidrug resistance. *Nanomedicine*, 2011; 8, 204–211.

[145] Meng, H., Liong, M., Xia, T., Li, Z., Ji, Z., Zink, J.I., Nel, A.E., 2010. Engineered design of mesoporous silica nanoparticles to deliver doxorubicin and P-glycoprotein siRNA to overcome drug resistance in a cancer cell line. *ACS Nano*, 4, 4539 -4550.

[146] Jiang J, Yang SJ, Wang JC, Yang, L.J., Xu, Z.Z., Yang, T., Liu, X.Y., Zhang, Q., 2010. Sequential treatment of drugre sistant tumors with RGD- modified liposomes containing siRNA or doxorubicin. *Eur. J. Pharm. Biopharm.*, 76, 170-178.

[147] Szybalski, W., Bryson, V., 1952. Genetic studies on microbial cross resistance to toxic agents. I. Cross resistance of Escherichia coli to fifteen antibiotics. *J. Bacteriol.*, 64, 489–499.

[148] Warr, J.R., Brewer, F., Anderson, M., Fergusson, J., 1986. Verapamil hypersensitivity of vincristine resistant Chinese hamster ovary cell lines. *Cell. Biol. Int. Rep.*, 10, 389–399.

[149] Perrotton, T., Trompier, D., Chang, X.B., Di Pietro, A., Baubichon-Cortay, H., 2007. (R)- and (S)-verapamil differentially modulate the multidrug-resistant protein MRP1. *J. Biol. Chem.*, 282, 31542–31548.

[150] Genoux-Bastide, E., Lorendeau, D., Nicolle, E., Yahiaoui, S., Magnard, S., Di Pietro, A., Baubichon-Cortay, H., Boumendjel, A., 2011. Identification of Xanthones as Selective Killers of Cancer Cells Overexpressing the ABC Transporter MRP1. ChemMedChem. 6, 1478–1484.

[151] Kaplan, O., Jaroszewski, J.W., Clarke, R., Fairchild, C.R., Schoenlein, P., Goldenberg, S., Gottesman, M.M., Cohen, J.S., 1991. The multidrug resistance phenotype: 31P nuclear magnetic resonance characterization and 2-deoxyglucose toxicity. *Cancer Res.*, 51, 1638–1644.

[152] Kaplan, O., Navon, G., Lyon, R.C., Faustino, P.J., Straka, E.J., Cohen, J.S., 1990. Effects of 2-deoxyglucose on drugsensitive and drug-resistant human breast cancer cells: toxicity and magnetic resonance spectroscopy studies of metabolism. *Cancer Res.*, 50, 544–551.

[153] Nagata, J., Kijima, H., Hatanaka, H., Asai, S., Miyachi, H., Abe, Y., Yamazaki, H., Nakamura, M., Watanabe, N., Mine, T., Kondo, T., Scanlon, K.J., Ueyama, Y., 2002. Reversal of drug resistance using hammerhead ribozymes against multidrug resistance-associated protein and multidrug resistance 1 gene. *Int. J. Oncol.*, 21, 1021-106.

[154] Nakagawa-Goto, K., Bastow, K.F., Chen, T.H., Morris-Natschke, S.L., Lee, K.H., 2008. Antitumor agents 260. New desmosdumotin B analogues with improved in vitro anticancer activity. *J. Med. Chem.*, 51, 3297–3303.

[155] Hall, M.D., Salam, N.K., Hellawell, J.L., Fales, H.M., Kensler, C.B., Ludwig, J.A., Szakacs, G., Hibbs, D.E., Gottesman, M.M., 2009b. Synthesis, activity, and pharmacophore development for isatin-betathiosemicarbazones with selective activity toward multidrug-resistant cells. *J. Med. Chem.*, 52, 3191–3204.

[156] Hall, M.D., Brimacombe, K.R., Varonka, M.S., Pluchino, K.M., Monda, J.K., Li, J., Walsh, M.J., Boxer, M.B., Warren, T.H., Fales, H.M., Gottesman, M.M., 2011. Synthesis and structure-activity evaluation of

isatin-betathiosemicarbazones with improved selective activity towards multidrug-resistant cells expressing P-glycoprotein. *J. Med. Chem.*, 54, 5878–5889.

[157] Whitnall, M., Howard, J., Ponka, P., Richardson, D.R., 2006. A class of iron chelators with a wide spectrum of potent antitumor activity that overcomes resistance to chemotherapeutics. Proc. *Natl. Acad. Sci. U S A.*, 103, 14901–14906.

[158] Goldsborough, A.S., Handley, M.D., Dulcey, A.E., Pluchino, K.M., Kannan, P., Brimacombe, K.R., Hall, M.D., Griffiths, G., Gottesman, M.M., 2011. Collateral Sensitivity of Multidrug-Resistant Cells to the Orphan Drug Tiopronin. *J. Med. Chem.*, 54, 4987–4997.

[159] Milinkovic, V., Bankovic, J., Rakic, M., Milosevic, N., Stankovic, T., Jokovic, M., Milosevic, Z., Skender-Gazibara, M., Podolski-Renic, A., Pesic, M., Ruzdijic, S., Tanic, N., 2012. Genomic instability and p53 alterations in patients with malignant glioma. *Exp. Mol. Pathol.*, 93, 200-206.

[160] Burger, H., van Tol, H., Boersma, A.W., Brok, M., Wiemer, E.A., Stoter, G., Nooter, K., 2004. Imatinib mesylate (STI571) is a substrate for the breast cancer resistance protein (BCRP)/ABCG2 drug pump. *Blood*, 104, 2940-2942.

[161] Brendel, C., Scharenberg, C., Dohse, M., Robey, R.W., Bates, S.E., Shukla, S., Ambudkar, S.V., Wang, Y., Wennemuth, G., Burchert, A., Boudriot, U., Neubauer, A., 2007. Imatinib mesylate and nilotinib (AMN107) exhibit high-affinity interaction with ABCG2 on primitive hematopoietic stem cells. *Leukemia*, 21, 1267-1275.

[162] Hegedus, C., Ozvegy-Laczka, C., Apáti, A., Magócsi, M., Német, K., Orfi, L., Kéri, G., Katona, M., Takáts, Z., Váradi, A., Szakács, G., Sarkadi, B., 2009. Interaction of nilotinib, dasatinib and bosutinib with ABCB1 and ABCG2: implications for altered anti-cancer effects and pharmacological properties. *Br. J. Pharmacol.*, 158, 1153-1164.

[163] Huang, W.C., Chen, Y.J., Li, L.Y., Wei, Y.L., Hsu, S.C., Tsai, S.L., Chiu, P.C., Huang, W.P., Wang, Y.N., Chen, C.H., Chang, W.C., Chang, W.C., Chen, A.J., Tsai, C.H., Hung, M.C., 2011. Nuclear translocation of epidermal growth factor receptor by Akt-dependent phosphorylation enhances breast cancer resistant protein expression in gefitinib resistant cells. *J. Biol. Chem.*, 286, 20558-20568.

[164] Balabanov, S., Gontarewicz, A., Keller, G., Raddrizzani, L., Braig, M., Bosotti, R., Moll, J., Jost, E., Barett, C., Rohe, I., Bokemeyer, C., Holyoake, T.L., Brümmendorf, T.H., 2011. Abcg2 overexpression

represents a novel mechanism for acquired resistance to the multiki nase inhibitor Danusertib in BCR-ABL positive cells in vitro. *PLoS One*, 6, e19164.

[165] Silva, K.L., de Souza, P.S., Nestal de Moraes, G., Moellmann-Coelho, A., Vasconcelos Fda, C., Maia, R.C., 2013. XIAP and P-glycoprotein co-expression is related to imatinib resistance in chronic myeloid leukemia cells.*Leuk. Res*, 37, 1350-1358.

[166] Mahon, F.X., Belloc, F., Lagarde, V., Chollet, C., Moreau-Gaudry, F., Reiffers, J., Goldman, J.M., Melo, J.V., 2003. MDR1 gene overexpression confers resistance to imatinib mesylate in leukemia cell line models. *Blood*, 101, 2368-2373.

[167] Czyzewski, K., Styczynski, J., 2009. Imatinib is a substrate for various multidrug resistance proteins. *Neoplasma*, 56, 202-207.

[168] Mahon, F.X., Hayette, S., Lagarde, V., Belloc, F., Turcq, B., Nicolini, F., Belanger, C., Manley, P.W., Leroy, C., Etienne, G., Roche, S., Pasquet, J.M., 2008. Evidence that resistance to nilotinib may be due to BCR-ABL, Pgp, or Src kinase overexpression. *Cancer Res.*, 68, 9809-9816.

[169] Shibayama, Y., Nakano, K., Maeda, H., Taguchi, M., Ikeda, R., Sugawara, M., Iseki, K., Takeda, Y., Yamada, K., 2011. Multidrug resistance protein 2 implicates anticancer drug-resistance to sorafenib. *Biol. Pharm. Bull.*, 34, 433-435.

[170] Mukai, M., Che, X.F., Furukawa, T., Sumizawa, T., Aoki, S., Ren, X.Q., Haraguchi, M., Sugimoto, Y., Kobayashi, M., Takamatsu, H., Akiyama, S., 2003. Reversal of the resistance to STI571 in human chronic myelogenous leukemia K562 cells. *Cancer Sci.*, 94, 557-563.

[171] Houghton, P.J., Germain, G.S., Harwood, F.C., Schuetz, J.D., Stewart, C.F., Buchdunger, E., Traxler, P., 2004. Imatinib mesylate is a potent inhibitor of the ABCG2 (BCRP) transporter and reverses resistance to topotecan and SN-38 in vitro. *Cancer Res.*, 64, 2333-2337.

[172] Tiwari, A.K., Sodani, K., Wang, S.R., Kuang, Y.H., Ashby, C.R.Jr., Chen, X., Chen, Z.S., 2009. Nilotinib (AMN107,Tasigna) reverses multidrug resistance by inhibiting the activity of the ABCB1/Pgp and ABCG2/BCRP/MXR transporters. *Biochem. Pharmacol.*, 78, 153-161.

[173] Shi, Z., Jain, S., Kim, I.W., Peng, X.X., Abraham, I., Youssef, D.T., Fu, L.W., El Sayed, K., Ambudkar, S.V., Chen, Z.S., 2007. Sipholenol A, a marine-derived sipholane triterpene, potently reverses P-glycoprotein (ABCB1)-mediated multidrug resistance in cancer cells. *Cancer Sci.*, 98,1373-1380.

[174] Nakagawa-Goto, K., Chang, P.C., Lai, C.Y., Hung, H.Y., Chen, T.H., Wu, P.C., Zhu, H., Sedykh, A., Bastow, K.F., Lee, K.H., 2010. Antitumor agents. 280. Multidrug resistance-selective desmosdumotin B analogues. *J. Med. Chem.,* 53, 6699–6705.

[175] Kitazaki, T., Oka, M., Nakamura, Y., Tsurutani, J., Doi, S., Yasunaga, M., Takemura, M., Yabuuchi, H., Soda, H., Kohno, S., 2005. Gefitinib, an EGFR tyrosine kinase inhibitor, directly inhibits the function of P-glycoprotein in multidrug resistant cancer cells. Lung Cancer, 49, 337-343.

[176] Hoffmann, K., Franz, C., Xiao, Z., , Mohr, E., Serba, S., Büchler, M.W., Schemmer, P., 2010. Sorafenib modulates the gene expression of multi-dr ug resistance mediating ATP binding cassette proteins in experimental hepatocellular carcinoma. Anticancer Res., 30, 4503-4508.

[177] Andjelkovic, T., Bankovic, J., Stojsic, J., Milinkovic, V., Podolski-Renic, A., Ruzdijic, S., Tanic, N., 2011. Coalterations of p53 and PTEN tumor suppressor genes in non-small cell lung carcinoma patients. *Transl. Res.*, 157, 19-28.

[178] Qi, X., Chang, Z., Song, J., Gao, G., Shen, Z., 2011. Adenovirus-mediated p53 gene therapy reverses resistance of breast cancer cells to adriamycin. *Anticancer Drugs.*, 22, 556-562.

[179] Michaelis, M., Rothweiler, F., Klassert, D., von Deimling, A., Weber, K., Fehse, B., Kammerer, B., Doerr, H.W., Cinatl, J.Jr., 2009. Reversal of P-glycoprotein-mediated multidrug resistance by the murine double minute 2 antagonist nutlin-3. *Cancer Res.*, 69, 416-421.

[180] Nguyen, H., Zhang, S., Morris, M.E., 2003. Effect of flavonoids on MRP1-mediated transport in Panc-1 cells. *J. Pharm. Sci.* 92, 250-257.

[181] Wang, W., McLeod, H. L., Cassidy, J., 2003. Disulfirammediated inhibition of NF-kappaB activity enhances cytotoxicity of 5-fluorouracil in human colorectal cancer cell lines. *Int. J. Canc.*, 104, 504–511.

[182] Serra, V., Markman, B., Scaltriti, M., Eichhorn, P. J., Valero, V., Guzman, M., Botero, M.L., Llonch, E., Atzori, F., Di Cosimo, S., Maira, M., Garcia-Echeverria, C., Parra, J.L., Arribas, J., Baselga, J., 2008. NVP-BEZ235, a dual PI3K/mTOR inhibitor, prevents PI3K signaling and inhibits the growth of cancer cells with activating PI3K mutations. *Cancer Res.*, 68, 8022–8030.

[183] Cleary, J.M., Shapiro, G.I., 2010. Development of phosphoinositide-3 kinase pathway inhibitors for advanced cancer. *Curr. Oncol. Rep.*, 12, 87–94.

[184] Han, Z., Hong, L., Wu, K., Han, S., Shen, H., Liu, C., Han, Y., Liu, Z., Han, Y., Fan, D., 2006. Reversal of multidrug resistance of gastric cancer cells by downregulation of Akt1 with Akt1 siRNA. *J. Exp. Clin. Cancer Res.*, 25, 601-6.

[185] Andjelkovic, T., Bankovic, J., Milosevic, Z., Stojsic, J., Milinkovic, V., Pesic, M., Ruzdijic, S., Tanic, N., 2011-2012. Concurrent alteration of p16 and PTEN tumor suppressor genes could be considered as potential molecular marker for specific subgroups of NSCLC patients. *Cancer Biomark.*, 10, 277-286.

[186] Cheng, Z., Yang, N., Liang, W., Yan, X., Li, L., Pan, L., 2012. Effect of phosphatase and tensin homology deleted on chromosome 10 (PTEN) gene transfection on reversal of multidrug resistance in K562/ADM cells. *Leuk. Lymphoma.*, 53, 1383-1389.

[187] van Vlerken, L.E., Duan, Z., Little, S.R., Seiden, M.V., Amiji, M.M., 2008. Biodistribution and pharmacokinetic analysis of Paclitaxel and ceramide administered in multifunctional polymer-blend nanoparticles in drug resistant breast cancer model. *Mol. Pharm.*, 5, 516–526.

[188] van Vlerken, L.E., Duan, Z., Seiden, M.V., Amiji, M.M., 2007. Modulation of intracellular ceramide using polymeric nanoparticles to overcome multidrug resistance in cancer. *Cancer Res.*, 67, 4843–4850.

[189] Gouaze, V., Liu, Y.Y., Prickett, C.S., Yu, J.Y., Giuliano, A.E., Cabot, M.C., 2005. Glucosylceramide synthase blockade down-regulates P-glycoprotein and resensitizes multidrug-resistant breast cancer cells to anticancer drugs. *Cancer Res.*, 65, 3861–3867.

[190] Gaber, M.H., 2002. Modulation of doxorubicin resistance in multidrug-resistance cells by targeted liposomes combined with hyperthermia. *J. Biochem. Mol. Biol. Biophys.* 6, 309–314.

[191] Rapoport, N., 2004. Combined cancer therapy by micellar-encapsulated drug and ultrasound. *Int. J. Pharm.*, 277, 155–162.

[192] Marin, A., Sun, H., Husseini, G.A., Pitt, W.G., Christensen, D.A., Rapoport, N.Y., 2002. Drug delivery in pluronic micelles: effect of high-frequency ultrasound on drug release from micelles and intracellular uptake. *J. Control. Release.*, 84, 39–47.

[193] Walther, W., Stein, U., 1994., Influence of cytokines on mdr1 expression in human colon carcinoma cell lines: increased cytotoxicity of MDR relevant drugs. *J. Cancer Res. Clin. Oncol.*, 120, 471–478.

[194] Grodzovski, I., Lichtenstein, M., Galski, H., Lorberboum-Galski, H., 2010., IL-2- granzyme A chimeric protein overcomes multidrug

resistance (MDR) through a caspase 3-independent apoptotic pathway. *Int. J. Cancer*, 128, 1966–1980.

[195] Thakur, N., Joshi, T., Shanmugam, R., Banerjee, R., 2013. Proapoptotic miltefosine nanovesicles show synergism with paclitaxel: implications for glioblastoma multiforme therapy. *Cancer Lett.*, 334, 274-283.

[196] Li, Z., Oh, D.Y., Nakamura, K., Thiele, C.J., 2011. Perifosine-induced inhibition of Akt attenuates brain-derived neurotrophic factor/TrkB-induced chemoresistance in neuroblastoma in vivo. *Cancer*, 117, 5412–5422.

[197] Block, M., Gründker, C., Fister, S., Kubin, J., Wilkens, L., Mueller, M.D., Hemmerlein, B., Emons, G., Günthert, A.R., 2012. Inhibition of the AKT/mTOR and erbB pathways by gefitinib, perifosine and analogs of gonadotropin-releasing hormone I and II to overcome tamoxifen resistance in breast cancer cells. *Int. J. Oncol.*, 41, 1845–1854.

[198] Podolski-Renić, A., Andelković, T., Banković, J., Tanić, N., Ruždijić, S., Pešić, M., 2011. The role of paclitaxel in the development and treatment of multidrug resistant cancer cell lines. *Biomed. Pharmacother.*, 65, 345-353.

[199] Pesic, M., Markovic, J.Z., Jankovic, D., Kanazir, S., Markovic, I.D., Rakic, L., Ruzdijic, S., 2006. Induced resistance in the human non small cell lung carcinoma (NCI-H460) cell line in vitro by anticancer drugs. *J. Chemother.*, 18, 66-73.

[200] Andjelkovic, T., Pesic, M., Bankovic, J., Tanic, N., Markovic, I.D., Ruzdijic, S., 2008. Synergistic effects of the purine analog sulfinosine and curcumin on the multidrug resistant human non-small cell lung carcinoma cell line (NCI-H460/R). *Cancer Biol. Ther.*, 7, 1024-1032.

[201] Pešić, M., Andjelković, T., Banković, J., Marković, I.D., Rakić, L., Ruzdijić, S., 2009. Sulfinosine enhances doxorubicin efficacy through synergism and by reversing multidrug resistance in the human non-small cell lung carcinoma cell line (NCI-H460/R). *Invest. New Drugs.*, 27, 99-110.

[202] Pešić, M., Podolski, A., Rakić, L., Ruzdijić, S., 2010. Purine analogs sensitize the multidrug resistant cell line (NCI-H460/R) to doxorubicin and stimulate the cell growth inhibitory effect of verapamil. *Invest. New Drugs.*, 28, 482-492.

[203] Podolski-Renić, A., Jadranin, M., Stanković, T., Banković, J., Stojković, S., Chiourea, M., Aljančić, I., Vajs, V., Tešević, V., Ruždijić, S., Gagos, S., Tanić, N., Pešić, M., 2013. Molecular and cytogenetic changes in

multi-drug resistant cancer cells and their influence on new compounds testing. Cancer Chemother. Pharmacol., 72, 683-697.

[204] Pešić, M., Banković, J., Aljančić, I.S., Todorović, N.M., Jadranin, M., Vajs, V.E., Tešević, V.V., Vučković, I., Momčilović, M., Marković, I.D., Tanić, N., Ruždijić, S., 2011. New anti-cancer characteristics of jatrophane diterpenes from Euphorbia dendroides. *Food Chem. Toxicol.*, 49, 3165-3173.

[205] Banković, J., Andrä, J., Todorović, N., Podolski-Renić, A., Milošević, Z., Miljković, D., Krause. J,, Ruždijić, S., Tanić, N., Pešić, M., 2013. The elimination of P-glycoprotein over-expressing cancer cells by antimicrobial cationic peptide NK-2: the unique way of multi-drug resistance modulation. *Exp. Cell Res.*, 319, 1013-1027.

[206] Rodrigues, N.R., Rowan, A., Smith, M.E., Kerr, I.B., Bodmer, W.F., Gannon, J.V., Lane, D.P., 1990. p53 mutations in colorectal cancer. *Proc. Natl. Acad. Sci. U S A.*, 87, 7555-7559.

[207] Lau, C.J., Koty, Z., Nalbantoglu, J., 2009. Differential response of glioma cells to FOXO1-directed therapy. *Cancer Res.*, 69, 5433-5440.

[208] Vasas A, Sulyok E, Rédei D, Forgo P, Szabó P, Zupkó I, Berényi Á, Molnár J, Hohmann J. Jatrophane diterpenes from Euphorbia esula as antiproliferative agents and potent chemosensitizers to overcome multidrug resistance. *J. Nat. Prod.* 2011 Jun 24;74(6):1453-61.

[209] Corea, G., Di Pietro, A., Dumontet, C., Fattorusso, E., Lanzotti, V., 2009. Jatrophane diterpenes from Euphorbia spp. as modulators of multidrug resistance in cancer therapy. *Phytochem. Rev.* 8, 431–447.

[210] Corea, G., Fattorusso, E., Lanzotti, V., Taglialatela-Scafati, O., Appendino, G., Ballero, M., Simon, P.-N., Dumontet, C., Di Pietro, A., 2003a. Jatrophane diterpenes as P-glycoprotein inhibitors. First insights of structure-activity relationships and discovery of a new, powerful lead. J. Med. Chem. 46, 3395–3402. Isolation and biological evaluation of jatrophane diterpenoids from Euphorbia dendroides.

[211] Aljančić IS, Pešić M, Milosavljević SM, Todorović NM, Jadranin M, Milosavljević G, Povrenović D, Banković J, Tanić N, Marković ID, Ruzdijić S, Vajs VE, Tešević VV. *J. Nat. Prod.* 2011 Jul 22;74(7):1613-20.

[212] Jadranin M, Pešić M, Aljančić IS, Milosavljević SM, Todorović NM, Podolski-Renić A, Banković J, Tanić N, Marković I, Vajs VE, Tešević VV. Jatrophane diterpenoids from the latex of Euphorbia dendroides and their anti-P-glycoprotein activity in human multi-drug resistant cancer cell lines. *Phytochemistry.* 2013 Feb;86:208-17.

[213] Miglietta A, Gabriel L, Appendino G, Bocca C. Biological properties of jatrophane polyesters, new microtubule-interacting agents. *Cancer Chemother Pharmacol.* 2003 Jan;51(1):67-74.

[214] McCubrey JA, Steelman LS, Chappell WH, Abrams SL, Wong EW, Chang F, Lehmann B, Terrian DM, Milella M, Tafuri A, Stivala F, Libra M, Basecke J, Evangelisti C, Martelli AM, Franklin RA. Roles of the Raf/MEK/ERK pathway in cell growth, malignant transformation and drug resistance. *Biochim. Biophys. Acta.* 2007 Aug;1773(8):1263-84.

[215] Burris HA 3rd. Overcoming acquired resistance to anticancer therapy: focus on the PI3K/AKT/mTOR pathway. Cancer Chemother Pharmacol. 2013 Apr;71(4):829-42.

[216] Sokoloski JA, Sartorelli AC (1987) Inhibition of the synthesis of glycoproteins and induction of the differentiation of HL-60 promyelocytic leukemia cells by 6- methylmercaptopurine ribonucleoside. *Cancer Res.*47: 6283–6287.

[217] Fontanini G, Vignati S, Boldrini L, Chine` S, Silvestri V, et al. (1997) Vascular endothelial growth factor is associated with neovascularization and influences progression of non-small cell lung carcinoma. *Clin. Cancer Res.*3: 861–865.

[218] Leonard, G.D., Fojo, T., Bates, S.E., 2003. The role of ABC transporters in clinical practice. *Oncologist.*, 8, 411-424.

[219] Revankar, G.R., Hanna, N.B., Imamura, N., Lewis, A.F., Larson, S.B., Finch, R.A., Avery, T.L., Robins, R.K., 1990. Synthesis and in vivo antitumor activity of 2-amino-9H-purine-6-sulfenamide, -sulfinamide, and -sulfonamide and related purine ribonucleosides. *J. Med. Chem.*, 33, 121-128.

[220] Avery, T.L., Finch, R.A., Vasquez, K.M., Radparvar, S, Hanna, N.B., Revankar, G.R., Robins, R.K., 1990. Chemotherapeutic characterization in mice of 2-amino-9-beta-D-ribofuranosylpurine-6-sulfinamide (sulfinosine), a novel purine nucleoside with unique antitumor properties. *Cancer Res.*, 50, 2625-2630.

[221] Dačević, M., Isaković, A., Podolski-Renić, A., Isaković, A.M., Stanković, T., Milošević, Z., Rakić, L., Ruždijić, S., Pešić, M., 2013. Purine nucleoside analog--sulfinosine modulates diverse mechanisms of cancer progression in multi-drug resistant cancer cell lines. *PLoS One.*, 8, e54044.

[222] Drabek, K., Pesić, M., Piperski, V., Ruzdijić, S., Medić-Mijacević, L., Pietrzkowski, Z., Rakić, L., 2000. 8-Cl-cAMP and tiazofurin affect vascular endothelial growth factor production and glial fibrillary acidic

protein expression in human glioblastoma cells. *Anticancer Drugs.*, 11, 765-770.

[223] Presta, M., Belleri, M., Vacca, A., Ribatti, D., 2002. Anti-angiogenic activity of the purine analog 6-thioguanine. *Leukemia.*, 16, 1490-1499.

[224] Janković, D., Pesić, M., Marković, J., Kanazir, S., Marković, I., Rakić, L., Ruzdijić, S., 2006. The combination of sulfinosine and 8-Cl-cAMP induces synergistic cell growth inhibition of the human neuroblastoma cell line in vitro. *Invest. New Drugs.*, 24, 15-25.

[225] Menon, S.G., Goswami, P.C., 2007. A redox cycle within the cell cycle: ring in the old with the new. *Oncogene.*, 26, 1101-1109.

[226] Banković, J., Podolski-Renić, A., Pešić, M., 2013. VEGF Signaling and Multi-drug Resistance Transporter (ABCB1): Perception of New Anti-cancer Therapeutic Strategy. Marcellus L. Parker (Ed.) Series: Protein Biochemistry, Synthesis, Structure and Cellular Functions. Nova Publishers. *Vascular Endothelial Growth Factor (VEGF): Biology, Regulation and Clinical Significance*, pp. 1-40.

[227] Yan, X.D., Li, M., Yuan, Y., Mao, N., Pan, L.Y., 2007. Biological comparison of ovarian cancer resistant cell lines to cisplatin and Taxol by two different administrations. *Oncol. Rep.*, 17, 1163–1169.

[228] Wani MC, Taylor HL, Wall ME, Coggon P, McPhail AT Plant antitumor agents. VI. The isolation and structure of taxol, a novel antileukemic and antitumor agent from Taxus brevifolia. *J. Am. Chem. Soc.* 1971 May 5;93(9):2325-7.

[229] McGrogan BT, Gilmartin B, Carney DN, McCann A Taxanes, microtubules and chemoresistant breast cancer. *Biochim. Biophys. Acta.* 2008 Apr;1785(2):96-132. Epub 2007 Nov 12.

[230] Brito DA, Yang Z, Rieder CL. Microtubules do not promote mitotic slippage when the spindle assembly checkpoint cannot be satisfied. *J. Cell Biol.* 2008 Aug 25;182(4):623-9.

[231] Stearns ME, Wang M. Taxol blocks processes essential for prostate tumor cell (PC-3 ML) invasion and metastases. *Cancer Res.* 1992 Jul 1;52(13):3776-81.

[232] Toiyama Y, Miki C, Inoue Y, Kawamoto A, Kusunoki M. Circulating form of human vascular adhesion protein-1 (VAP-1): decreased serum levels in progression of colorectal cancer and predictive marker of lymphatic and hepatic metastasis. *J. Surg. Oncol.* 2009 May 1;99(6):368-72.

[233] Banković, J., Podolski-Renić, A., Pešić, M., 2013. Paclitaxel Resistance and Overcoming Strategies with Structurally- or Functionally-Related

Drugs. Diego Morales (Ed.) Series:Pharmacology - Research, Safety Testing and Regulation Cancer Etiology, Diagnosis and Treatments. Nova Publishers. *Paclitaxel: Biosynthesis, Mechanisms of Action and Clinical Uses*, pp. 1-58.

[234] Leuschner, C., Hansel, W., 2004. Membrane disrupting lytic peptides for cancer treatments. *Curr. Pharm. Des.*, 10, 2299–2310.

[235] Bechinger, B., Lohner, K., 2006. Detergent-like actions of linear amphipathic cationic antimicrobial peptides. *Biochim. Biophys. Acta*, 1758, 1529–1539.

[236] Chen, Y.Q., Min, C., Sang, M., Han, Y.Y., Ma, X., Xue, X.Q., Zhang, S.Q., 2010. A cationic amphiphilic peptide ABP-CM4 exhibits selective cyto- toxicity against leukemia cells. *Peptides*, 31, 1504–1510.

[237] Cruciani, R.A., Barker, J.L., Zasloff, M., Chen, H.C., Colamonici, O., 1991. Antibiotic magainins exert cytolytic activity against transformed cell lines through channel formation, *Proc.Natl.Acad.Sci.USA*, 88, 3792–3796.

[238] Hui, L., Leung, K., Chen, H.M., 2002. The combined effects of antibacterial peptide cecropin A and anti-cancer agents on leukemia cells. *Anticancer Res.*, 22, 2811–2816.

[239] Hammer, M., Brauser, A., Olak, C., Brezesinski, G., Goldmann, T., Gutsmann, T., Andrä, J., 2010. Lipopolysaccharide interaction is decisive for the activity of the antimicrobial peptide NK-2 against Escherichia coli and Proteus mirabilis. *Biochem. J.*, 427, 477–488.

[240] Zwaal, R., Schroit, A., 1997. Pathophysiologic implications of membrane phospholipid asymmetry in blood cells. *Blood*, 89, 1121–1132.

[241] Manno, S., Takakuwa, Y., Mohandas, N., 2002. Identification of a functional role for lipid asymmetry in biological membranes: phosphatidylserine–skeletal protein interactions modulate mem- brane stability. *Proc. Natl. Acad. Sci. USA*, 99, 1943–1948.

[242] Schroit, A.J., Madsen, J.W., Tanaka, Y., 1985. In vivo recognition and clearance of red blood cells containing phosphatidylserine in their plasma membranes. *J. Biol. Chem.*, 260, 5131–5138.

[243] Fadok, V.A., Voelker, D.R., Campbell, P.A., Cohen, J.J., Bratton, D.L., Henson, P.M., 1992. Exposure of phosphatidylserine on the surface of apoptotic lymphocytes triggers specific recognition and removal by macrophages. *J. Immunol.*, 148, 2207–2216.

[244] Utsugi, T., Schroit, A.J., Connor, J., Bucana, C.D., Fidler, I.J., 1991. Elevated expression of phosphatidylserine in the outer membrane leaflet

of human tumor cells and recognition by activated human blood monocytes, *Cancer Res.,* 51, 3062–3066.

[245] Ran, S., Downes, A., Thorpe, P.E., 2002. Increased exposure of anionic phospholipids on the surface of tumor blood vessels. *Cancer Res.*, 62 , 6132–6140.

[246] Schröder-Borm a, H., Bakalova, R., Andrä, J., 2005. The NK-lysin derived peptide NK-2 preferentially kills cancer cells with increased surface levels of negatively charged phosphatidylserine. *FEBS Lett.*, 579, 6128–6134.

[247] Riedl, S., Rinner, B., Asslaber, M., Schaider, H., Walzer, S., Novak, A., Lohner, K., Zweyticka, D., 2011. In search of a novel target—phosphatidylserine exposed bynon-apoptotic tumor cells and metastases of malignancies with poor treatment efficacy. *Biochim.Biophys.Acta*, 1808, 2638–2645.

[248] Nguyen, M., Marcellus, R.C., Roulston, A., Watson, M., Serfass, L., Murthy Madiraju, S. R., Goulet, D., Viallet, J., Bélec, L., Billot, X., Acoca, S., Purisima, E., Wiegmans, A., Cluse, L., Johnstone, R.W., Beauparlant, P., Shore, G.C., 2007. Small molecule obatoclax (GX15-070) antagonizes MCL-1 and overcomes MCL-1- mediated resistance to apoptosis. *Proc. Natl. Acad. Sci. U S A*., 104, 19512–19517.

[249] Pohl, A., Lage, H., Müller, P., Pomorski, T., Herrmann, A., 2002. Transport of phosphatidylserine via MDR1 (multidrugresistance 1) P-glycoprotein in a human gastric carcinoma cell line. *Biochem. J.*, 365, 259–268.

[250] May, G.L., Wright, L.C., Dyne, M., Mackinnon, W.B., Fox, R.M., Mountford, C.E., 1988. Plasma membrane lipid composition of vinblastine sensitive and resistant human leukaemic lymphoblasts.*Int .J. Cancer*, 42, 728-733.

[251] Mazzoni, A., Trave, F., 1993. Cytoplasmic membrane cholesterol and doxorubicin cytotoxicity in drug-sensitive and multidrug-resistant human ovarian cancer cells. *Oncol. Res.*, 5,75-82.

[252] Peterson, R.H., Meyers, M.B., Spengler, B.A., Biedler, J.L., 1983. Alteration of plasma membrane glycopeptides and gangliosides of Chinese hamster cells accompanying development of resistance to daunorubicin and vincristine. *Cancer Res.*, 43,222-228.

[253] Yunomae, K., Arima, H., Hirayama, F., Uekama, K., 2003. Involvement of cholesterol in the inhibitory effect of dimethyl-beta-cyclodextrin on P-glycoprotein and MRP2 function in Caco-2 cells. *FEBS Lett.*, 536,225-231.

[254] Plo, I., Lehne, G., Beckstrøm, K.J., Maestre, N., Bettaïeb, A., Laurent, G., Lautier, D., 2002. Influence of ceramide metabolism on P-glycoprotein function in immature acute myeloid leukemia KG1a cells. *Mol. Pharmacol.*, 62,304-312.

[255] Sinicrope, F.A., Dudeja, P.K., Bissonnette, B.M., Safa, A.R., Brasitus, T.A., 1992. Modulation of P-glycoprotein-mediated drug transport by alterations in lipid fluidity of rat liver canalicular membrane vesicles.*J. Biol. Chem.*, 267,24995-25002.

[256] Doige, C.A., Yu, X., Sharom, F.J., 1993. The effects of lipids and detergents on ATPase-active P-glycoprotein. *Biochim. Biophys. Acta*, 1146,65-72.

[257] Bucher, K.,Belli, S., Wunderli-Allenspach, H., Krämer, S.D., 2007. P-glycoprotein in proteoliposomes with low residual detergent: the effects of cholesterol. *Pharm. Res.*, 24,1993-2004.

[258] Romsicki, Y., Sharom, F.J., 1999. The membrane lipid environment modulates drug interactions with the P-glycoprotein multidrug transporter. *Biochemistry*, 38, 6887-6896.

[259] Hinrichs, J.W., Klappe, K., Hummel, I., Kok, J.W., 2004. ATP-binding cassette transporters are enriched in non-caveolar detergent-insoluble glycosphingolipid-enriched membrane domains (DIGs) in human multidrug-resistant cancer cells. *J. Biol. Chem.*, 279, 5734-5738.

[260] Hinrichs, J.W., Klappe, K., van Riezen, M., Kok, J.W., 2005. Drug resistance-associated changes in sphingolipids and ABC transporters occur in different regions of membrane domains. *J. Lipid. Res.*, 46, 2367-2376.

[261] Ghetie, M.A., Marches, R., Kufert, S., Vitetta, E.S., 2004. An anti-CD19 antibody inhibits the interaction between P-glycoprotein (P-gp) and CD19, causes P-gp to translocate out of lipid rafts, and chemosensitizes a multidrug-resistant (MDR) lymphoma cell line. *Blood*, 104, 178-183.

[262] Parmryd, I., Adler, J., Patel, R., Magee, A.I., 2003. Imaging metabolism of phosphatidylinositol 4,5-bisphosphate in T-cell GM1-enriched domains containing Ras proteins. *Exp. Cell Res.*, 285, 27-38.

[263] Nakamura, Y., Oka, M., Soda, H., Shiozawa, K., Yoshikawa, M., Itoh, A., Ikegami, Y., Tsurutani, J., Nakatomi, K., Kitazaki, T., Doi, S., Yoshida, H., Kohno, S., 2005. Gefitinib ("Iressa", ZD1839), an epidermal growth factor receptor tyrosine kinase inhibitor, reverses breast cancer resistance protein/ABCG2-mediated drug resistance. Cancer Res., 65, 1541-1546.

[264] Dinic, J., Ashrafzadeh, P. Parmryd, I. 2013. Actin filaments attachment at the plasma membrane in live cells cause the formation of ordered lipid domains. *Biochim. Biophys. Acta*, 1828, 1102-1111.

[265] Mahammad, S., Dinic, J., Adler, J., Parmryd, I., 2010. Limited cholesterol depletion causes aggregation of plasma membrane lipid rafts inducing T cell activation. *Biochim. Biophys. Acta*, 1801, 625-634.

[266] von Haller, P.D., Donohoe, S., Goodlett, D.R., Aebersold, R., Watts, J.D., 2001. Mass spectrometric characterization of proteins extracted from Jurkat T cell detergent-resistant membrane domains. *Proteomics*, 1, 1010-1021.

[267] Bacso, Z., Nagy, H., Goda, K., Bene, L., Fenyvesi, F., Matkó, J., Szabó, G., 2004. Raft and cytoskeleton associations of an ABC transporter: P-glycoprotein. *Cytometry A*, 61, 105-116.

[268] Shai Y., Mechanism of the binding, insertion and destabilization of phospholipid bilayer membranes by alpha-helical antimicrobial and cell non-selective membrane-lytic peptides, *Biochim. Biophys. Acta* 1462 (1999) 55–70.

[269] Schröder-Borm b, H., Willumeit, R., Brandenburg, K., Andrä, J., 2003. Molecular basis for membrane selectivity of NK-2, a potent peptide antibiotic derived from NK-lysin. *Biochim.Biophys.Acta*, 1612, 164–171.

[270] DeMilito, A., Fais, S., 2005. Tumor acidity, chemoresistance and proton pump inhibitors. *Future Oncol*, 1, 779–786.

[271] Thews, O., Gassner, B., Kelleher, D.K., Schwerdt, G., Gekle, M., 2006. Impact of extracellular acidity on the activity of P-glycoprotein and the cytotoxicity of chemotherapeutic drugs. *Neoplasia*, 8, 143–152.

[272] Harguindey, S., Arranz, J.L., Wahl, M.L., Orive, G., Reshkin, S.J., 2009. Proton transport inhibitors as potentially selective anticancer drugs. *Anticancer Res.*, 29, 2127–2136.

Reviewed by:

Dr. Miljana Tanić
Laboratory for molecular genetics
Institute for oncology and radiology -
Serbian National Cancer Research Center
Pasterova 14,
11000 Belgrade, Serbia
e-mail: tanic.miljana@ncrc.ac.rs

In: Advances in Drug Resistance Research ISBN: 978-1-63117-131-4
Editor: Christudas Morais

Chapter 3

Tumor Fibroblasts: Pivotal Players in Drug Resistance

*Ivy Chung**
University of Malaya Cancer Research Institute,
Department of Pharmacology, Faculty of Medicine,
University of Malaya, Kuala Lumpur, Malaysia

Abstract

Chemotherapy remains one of the mainstay options for treating cancer. The dawn of the post-genomic era has witnessed several major breakthroughs in personalized medicine, and it has been an exciting time for the emergence of targeted chemotherapy for cancers with distinctive molecular characteristics. Yet, the development of drug resistance continues to hinder the success of chemotherapy, and it is often viewed as the outcome of cancer cell-autonomous processes. In fact, recent evidence points to the fact that the host environment itself can be equally guilty. Tumor fibroblasts - one of the responsible perpetrators - cooperate with the tumor cells to initiate and drive tumor progression. These cells

---

* University of Malaya Cancer Research Institute, Department of Pharmacology, Faculty Medicine, University of Malaya, Lembah Pantai, 50603 Kuala Lumpur, Malaysia. E-mail: ivychung@ummc.edu.my. This work was funded by UM/HIR/MOHE/MED-12 and RG492/13HTM.

are prominent members in most carcinoma tissues, and they provide a protective niche for tumor cells to escape from cytotoxic effects of chemotherapy. This chapter discusses the different types and origins of fibroblast population that exist within solid tumors, and their roles in dictating the response of tumors to therapies. The underlying key mechanisms by which the dynamic tumor-fibroblast cell interaction allow escape from therapeutic drugs and the eventual development of drug resistance are also discussed. This evidence supports the notion that tumor fibroblasts can potentially be a good target in overcoming drug resistance, and such tumor-fibroblast cell interaction should be targeted for designing more effective and less resistance-prone anti-cancer therapies.

Keywords: Tumor microenvironment, fibroblast, myofibroblasts, extracellular matrix remodeling, epithelial-mesenchymal transition, chemoresistance

Challenges in Cancer Chemotherapy

Chemotherapy remains one of the important therapeutic options for most patients with cancer. This field has grown tremendously over the past years, from "one drug-fits-all" strategy to targeted therapy using small molecule inhibitors that focus on "addicted" oncogenic pathways utilized by the tumor cells. Encouraging clinical results were observed with the use of epidermal growth factor (EGF) receptor inhibitors in non-small cell lung cancer [1], Bcr-Abl inhibitors in chronic myeloid leukemia [2] and c-KIT inhibitors in gastrointestinal stromal tumors [3]. Yet, the efficacy of chemotherapy, whether the conventional cytotoxic drugs or targeted small molecule inhibitors, in a single-agent setting or in drug combination, is severely hampered by the emergence of drug resistance [4, 5]. Drug resistance can be classified into two categories: intrinsic (also known as innate or *de novo*) resistance and acquired (or extrinsic) resistance. Patients with intrinsic drug resistance do not respond to the therapy from the start of treatment. In contrast, patients with acquired resistance responded initially to the treatment, but continued treatment ultimately leads to tumor recurrence and metastasis [6].

Development of drug resistance is often thought as the outcome of cancer cell-autonomous processes. Many studies elegantly demonstrate the acquisition of drug resistance through expression of ATP-binding cassette receptors which pump out drugs from the cancer cells [7]. Others suggest that the increased drug metabolism in cancer cells leads to increased detoxification and reduced cytotoxic activities [8]. Cancer cells can also strengthen their defense signaling pathways to overcome drug-induced apoptosis [8]. All these processes are partly attributable to the development of acquired drug resistance, which require exposure to chemotherapeutic drugs.

The factors contributing to the development of innate drug resistance are less clear; however, accumulating evidence is pointing to the tumor microenvironment as a major player. Interaction of cancer cells with the surrounding extracellular matrix, via cell surface integrins, dramatically improved the survival of cancer cells at both primary and secondary sites, and when exposed to chemotherapeutic drugs [9]. Recently, the fibroblast population within the tumor microenvironment has emerged as another key player in contributing to the drug-resistant phenotype of cancer cells. This is especially apparent in tumors with evident desmoplastic reaction such as pancreatic cancer, which is well-known for its lethality due to limited response to conventional chemotherapy [10]. An understanding of the molecular mechanisms underlying fibroblasts-mediated drug resistance might help in devising novel strategies to overcome such resistance. This review summarizes the significance of several key mechanisms associated with fibroblasts-mediated drug resistance in cancer therapy.

Types and Origins of Tumor Fibroblasts

To date, it is unclear how many types of tumor fibroblasts exist within the tumor microenvironment. This is probably due to the lack of specific markers which can identify different subtypes of this cell population [11]. Tumor fibroblasts in general share similar phenotypes with myofibroblasts– the type of fibroblasts that are activated during wound healing [12]. These fibroblasts are thought to derive from resident fibroblasts undergoing transdifferentiation after stimulation by tumor secreted growth factors, which probably mimic the trigger of a wound healing-like process [13]. Unlike resident or benign fibroblasts, tumor fibroblasts show increased expression of fibronectin, fibroblast activation protein (FAP), tenascin-C, desmin and alpha-smooth muscle actin (α-SMA) [11, 14]. These fibroblasts are responsible for synthesizing and depositing various growth factors and extracellular matrix (ECM) proteins, including matrix metalloproteinases (MMPs), fibrin, heparanase and collagen, which are important for extracellular remodeling [11, 13].

Growing evidence is now indicating that these tumor fibroblasts may be transformed by the tumor cells. For example, *TP53* and *PTEN* somatic mutations were observed in the fibroblast within the breast carcinoma tissues [15]. These mutations are well-known for their roles in tumor progression and response to chemotherapy if found expressed in the tumor cells. Indeed, high frequency of stromal *TP53* mutation is associated with lymph node metastases in sporadic breast cancers [16], and loss of *PTEN* function in mouse mammary stroma accelerates initiation, progression and malignant transformation of mammary epithelial tumor cells [17]. In hormone (progesterone)-sensitive endometrial cancer, loss of progesterone receptor expression in the stromal fibroblasts renders resistance to the therapy [18]. Using genetically modified animal model, the progesterone receptor was shown to be epigenetically silenced by tumor cells harboring activated *KRAS* and loss of *PTEN*. While it remains unclear how the tumor cells transform the tumor fibroblasts, these once thought tumor-specific mutations are now found to have critical roles in the fibroblast biology and may therefore affect the response of tumors to drug therapy.

It is possible that tumor cells reprogram the fibroblasts phenotype at the genetic level, especially if these fibroblasts are derived from multi-lineage cells such as mesenchymal stem cells (MSCs). There have been suggestions that tumor fibroblasts may originate from distant sources such as bone marrow-derived MSCs [19]. MSCs may act as a tumor fibroblast precursor cell lineage, as these cells can be mobilized into the tumor by tumor-secreted chemotaxis factors such as chemokine C-C motif ligand 2 (CCL2), vascular endothelial growth factor (VEGF) and epidermal growth factor (EGF)[20]. Such niche promotes MSCs transdifferentiation into highly proliferative myofibroblasts that express activation markers α-SMA, fibronectin and tenascin [19, 20]. Through the milieu of secreted factors (including fatty acids), these MSCs-transdifferentiated fibroblasts were shown to induce tumor chemoresistance [21, 22].

Besides MSCs, there are evidence that tumor fibroblasts can be transdifferentiated from tumor and endothelial cells, via epithelial-mesenchymal transition (EMT) and endothelial-mesenchymaltransition (EndMT), respectively [23, 24]. Again, these processes require certain signaling cues from the tumor microenvironment, which involve dynamic activation of multiple growth factor pathways. Transforming growth factor (TGF)-beta, in particular, can almost single-handedly activates pathways implicated in EMT including PI3K/AKT, Smad and RhoA which in turn lead to the loss of epithelial E-cadherin and gain of mesenchymalα-SMA, desmin and vimentin markers [25]. Yet, the presence of other growth factors such as epidermal growth factor (EGF), hepatocyte growth factor (HGF) and fibroblast growth factor (FGF) within the tumor microenvironment can further collaborate to enhance the transdifferentiation process [26], and this further complicates the effort in delineating the underlying mechanisms. Although observed only in limited models, transdifferentiation of fibroblasts from endothelial cells underscores the plasticity of cells within the tumor microenvironment. Following treatment with TGF-beta and bone morphogenetic protein (BMP), endothelial cells undergo an incomplete mesenchymal transition, expressing mesenchymal markers and retaining endothelial markers such as VE-cadherin, CD31, EGF-like domains 1 (TIE1) and cytokeratins [24]. More intriguingly, these endothelial-derived fibroblasts are predominantly found at the invasive front of the tumors [24], suggesting important roles in tumor aggressiveness.

All these evidence point to the potentially diverse origins of tumor fibroblasts; this may reflect the heterogeneity of fibroblasts expressing different markers, and within different tumor types. Nevertheless, the presence of fibroblast population is difficult to ignore as it constitutes a large proportion of some tumor tissues such as pancreatic adenocarcinoma [27]. Their plasticity and multi-functional properties almost mirror the characteristics of tumor cells, which may serve as the underlying principles for their role in contributing to chemoresistance.

Tumor Fibroblasts Shape the Architecture of Chemoresistance

As in wound healing, fibroblasts in the tumor microenvironment are the primary cells that produce extracellular matrix proteins (e.g. fibronectin and laminin) and matrix regulators (eg. matrix metalloproteinases and matrix protein inhibitors) [9]. These factors are responsible mainly for remodeling the tumor ECM, and hence serve as messengers to relay information between tumor cells and their surroundings. Such communication is dynamic, both in the form of cell-to-cell and cell-to-matrix. Different composition of ECM affects various physical properties such as interstitial fluid pressure and gradients in oxygen and drug concentrations, all of which have been associated with development of chemoresistance [9]. It is well established that tumor cells when grown in 3D matrix show reduced sensitivity to chemotherapy agents as compared to those that are grown in monolayer culture. This occurs through activation of integrin- and other cell adhesion molecules-mediated survival pathways [9, 28]. In a recent study in lung cancer and squamous cell carcinoma, unbiased genome-wide analysis revealed a unique signature of alteration in gene expression, whereby genes associated with cell adhesion and defense mechanisms, rather than DNA repair, were affected when tumor cells were grown in 3D as compared to 2D culture [29]. Consequently, this yields a significant increase in radio- and chemo-resistance in tumor cells grown in ECM-enriched environment. In some cases, the support provided by the ECM affects mainly the survival of tumor cells, rather than other cellular processes such as cell proliferation and migration. When myeloma cells were cultured on fibronectin, β integrin-mediated amplification of interleukin-6 (IL-6) resulted in an increase of anti-apoptotic Bcl-2 and a decreased of pro-apoptotic Bim protein expression, suggestive of enhanced survival of the tumor cells [30]. Endometrial cancer cells grew very slowly on Matrigel as shown by reduced BrdU incorporation, but their response to progesterone was diminished markedly [31].

The process by which ECM regulates tumor cells response to chemotherapy may be protein-specific. In a leukemia model, β1 integrin induced resistance to doxorubicin through binding to collagen but not fibrin, by upregulating the expression of ATP-binding cassette C1 (ABCC1) protein [32]. Similarly, partnership between β1 integrin and fibronectin results in p27-mediated G1 arrest, and hence development of resistance to etoposide in myeloma cells [33]. It is quite clear that fibroblasts-secreted ECM provides not only biomechanical support, but also information channels for the tumor cells to communicate with their surroundings.

Tumor Fibroblasts-Derived Soluble Factors Confer to Increased Tumor Cell Survival

One of the key activities of fibroblasts is to produce a reservoir of soluble growth factors and cytokines that act in an autocrine or paracrine fashion. These factors are well known for their multiple effects on the epithelial cell survival, including the tumor cells [14]. Although these factors may have overlapping functions, their mechanisms in mediating chemoresistance could be tumor type-specific. In pancreatic cancer, fibroblasts-produced CXCL12 (also known as stroma-derived factor-1, SDF-1) induced transcription of sonic hedgehog (SHH) expression through nuclear factor kappa B (NFκB) activity [34], and hedgehog inhibition by a cyclopamine analog (IPI-296) depleted the stromal tissue and markedly improved delivery of gemcitabine in an animal model [35]. Moreover, abrogation of hedgehog signaling is associated with reduced *stemness* potential of pancreatic tumorspheres and this translated to decreased chemoresistance [36]. Targeting hedgehog signaling in pancreatic cancer may not appear as effective if the tumor tissue is hypoxic, as decreased sensitivity to gemcitabine and 5-fluorouracil was observed when used in combination with hedgehog inhibitors [37]. In cholangiocarcinoma, however, hedgehog signaling was activated by fibroblasts-secreted platelet growth factor BB (PDGF-BB), which rendered reduced cytotoxicity to TRAIL [38]. Hence, the action of soluble factors secreted by tumor fibroblasts may depend greatly on the biology of the tumor cells. It is, therefore, important to determine the exact mechanisms by which these fibroblasts secretion can affect the response of tumor cells to different therapy. As most studies were focusing on selected one or two factors found abundantly in their model, it is worthwhile to note that the synergistic effects between multiple secretory factors may render a different landscape of mechanisms to induce chemoresistance.

Due to many resemblances in function between tumor fibroblasts and activated fibroblasts from benign, inflammatory conditions, it is reasonable to think that benign fibroblasts secretion may exert similar pro-tumorigenic effects including inducing chemoresistance. However, there is accumulating evidence stating otherwise. A classic example was shown in prostate cancer, whereby non-tumorigenic benign prostatic hyperplasia (BPH) cells become tumorigenic after co-inoculated with tumor fibroblasts in a renal capsule implantation, but not when inoculated with benign fibroblasts [39]. Data from our laboratory and others showed that endometrial cancer cells increased their proliferation and resistance to hormonal therapy after exposed to the secretion from tumor fibroblasts, while contrasting effects were seen with the secretion from the benign counterparts [40, 41]. The pro-survival effects were mediated by activation of phosphoinositide 3-kinase (PI3K)/AKT and MAPK signaling, as antagonism using specific inhibitors reversed the tumor fibroblasts-mediated cell proliferation [41]. Such contrasting phenotypes may be explained by the increase levels of pro-inflammatory cytokines (IL-6, IL-8 and macrophage chemoattractant protein (MCP-1)) secreted by these primary fibroblasts established from individual tumor tissues, which were secreted at much lower levels by those from benign tissues [41]. The magnitude of secretory factor levels may be one of the reasons, but temporal effects and readiness in recipient (tumor) cells to be activated by these factors may also be possible [42]. Hence, it is crucial to first critically characterize the secretome profile in fibroblasts from different pathological conditions. Then, delineation of the signaling pathways orchestrated by these co-existing factors in the tumor microenvironment may potentially provide venues for understanding the development of chemoresistance by tumor fibroblasts. Some of the studies using co-culture studies that demonstrate the role of fibroblast secretion in mediating chemotherapy resistance are summarized in Table 1.

Table 1. Fibroblast-mediated resistance to chemotherapy

Tumor	Cell type	Chemotherapeutic agent	Reference
Pancreas	T3M4, PT45-P1	etoposide	[43]
Melanoma	1205Lu	cisplatin	[30]
Breast	MCF-7	tamoxifen, fulvestrant doxorubicin, PARP inhibitor	[44]
Multiple myeloma	U266, NCI-H929	bortezomib	[22]
Cholangio carcinoma	KMCH-1, KMBC, HuCCT-1, TFK-1, Mz-ChA-1	TRAIL	[38]
Colon	Primary cells	irinotecan, IL-1 beta	[45]
Lung	NCI-H460	VP-16	[46]
Various tumor types	45 cell lines	16 agents	[47]

Tumor Fibroblasts Contribute to EMT Induction

Epithelial-mesenchymal transition (EMT) is an important process during development by which epithelial cells acquire mesenchymal, fibroblast-like properties and show reduced intercellular adhesion and increased motility. Accumulating evidence points to a critical role of EMT in tumor progression, via which tumor cells acquired aggressive properties including resistance to therapy [48, 49]. EMT induction is mainly mediated by selected differentiation-related transcription factors, including Snail, Twist and zinc finger E-box-binding homeobox (ZEB)[49]. While activation of these transcription factors are thought to be regulated by oncogenic pathways, such as Ras, Src and Wnt [50-52], recent evidence suggests that tumor fibroblasts-secreted growth factors and cytokines may also induce EMT [53-55].

In an *in vitro* direct co-culture model, fibroblasts derived from the interface zone of breast cancer tissues in comparison to those from adjacent benign area, demonstrated greater capacity in inducing an EMT in MCF-7 breast cancer cell line, as indicated by decreased E-cadherin and increased vimentin and N-cadherin expression [56]. In a prostate carcinoma model, tumor fibroblasts induced EMT via a pro-inflammatory signature that is highly dependent on cycloxygenase (COX)-2 activities [53]. Similarly, tumor fibroblasts-induced inflammatory reaction was accounted for the EMT observed in a transgenic pancreatic adenocarcinoma mouse model [54]. In this particular work, EMT and invasiveness were most abundant at inflammatory foci and that leads to increased circulating cancer cells. Although induction of chemoresistance was not the main focus in this work, it is evident that the presence of tumor fibroblasts at close proximity was necessary to induce EMT at both the benign and cancer stages [54]. In fact, tumor fibroblasts exerted greater potency in inducing EMT via direct cells contact, rather than via paracrine signaling molecules, although a reduced proliferation was observed in the tumor cells [57].

Despite extensive studies on EMT in cancer, the role of EMT in tumor progression and chemoresistance *in vivo* remains debatable, as we lack pathological evidence from clinical samples to correlate with the molecular alterations observed in pre-clinical models [58]. More studies are warranted to explore if correlation exists between tumor cells with EMT markers and their response to chemotherapy in cancer patients.

Strategies to Overcome Tumor Fibroblasts-Mediated Chemoresistance

Given the different attributes by which tumor fibroblasts mediate chemoresistance, it is attractive to develop treatment strategies that abrogate the communication between tumor and fibroblast cells. The different chemoresistance-induced mechanisms exploited by the tumor fibroblasts offer many potential ways to re-structure the network. One obvious strategy is to remove the fibroblasts from the microenvironment. Extensive proliferation of tumor fibroblasts (also known as desmoplasia) can affect delivery of chemotherapy agent into the tumor. Depletion of stromal fibroblasts, via blocking of hedgehog cellular signaling pathway with IPI-926, leads to a transient increase in intratumoral concentration of gemcitabine and hence, a transient stabilized disease in the gemcitabine-resistant KrasLSL.G12D/ +;p53R172H/+; Pdx-Cretg/+ (KPC) pancreatic tumor mouse model [35].

However, not all hedgehog inhibitors resulted in an attenuation of tumor stroma, despite remarkably inhibited tumor growth [59]. There are ongoing attempts to translate this promising strategy to the clinic. Despite some encouraging Phase I clinical data, a Phase II trial of gemcitabine plus saridegib, a hedgehog inhibitor, in metastatic pancreatic cancer showed a higher rate of progressive disease and a shorter overall survival in the intervention arm, leading to an early halt [60]. Clinical evidence for nab-paclitaxel in combination with gemcitabine offered a more promising strategy to eliminate desmoplasia in pancreatic tumors, targeting SPARC protein expressed by both the tumor and endothelial cells [61]. Taken together, activated tumor fibroblasts within the pancreatic tissues may be relying on redundant pathways to survive and proliferate, and we may be still far from perfecting our clinical skills to design and interpret potential determinants and predictors of efficacy when targeting the fibroblasts within the tumors.

Following a challenge with cytotoxic agents or small molecule inhibitors, tumor fibroblasts may release various pro-survival growth factors that allow rapid adaptation to overcome the therapy-induced cytotoxicity. For example, treatment of triple negative breast cancer with MEK inhibitor was associated with increased signaling by platelet-derived growth factor receptor (PDGFR), vascular endothelial growth factor receptor (VEGFR) and HER2 [62]. Activation of different receptor kinase receptors simultaneously may indicate the crucial role of a common downstream effector that is critical for that particular tumor cells to survive. Designing activators/inhibitors that selectively target this common effector may be proven useful. A recent study has utilized a large scale RNAi screen to identify MED12, a regulator of TGF beta signaling, to be the common mediator of resistance to multiple kinase inhibitors including BRAF, ALK and MEK inhibitors [63]. Loss of MED12 was associated with increased TGF beta signaling, which thought to induce EMT and confer resistance to therapy [63]. Hence, it is reasonably possible to determine potential drug target despite the complexity from activation of redundant signaling pathways. Detailed investigation is therefore necessary to understand the step-by-step mechanistic events leading to the development of chemoresistance for different therapy in different tumor type.

Recently, nanomedicine or therapeutic nanoparticles have emerged as an innovative and promising alternative to overcome drug resistance [64]. Due to the almost indefinite chemical properties of nanovehicle, it is possible to load various targeted agents into such nanometric delivery system.

Shapira et al. has recently proposed a quadrugnostic platform, whereby an ideal nanomedicine will contain a selective targeting moiety to the tumor tissue, a diagnostic imaging aid to localize the tumor tissue, a cytotoxic small molecule or therapeutic biological, and lastly, a chemosensitizing agent aimed to neutralize any chemoresistance induced by the tumor microenvironment [64].

Such strategy is exploiting the nano-properties of the vehicle to accumulate in the tumor microenvironment, before releasing the therapeutic cargoes that can interfere with the tumor-fibroblast cells communication. A good example for targeting tumor fibroblasts was recently shown using a simpler nanotherapeutic approach. Docetaxel-conjugate nanoparticles, also known as Cellax, are 120 nm particles containing docetaxel and polyethylene glycol (PEG) conjugated to acetylated carboxymethycellulose. In two different orthotopic breast tumor models, treatment with Cellax remarkably depleted up to 80% of alpha-SMA-expressing fibroblasts within the tumor tissues, a significantly greater anti-stroma effect compared to native docetaxel and nab-paclitaxel [65].

Both tumor perfusion and vascular permeability were enhanced significantly, accompanied with a considerable reduction in tumor matrix and tumor interstitial fluid pressure [65]. At least 85% of Cellax administered were delivered to α-SMA-positive fibroblasts, resulting in a rapid depletion of tumor stroma (within 24-hours) and a significant reduction in metastatic lesions [65].

These effects were not seen with docetaxel alone or nab-paclitaxel treatment, strongly suggesting that co-targeting the tumor fibroblasts can impact the drug delivery and hence the efficacy of the cytotoxic agents.

It should be emphasized that tumor fibroblasts are not the only non-tumor component within the tumor microenvironment. Although not covered in this review, overcoming fibroblasts-mediated chemoresistance may require concurrent strategies to target other host-derived factors, for example the macrophages and lymphocytes.

Given the emerging enthusiasm in cancer immunotherapy, it is anticipated that development of fibroblasts- and immune-modulatory agents to complement tumor-targeted therapies will be an exciting area of research.

Conclusion

All anti-cancer drugs used in the clinic are capable of noticeably suppressing tumor growth; yet, each suffers from rapid development of resistance programs. Distinct microenvironment landscaped by tumor fibroblasts can provide sanctuary to the tumors, which contributes substantially to tumor cell survival and eventually relapse and therapy failure. Consequently, tumor cells are no longer the only player responsible for the induction of chemoresistance. Addition of tumor fibroblasts into the paradigm has change the way we look at the failed chemotherapy. Our own body cells, although unwillingly, are partly responsible for the lack of therapeutic efficacy. Strategies to target the bi-directional communication between tumor and fibroblast cells should be emphasized and considered in future cancer drug design and development.

References

[1] Lee C, Brown C, Gralla R, Hirsh V, Thongprasert S, Tsai C-M, et al. Impact of EGFR inhibitor in non-small cell lung cancer on progression-free and overall survival: a meta-analysis. *Journal of the National Cancer Institute.* 2013;105(9):595-605.

[2] O'Hare T, Zabriskie M, Eiring A, Deininger M. Pushing the limits of targeted therapy in chronic myeloid leukaemia. *Nature reviews Cancer.* 2012;12(8):513-26.

[3] Blay J-Y. A decade of tyrosine kinase inhibitor therapy: Historical and current perspectives on targeted therapy for GIST. *Cancer treatment reviews.* 2011;37(5):373-84.

[4] Remon J, Moran T, Majem M, Reguart N, Dalmau E, Marquez-Medina D, et al. Acquired resistance to epidermal growth factor receptor tyrosine kinase inhibitors in EGFR-mutant non-small cell lung cancer: A new era begins. *Cancer treatment reviews.* 2013.

[5] Lambert G, Duhme-Klair A-K, Morgan T, Ramjee M. The background, discovery and clinical development of BCR-ABL inhibitors.*Drug discovery today*. 2013.

[6] Szakacs G, Paterson J, Ludwig J, Booth-Genthe C, Gottesman M. Targeting multidrug resistance in cancer. Nature reviews *Drug discovery*. 2006;5(3):219-34.

[7] Takara K, Sakaeda T, Okumura K. An update on overcoming MDR1-mediated multidrug resistance in cancer chemotherapy.*Current pharmaceutical design*. 2006;12(3):273-86.

[8] Lonning P, Knappskog S. Mapping genetic alterations causing chemoresistance in cancer: identifying the roads by tracking the drivers. *Oncogene*. 2013.

[9] Correia A, Bissell M. The tumor microenvironment is a dominant force in multidrug resistance. *Drug resistance updates : reviews and commentaries in antimicrobial and anticancer chemotherapy*. 2012;15(1-2):39-49.

[10] Li X, Ma Q, Xu Q, Duan W, Lei J, Wu E. Targeting the cancer-stroma interaction: a potential approach for pancreatic cancer treatment. *Current pharmaceutical design*. 2012;18(17):2404-15.

[11] Kalluri R, Zeisberg M. Fibroblasts in cancer. *Nat Rev Cancer*. 2006 May;6(5):392-401.

[12] Dvorak H. Tumors: wounds that do not heal. Similarities between tumor stroma generation and wound healing.*The New England journal of medicine*. 1986;315(26):1650-9.

[13] Tomasek JJ, Gabbiani G, Hinz B, Chaponnier C, Brown RA. Myofibroblasts and mechano-regulation of connective tissue remodelling. *Nat Rev Mol Cell Biol*. 2002 May;3(5):349-63.

[14] Xing F, Saidou J, Watabe K. Cancer associated fibroblasts (CAFs) in tumor microenvironment. *Frontiers in bioscience* (Landmark edition). 2010;15:166-79.

[15] Kurose K, Gilley K, Matsumoto S, Watson PH, Zhou XP, Eng C. Frequent somatic mutations in PTEN and TP53 are mutually exclusive in the stroma of breast carcinomas. *Nat Genet*. 2002 Nov;32(3):355-7.

[16] Patocs A, Zhang L, Xu Y, Weber F, Caldes T, Mutter G, et al. Breast-cancer stromal cells with TP53 mutations and nodal metastases. *The New England journal of medicine*. 2007;357(25):2543-51.

[17] Trimboli A, Cantemir-Stone C, Li F, Wallace J, Merchant A, Creasap N, et al. Pten in stromal fibroblasts suppresses mammary epithelial tumours. *Nature*. 2009;461(7267):1084-91.

[18] Janzen D, Rosales M, Paik D, Lee D, Smith D, Witte O, et al. Progesterone receptor signaling in the microenvironment of endometrial cancer influences its response to hormonal therapy. *Cancer research.* 2013.

[19] Mao Y, Keller E, Garfield D, Shen K, Wang J. Stromal cells in tumor microenvironment and breast cancer. *Cancer metastasis reviews.* 2013;32(1-2):303-15.

[20] Hanahan D, Coussens L. Accessories to the crime: functions of cells recruited to the tumor microenvironment. *Cancer cell.* 2012;21(3):309-22.

[21] Roodhart J, Daenen L, Stigter E, Prins H-J, Gerrits J, Houthuijzen J, et al. Mesenchymal stem cells induce resistance to chemotherapy through the release of platinum-induced fatty acids. *Cancer cell.* 2011;20(3): 370-83.

[22] Hao M, Zhang L, An G, Meng H, Han Y, Xie Z, et al. Bone marrow stromal cells protect myeloma cells from bortezomib induced apoptosis by suppressing microRNA-15a expression. *Leukemia & lymphoma.* 2011;52(9):1787-94.

[23] Petersen O, Nielsen H, Gudjonsson T, Villadsen R, Rank F, Niebuhr E, et al. Epithelial to mesenchymal transition in human breast cancer can provide a nonmalignant stroma. *The American journal of pathology.* 2003;162(2):391-402.

[24] Medici D, Kalluri R. Endothelial-mesenchymal transition and its contribution to the emergence of stem cell phenotype. *Seminars in cancer biology.* 2012;22(5-6):379-84.

[25] Heldin C-H, Vanlandewijck M, Moustakas A. Regulation of EMT by TGF尾 in cancer. *FEBS letters.* 2012;586(14):1959-70.

[26] Smalley K, Brafford P, Herlyn M. Selective evolutionary pressure from the tissue microenvironment drives tumor progression. *Seminars in cancer biology.* 2005;15(6):451-9.

[27] Feig C, Gopinathan A, Neesse A, Chan D, Cook N, Tuveson D. The pancreas cancer microenvironment. Clinical cancer research: an official *journal of the American Association for Cancer Research.* 2012;18(16):4266-76.

[28] Sutherland R, Eddy H, Bareham B, Reich K, Vanantwerp D. Resistance to adriamycin in multicellular spheroids. *International journal of radiation oncology, biology, physics.* 1979;5(8):1225-30.

[29] Zschenker O, Streichert T, Hehlgans S, Cordes N. Genome-wide gene expression analysis in cancer cells reveals 3D growth to affect ECM and

processes associated with cell adhesion but not DNA repair. *PLoS One*. 2012;7(4).

[30] Flach E, Rebecca V, Herlyn M, Smalley K, Anderson A. Fibroblasts contribute to melanoma tumor growth and drug resistance. *Molecular pharmaceutics*. 2011;8(6):2039-49.

[31] Arnold JT, Kaufman DG, Seppala M, Lessey BA. Endometrial stromal cells regulate epithelial cell growth in vitro: a new co-culture model. *Hum Reprod*. 2001 May;16(5):836-45.

[32] El Azreq M-A, Naci D, Aoudjit F. Collagen/尾1 integrin signaling up-regulates the ABCC1/MRP-1 transporter in an ERK/MAPK-dependent manner. *Molecular biology of the cell*. 23(17):3473-84.

[33] Hazlchurst L, Enkcmann S, Beam C, Argilagos R, Painter J, Shain K, et al. Genotypic and phenotypic comparisons of de novo and acquired melphalan resistance in an isogenic multiple myeloma cell line model. *Cancer research*. 2003;63(22):7900-6.

[34] Singh A, Arora S, Bhardwaj A, Srivastava S, Kadakia M, Wang B, et al. CXCL12/CXCR4 protein signaling axis induces sonic hedgehog expression in pancreatic cancer cells via extracellular regulated kinase- and Akt kinase-mediated activation of nuclear factor 魏B: implications for bidirectional tumor-stromal interactions. *The Journal of biological chemistry*. 2012;287(46):39115-24.

[35] Olive K, Jacobetz M, Davidson C, Gopinathan A, McIntyre D, Honess D, et al. Inhibition of Hedgehog signaling enhances delivery of chemotherapy in a mouse model of pancreatic cancer. *Science* (New York, NY). 2009;324(5933):1457-61.

[36] Huang F-T, Zhuan-Sun Y-X, Zhuang Y-Y, Wei S-L, Tang J, Chen W-B, et al. Inhibition of hedgehog signaling depresses self-renewal of pancreatic cancer stem cells and reverses chemoresistance. *International journal of oncology*. 2012;41(5):1707-14.

[37] Onishi H, Morifuji Y, Kai M, Suyama K, Iwasaki H, Katano M. Hedgehog inhibitor decreases chemosensitivity to 5-fluorouracil and gemcitabine under hypoxic conditions in pancreatic cancer. *Cancer science*. 2012;103(7):1272-9.

[38] Fingas C, Bronk S, Werneburg N, Mott J, Guicciardi M, Cazanave S, et al. Myofibroblast-derived PDGF-BB promotes Hedgehog survival signaling in cholangiocarcinoma cells. *Hepatology* (Baltimore, Md). 2011;54(6):2076-88.

[39] Hayward S, Wang Y, Cao M, Hom Y, Zhang B, Grossfeld G, et al. Malignant transformation in a nontumorigenic human prostatic epithelial cell line. *Cancer research*. 2001;61(22):8135-42.

[40] Arnold JT, Lessey BA, Seppala M, Kaufman DG. Effect of normal endometrial stroma on growth and differentiation in Ishikawa endometrial adenocarcinoma cells. *Cancer Res*. 2002 Jan 1;62(1):79-88.

[41] Subramaniam K, Tham S, Mohamed Z, Woo Y, Mat Adenan N, Chung I. Cancer-associated fibroblasts promote proliferation of endometrial cancer cells. *PLoS One*. 2013;8(7).

[42] Szabo P, Valach J, Smetana K, Dvo艜谩nkov谩 B. Comparative Analysis of IL-8 and CXCL-1 Production by Normal and Cancer Stromal Fibroblasts. *Folia biologica*. 2013;59(3):134-7.

[43] Muerkoster S, Wegehenkel K, Arlt A, Witt M, Sipos B, Kruse M-L, et al. Tumor stroma interactions induce chemoresistance in pancreatic ductal carcinoma cells involving increased secretion and paracrine effects of nitric oxide and interleukin-1beta. *Cancer research*. 2004;64(4):1331-7.

[44] Martinez-Outschoorn U, Goldberg A, Lin Z, Ko Y-H, Flomenberg N, Wang C, et al. Anti-estrogen resistance in breast cancer is induced by the tumor microenvironment and can be overcome by inhibiting mitochondrial function in epithelial cancer cells. *Cancer biology* & therapy. 2011;12(10):924-38.

[45] Paduch R, Jakubowicz-Gil J, Niedziela P. Hepatocyte growth factor (HGF), heat shock proteins (HSPs) and multidrug resistance protein (MRP) expression in co-culture of colon tumor spheroids with normal cells after incubation with interleukin-1beta (IL-1beta) and/or camptothecin (CPT-11). *Indian journal of experimental biology*. 2011;48(4):354-64.

[46] Hao Y, Zhang L, He J, Guo Z, Ying L, Xu Z, et al. Functional investigation of NCI-H460-inducible myofibroblasts on the chemoresistance to VP-16 with a microfluidic 3D co-culture device. *PLoS One*. 2013;8(4).

[47] Straussman R, Morikawa T, Shee K, Barzily-Rokni M, Qian Z, Du J, et al. Tumour micro-environment elicits innate resistance to RAF inhibitors through HGF secretion. *Nature*. 2010;487(7408):500-4.

[48] Iwatsuki M, Mimori K, Yokobori T, Ishi H, Beppu T, Nakamori S, et al. Epithelial-mesenchymal transition in cancer development and its clinical significance. *Cancer science*. 2010;101(2):293-9.

[49] Kalluri R. EMT: when epithelial cells decide to become mesenchymal-like cells. *The Journal of clinical investigation*. 2009;119(6):1417-9.

[50] Larue L, Bellacosa A. Epithelial-mesenchymal transition in development and cancer: role of phosphatidylinositol 3' kinase/AKT pathways. *Oncogene*. 2005;24(50):7443-54.

[51] Nagathihalli N, Merchant N. Src-mediated regulation of E-cadherin and EMT in pancreatic cancer. *Frontiers in bioscience* (Landmark edition). 2012;17:2059-69.

[52] Wang Z, Li Y, Ahmad A, Banerjee S, Azmi A, Kong D, et al. Pancreatic cancer: understanding and overcoming chemoresistance. Nature reviews *Gastroenterology &hepatology*. 2011;8(1):27-33.

[53] Giannoni E, Bianchini F, Calorini L, Chiarugi P. Cancer associated fibroblasts exploit reactive oxygen species through a proinflammatory signature leading to epithelial mesenchymal transition and stemness. *Antioxidants & redox signaling*. 2011;14(12):2361-71.

[54] Rhim A, Mirek E, Aiello N, Maitra A, Bailey J, McAllister F, et al. EMT and dissemination precede pancreatic tumor formation. *Cell*. 2012;148(1-2):349-61.

[55] Soon P, Kim E, Pon C, Gill A, Moore K, Spillane A, et al. Breast cancer-associated fibroblasts induce epithelial-to-mesenchymal transition in breast cancer cells. *Endocrine-related cancer*. 2013;20(1): 1-12.

[56] Gao M-Q, Kim B, Kang S, Choi Y, Park H, Kang K, et al. Stromal fibroblasts from the interface zone of human breast carcinomas induce an epithelial-mesenchymal transition-like state in breast cancer cells in vitro. *Journal of cell science*. 2010;123(Pt 20):3507-14.

[57] Choe C, Shin Y-S, Kim S-H, Jeon M-J, Choi S-J, Lee J, et al. Tumor-stromal Interactions with Direct Cell Contacts Enhance Motility of Non-small Cell Lung Cancer Cells Through the Hedgehog Signaling Pathway. *Anticancer research*. 2013;33(9):3715-23.

[58] Stewart C, McCluggage W. Epithelial-mesenchymal transition in carcinomas of the female genital tract. H*istopathology*. 2013;62(1): 31-43.

[59] Chang Q, Foltz W, Chaudary N, Hill R, Hedley D. Tumor-stroma interaction in orthotopic primary pancreatic cancer xenografts during hedgehog pathway inhibition. *International journal of cancer Journal international du cancer*. 2013;133(1):225-34.

[60] Ruch J, Kim E. Hedgehog signaling pathway and cancer therapeutics: progress to date. *Drugs*. 2013;73(7):613-23.

[61] Heinemann V, Reni M, Ychou M, Richel D, Macarulla T, Ducreux M. Tumour-stroma interactions in pancreatic ductal adenocarcinoma: Rationale and current evidence for new therapeutic strategies. *Cancer treatment reviews.* 2013.

[62] Duncan JS, Whittle MC, Nakamura K, Abell AN, Midland AA, Zawistowski JS, et al. Dynamic reprogramming of the kinome in response to targeted MEK inhibition in triple-negative breast cancer.*Cell.* 2012;149(2):307-21.

[63] Huang S, Halzel M, Knijnenburg T, Schlicker鈥 A. MED12 controls the response to multiple cancer drugs through regulation of TGF-尾 receptor signaling. *Cell.* 2012.

[64] Shapira A, Livney Y, Broxterman H, Assaraf Y. Nanomedicine for targeted cancer therapy: towards the overcoming of drug resistance. Drug resistance updates: *reviews and commentaries in antimicrobial and anticancer chemotherapy*. 2013;14(3):150-63.

[65] Murakami M, Ernsting M, Undzys E, Holwell N, Foltz W, Li S-D. Docetaxel Conjugate Nanoparticles That Target 伪-Smooth Muscle Actin-Expressing Stromal Cells Suppress Breast Cancer Metastasis. *Cancer research*. 2013;73(15):4862-71.

In: Advances in Drug Resistance Research ISBN: 978-1-63117-131-4
Editor: Christudas Morais

Chapter 4

Erythropoiesis Stimulating Agent Resistance

***Stacey O'Shea*[1], *Sunil V. Badve*[1,2] *and David W. Johnson*[1,2*]**

[1] Department of Nephrology, Princess Alexandra Hospital, Brisbane, Australia

[1,2] Centre for Kidney Disease Research, Translational Research Institute, University of Queensland, Brisbane, Australia

Abstract

Erythropoietin is produced by the kidney and stimulates growth and differentiation of red blood cells. Loss of this hormone production with renal failure is the major mechanism behind anaemia of chronic kidney disease (CKD). Severe anaemia is known to be associated with increased cardiovascular events and mortality in renal failure and thus the development of recombinant erythropoietin revolutionised the management of anaemia in CKD. Erythropoiesis stimulating agent (ESA) administration became widespread without randomised trial data to generate parameters for use. The use of these agents to minimise blood

* Address for Correspondence: Professor David Johnson, Department of Renal Medicine,Level 2, Ambulatory Renal and Transplant Services Building, Princess Alexandra Hospital Ipswich Road, Woolloongabba, Brisbane Qld 4102 AUSTRALIATel: +61 7 3240 5080, Fax: +61 7 3240 5480; Email: david_johnson@health.qld.gov.au.

transfusions and correct severe anaemia is appropriate. Although observational data demonstrated that using ESAs to target normal haemoglobin and haematocrit was associated with improved outcomes, four large randomised trials demonstrated harm using these agents to aggressively correct anaemia. Subsequent analyses of these trials revealed that it may not have been the high haemoglobin per se that resulted in high adverse event rates, but rather the high doses of ESA required in a subset of patients. ESA resistance has emerged as an independent risk factor for morbidity and mortality in CKD patients and is an indicator of significant underlying comorbidity. Common causes of ESA resistance include iron deficiency, inflammation, infection, malnutrition, hyperparathyroidism and inadequate dialysis. Erythropoietin resistance as a risk factor for poor outcomes persists into transplantation, and thus the identification of this should prompt investigation and treatment for underlying causes. Treatment with ESA should be individualised to avoid excessive dosing or high haemoglobin. This review discusses the epidemiology, clinical sequelae and causes of ESA resistance. A suggested plan for the investigation and management of such patients is also provided.

Keywords: Anaemia, chronic kidney disease, erythropoietin resistance

Introduction

Anaemia is a common complication of chronic kidney disease (CKD) and is associated with increased risks of adverse outcomes, including all-cause mortality, cardiovascular events, impaired cognitive function, sleep disturbance, sexual dysfunction and impaired quality of life [1-5]. For example, a study in haemodialysis patients demonstrated that every 10 g/L drop in haemoglobin level was associated with increased LV diameter (relative risk [RR] 1.42; $p = 0.018$) and heightened risks of new cardiac failure (RR 1.28; $p = 0.017$), recurrent heart failure (RR 1.2, $p = 0.046$), and mortality on dialysis therapy (RR = 1.14, $p = 0.024$) [6]. Studies have also consistently demonstrated that the prevalence and severity of anaemia progressively increase as kidney function declines. The incidence of anaemia is less than 2% in CKD stage 1-2, 5% in CKD stage 3, 44% in CKD stage 4 and more than 70% in end stage kidney disease [7]. Historically, people with end stage kidney disease were profoundly anaemic with an average haemoglobin of 60-80g/L, and were heavily transfusion dependent, with concomitant transfusion-related risks including transmitted infections, iron overload and allosensitisation [8].

The contributing causes to anaemia of CKD are multifactorial, although a major aetiologic factor is impaired production of erythropoietin, a glycoprotein hormone that stimulates growth and differentiation of erythroid progenitors in the bone marrow and is produced by type 1 cortical fibroblasts in the kidneys [9; 10]. The subsequent development of recombinant erythropoietin in the 1980s revolutionised the treatment of anaemia in patients with CKD. Multiple studies in the 1980s and 1990s demonstrated the efficacy, safety and tolerability of erythropoietin. The Food and Drug Administration approved the use of erythropoietin in 1989 and its use became widespread. Over the ensuing decades, other types of erythropoiesis stimulating agents (ESAs) have been developed commercially and introduced into routine clinical practice.

Unfortunately, up to 10% of CKD patients exhibit a suboptimal haematologic response to ESAs [11; 12], which in turn is associated with increased risks of adverse effects, including mortality [12; 13]. The aim of this paper is to review the definition, prevalence, recognised causes and adverse outcomes of ESA resistance in patients with CKD. A suggested plan for the investigation and management of such patients is also provided.

What is ESA Resistance?

There is no agreed definition of ESA resistance in the literature. The Kidney Disease Improving Global Outcomes (KDIGO) Guidelines divide the issue into initial and subsequent ESA hyporesponsiveness [14]. Initial ESA hyporesponsiveness is defined as no increase in haemoglobin concentration from baseline after one month of ESA weight-based dosing. Subsequent ESA hyporesponsiveness is defined as patients previously on a stable ESA dose who require two increases in ESA dose more than 50% beyond the initial stable dose. On the other hand, the National Kidney Foundation (NKF) Kidney Disease Outcomes Quality Initiative (KDOQI) suggests ESA resistance is present when there is a significant decrease in haemoglobin level at a constant ESA dose, a requirement for a significant increase in ESA dose to maintain a certain haemoglobin level, or failure to increase the haemoglobin level to greater than11g/L despite an ESA dose of greater than 500 U/kg/week [15]. The European Guidelines suggest ESA resistance is present if a patient requires ≥ 300 U/kg/wk of ESA or 1.5 μg/kg/wk of darbepoetin alpha [16].

The Erythropoieitin Resistance Index (ERI) has been proposed as an alternative measurement and is derived by the equation erythropoietin dose (IU/kg/week) divided by haemoglobin level in grams [17]. A value of > 0.02 U/kg/wk/gHb is indicative of erythropoietin resistance.

Why is ESA Resistance Clinically Important?

Erythropoietin stimulating agents are expensive. For example, epoetin alpha is the single greatest drug expenditure paid for by US Medicare such that in 2010 Medicare spent $2 billion on this drug [18]. ESAs were introduced to improve adverse outcomes associated with anaemia and to prevent the need for blood transfusion. In a study comparing a cohort of ESRD patients receiving ESAs to a historical simulated group relying on blood transfusion, estimated total costs were comparable between the two groups, as were the quality adjusted life years (QALYs). The incremental cost-effectiveness ratio (ICER) of using ESAs compared to transfusion was $873 per QALY gained [19]. However, Clement et al compared the cost effectiveness of using ESAs vs. no ESAs and found a cost per QALY of $96,270, which is significant [20]. None of these analyses considered the increased costs that must necessarily be associated with an ESA hyporesponsive patient who requires escalating doses of these drugs.

Aside from pure cost considerations, recent evidence has highlighted that resistance to ESAs may confer an increased risk of adverse clinical outcomes. For example, the Correction of Haemoglobin and Outcomes in Renal Insufficiency [21] trial compared the effects of targeting haemoglobin values 135g/L vs. 113g/L on death and the composite cardiovascular outcomes of congestive cardiac failure, stroke and acute myocardial infarction in ESA-treated CKD patients [22]. This trial was terminated early due to excess death and heart failure in the high haemoglobin group, which also had a significantly higher ESA dose requirement. Subset analysis showed the composite event rates were not statistically significant when corrected for failure to achieve target haemoglobin and requirement for high dose ESA, thereby suggesting that the adverse events could have been due to toxicities in high dose ESA treatment or factors attributable to ESA hyporesponsiveness [23]. Although other randomised controlled trials [24; 25] and systematic reviews [13; 26] have also consistently demonstrated increased risks of adverse events (stroke, vascular thrombosis, hypertension and mortality) when ESAs were administered to target higher haemoglobin values, post hoc analyses have suggested that poor response to ESA therapy rather than achieved high haemoglobin values may have been responsible for the deleterious outcomes associated with ESA therapy [23; 27-30]. Indeed, at any given haemoglobin level, higher required ESA dosage was associated with increased mortality. Another study by Kilpatrick et al demonstrated that poor ESA responsiveness and the use of high ESA doses was a strong, independent predictor of increased risks of mortality, myocardial infarction, congestive heart failure and stroke [27]. Thus, it is possible that the excess morbidity and mortality observed in these ESA trials arose from the patients requiring higher ESA doses to push their haemoglobin to higher targets, and was not a reflection of the high haemoglobin achieved. Alternatively, the requirement for high erythropoietin doses may have reflected underlying comorbid medical conditions, intercurrent illnesses and inflammation, which in turn generated increased risks of mortality. Erythropoietin resistance is also an independent risk factor for death after renal transplantation [31; 32].

What Causes ESA Resistance?

The contributing factors to ESA resistance are manifold (Figure 1).

Iron Deficiency

CKD patients are at risk for absolute, inflammatory and functional iron deficiency. Absolute iron deficiency may occur through repeated blood tests, blood retention in the dialyser circuit, needle puncture site losses, increased gastrointestinal blood loss and impaired gastrointestinal iron absorption [33]. Inflammatory iron deficiency resulting in anaemia of chronic disease occurs with inflammation and upregulation of hepcidin to cause decreased iron absorption and prevention of iron mobilisation from the reticuloendothelial system, resulting in hypoferraemia and iron restricted erythropoiesis [34; 35]. Functional iron deficiency occurs when iron stores are adequate but unable to be mobilised when stimulated by an ESA [34; 36].

Intravenous (IV) iron supplementation is safe (major side effect is 0.3-0.7% rate of Arthralgia-myalgia syndrome) [37] and remains the most efficacious and cost beneficial way of improving iron stores in CKD patients

[38]. The Dialysis Patients' Response to IV Iron with Elevated Ferritin (DRIVE) [39] and DRIVE II [40] studies showed that high dose iron can improve haemoglobin targets without increased ESA use, even in the setting of seemingly adequate or even high serum ferritin levels. Indeed, DRIVE II demonstrated a reduction of ESA dose required over time. Nevertheless, caution should be exercised as these studies were relatively short in duration and the long-term safety of IV iron administration in the setting of normal or elevated iron studies has not been established.

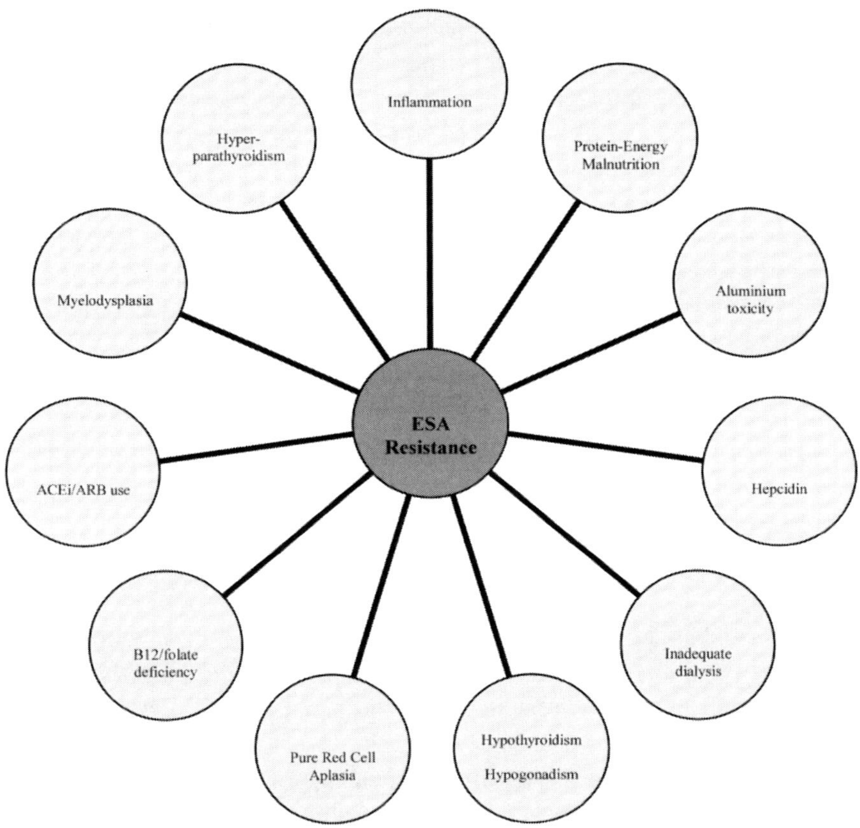

Figure 1. Causes of ESA resistance.

Moreover, serum iron markers are a poor reflection of total body iron stores, particularly in inflammatory states, such as CKD. A study by Ferrari et al using FerriScan technology (magnetic resonance imaging relaxometry) demonstrated that transferrin saturation (TSAT) and ferritin measures were poor predictors of total body iron in haemodialysis patients, and that some patients had liver iron concentrations equivalent to those observed in patients with haemochromatosis [41]. Thus, while increased IV iron is safe and may overcome some ESA resistance in some cases, patients may develop occult iron overload.

IV iron may also be potentially associated with other hazards, such as infection and mortality. Although earlier data were conflicting, large prospective observational trials have shown that IV iron was not associated with increased risk of bacterial infections in hemodialysis patients [37]. Earlier association data between high ferritin and risk of death or hospitalization were also refuted by a subsequent large prospective haemodialysis cohort, which found that the association was dramatically reduced or eliminated after adjustment for inflammation and malnutrition [42].

Hepcidin

Iron physiology, ESA resistance and inflammation-associated anaemia may share a common denominator in the protein hepcidin. Hepcidin is a negative iron regulating protein produced mostly by the liver and in small parts by kidney tubular cells. Hepcidin regulates iron homeostasis by reducing ferroportin, an intracellular iron transporting molecule, thereby reducing both iron absorption and iron recycling [36]. Hepcidin also acts in the kidneys to regulate iron excretion via divalent metal transporter 1 (DMT1) [43]. Hepcidin production is stimulated by iron overload, hypoxia, inflammation and cytokines like interleukin-1 (IL-1) and interleukin-6 (IL-6) [43]. Hepcidin levels are significantly elevated in dialysis patients, particularly those with elevated CRP levels, are lower in patients receiving ESA therapy, and are inversely correlated with ESA dosage [36; 43; 44]. However, the data is not consistent as evaluation of a large cohort of chronic haemodialysis patients enrolled in the Convective Transport Study (CONTRAST) demonstrated elevated hepcidin levels were associated with markers of iron storage, erythropoiesis and inflammation, but not with ESA dosage [45]. In contrast, Won et al reviewed a cohort of ESA resistant dialysis patients and found no relationship between hepcidin, inflammatory markers or iron status [46]. Others have found hepcidin not to be predictive of response to iron loading or ESA dose and to fall with dialysis initiation [44; 47; 48]. Additionally, hepcidin assays are variable and lack standardization and hepcidin has a high intra-patient coefficient of variation [43]. It is possible therefore that excess hepcidin or hepcidin resistance may be a major contributor to ESA resistance in subgroup of CKD patients, and is probably related to underlying inflammatory state.

Inflammation

Inflammation plays a role in ESA resistance via multiple mechanisms. CKD is an inflammatory state and patients have elevated levels of C-reactive protein (CRP) and circulating cytokines, such as IL-1, IL-6 and tumour necrosis factor-α (TNF-α) [49]. In addition to upregulating hepcidin production, these cytokines can suppress bone marrow erythropoiesis directly [49]. However, the relationship is not consistent across the literature. In a cohort of 68 prevalent dialysis patients, IL-6 was an independent risk factor for ESA resistance, although the relationship with CRP was not significant [46]. The RISchio CArdiovascolare nei pazienti afferenti all' Area Vasta In Dialisi (RISCAVID) study explored the interaction between ESAs, inflammation, anaemia and cardiovascular events and mortality in 757 haemodialysis patients and demonstrated that patients with haemoglobin levels below 11g/L were at increased risk of cardiovascular events and mortality, while those with haemoglobin levels above 11g/L were protected [50]. When patients were categorised according to quartiles of ESA resistance, there was a linear rise in risk with increasing ESA resistance quartiles, which in turn correlated independently with reduced albumin, high CRP & high IL-6. Pro-inflammatory cytokines have also recently been reported to promote increased levels of soluble erythropoietin receptor (an inhibitor of erythropoiesis signalling) in haemodialysis patients [51].

ESA resistance in patients should therefore prompt a search for inflammation. Common causes of inflammation in this setting include occult infection, tunnelled dialysis catheters, arteriovenous grafts, periodontal disease and poor water quality [52]. Inflammation is associated with poor outcome measures, such as hypoalbuminaemia, and is itself a predictor of hospitalisation, cardiovascular events and mortality [52]. While there are physiological mechanisms by which inflammation can directly contribute to ESA resistance, the poor outcomes observed are likely a reflection of this comorbidity.

Malnutrition

Protein-energy malnutrition (PEM) is a state of decreased body protein with or without fat depletion or a state of diminished functional capacity, in which the need for protein or energy cannot be satisfied by the diet [42]. Like inflammation, malnutrition is a significant predictor of morbidity, mortality and erythropoiesis hyporesponsiveness. Indeed, it is often difficult to separate PEM from inflammation as the biomarkers overlap and the conditions often occur concurrently and coexist in the same patient [42]. The low body mass index (BMI), low serum cholesterol and low serum albumin concentrations that are part of this syndrome are strong independent predictors of adverse outcome in haemodialysis. The terms malnutrition-inflammation complex syndrome (MICS) or malnutrition, inflammation and atherosclerosis syndromes have been proposed to cover the combination of the conditions [42]. It is likely that in PEM/inflammation/MICS, the same processes are underpinning ESA hyporesponsiveness.

Hyperparathyroidism

Secondary hyperparathyroidism is a recognised risk factor for erythropoietin resistance. Hyperparathyroidism induces bone marrow fibrosis, reducing the effectiveness of ESA stimulation. Parathyroid hormone (PTH) also inhibits the actions of ESAs in the marrow [49]. Treatment of hyperparathyroidism by calcitriol suppression or parathyroidectomy has been shown to improve haemoglobin and reduce ESA requirements [49]. Studies using cinacalcet to reduce PTH have also been shown to reduce ESA dose requirements without any change in haemoglobin [53]. Similarly, multiple evaluations of dialysis patient cohorts have shown that low serum vitamin D levels are independently associated with ESA resistance and anaemia [54].

Inadequate Dialysis

Poor response to ESA therapy is a recognised consequence of poor dialysis. While there is no universal parameter to measure dialysis adequacy, low Kt/V and poor urea reduction ratios have each been shown to be associated with higher ESA requirements [49]. On the other hand, Movilli et al showed that increasing the Kt/V above 1.3 did not affect ESA responsiveness in iron replete haemodialysis patients [55], thereby indicating that increasing dialysis adequacy above standard targets does not improve ESA responsiveness. Conversely, observational data has shown extended hour, nocturnal and short daily dialysis regimens are associated with reduced erythropoietin requirements. A small randomised controlled trial comparing the use of low flux haemodialysis to online convective dialysis did not find significant differences in haemoglobin levels or ESA resistance [56]. The mechanism by which inadequate dialysis causes ESA resistance is multifactorial, and includes increased inflammation, inhibition of erythropoiesis by uraemic bone marrow suppression, and hyper-parathyroidism. The evidence for type and duration of dialysis influencing this association is not conclusive.

ACE Inhibitors & AR Blockers

The use of angiotensin-converting enzyme inhibitors (ACEi) and angiotensin receptor blockers (ARB) has been associated with ESA hyporesponsiveness. Angiotensin II may increase proliferation of erythroid progenitors and induce EPO release, such that use of these agents has been found to correlate with higher ESA dose requirements [49]. Several studies have identified genetic polymorphisms in the ACE gene which may determine the responsiveness of these patients to ESAs [49]. The use of ACEi/ARB is extremely widespread in CKD as the data for nephroprotection in the setting of proteinuria are compelling. Although ACEi/ARB use is not consistently identified across studies as a risk factor for ESA resistance, it may represent a ubiquitous and potentially modifiable risk factor for ESA resistance. Alternatively, it may be a reflection of the underlying comorbidity (e.g. heart disease, diabetes and heart failure) in patients on ACEi/ARB therapy.

Other Causes

Multiple other comorbidities may contribute to erythropoietin resistance in a patient and must be considered, investigated and treated

- Occult malignancy,
- Other bone marrow pathology such as multiple myeloma, myelofibrosis, aluminium toxicity, severe renal bone disease,
- Inherited haemoglobinopathies such as the thalassaemias and sickle cell anaemia ,
- Pure red cell aplasia,
- Other drug interactions e.g. sevelamer [57],

- Hypothyroidism,
- Hypogonadism (testosterone is an inhibitor of hepcidin testosterone was used historically to treat renal anaemia),
- Vitamin B12/folate deficiency (water soluble vitamins that are removed by dialysis & are important cofactors in erythrogenesis).

How Should ESA Resistance Be Managed?

The identification, investigation and management of patients with ESA resistances is important as it is a potentially modifiable risk factor for adverse outcomes. First occult blood loss must be excluded, and then iron deficiency (absolute or functional), vitamin B12 and folate deficiency must be treated.

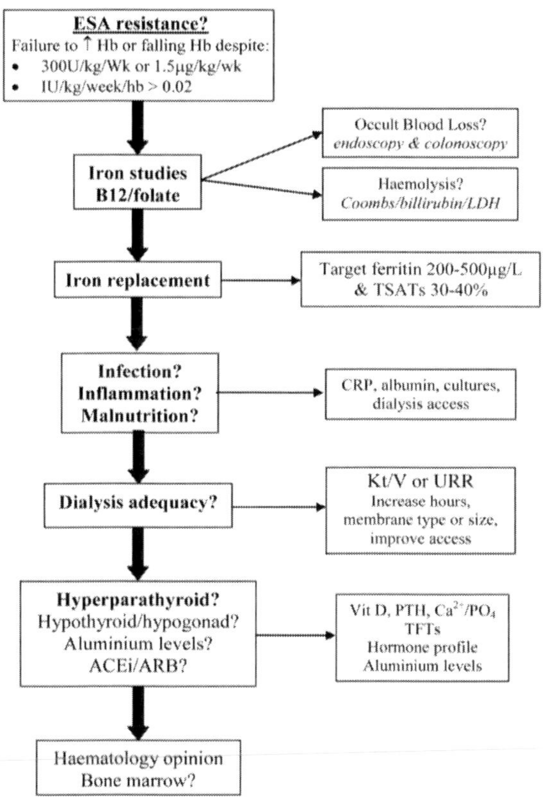

Figure 2. Algorithm for management of ESA resistance.

A target for iron studies during ESA therapy is suggested as serum ferritin 200-500μg/L and TSATs 30-40% [58]. Next inflammation, infection and malnutrition must be considered, and assessed by measurement of CRP and albumin; examination for source of infection, including consideration of type of dialysis access; removal of old renal allografts and review by a renal dietician.

Once iron deficiency and inflammation are excluded or treated, dialysis adequacy must be assessed and consideration given to maximising dialysis adequacy by increased hours, membrane size and biocompatibility, improved access, etc [9; 59]. Hyperparathyroidism, hypothyroidism, aluminium toxicity and hypogonadism should be evaluated. If all of the above have been excluded, novel approaches such as ascorbic acid therapy [60], polysulphone high-flux dialyzer [61], vitamin E supplementation [59], statins [9], L-carnitine [9; 49] or oxypentifylline administration [59] should be considered. In the absence of strong indications for ACEi/ARB therapy, a trial of cessation of these drugs should also be considered. Ongoing ESA hyporesponsiveness, particularly if resistant to the aforementioned measures, should prompt a bone marrow examination to exclude pathology and bone marrow disorders (Figure 2).

Conclusion

Anaemia is a common complication of renal failure and is independently associated with increased morbidity and mortality. The use of erythropoietin stimulating agents (ESA) to treat anaemia whilst minimising blood transfusions is appropriate. While the target for haemoglobin is controversial, it is clear that the minimum dose of ESA should be used to achieve appropriate haemoglobin levels. Therapy clearly needs to be prescribed in an individualised manner.

A patient failing to achieve target haemoglobin with appropriate iron supplementation should prompt consideration, investigation and treatment of underlying comorbidities, particularly inflammation. Erythropoiesis resistance remains a significant predictor of morbidity and mortality in this population.

References

[1] Parfrey, P. S. (2013). Why does the treatment of anaemia not improve cardiac outcomes in CKD? *Nat Rev Nephrol,* Vol.9, No.1, 59-61.

[2] Parfrey, P. S., et al. (2009). Erythropoietin therapy and left ventricular mass index in CKD and ESRD patients: a meta-analysis. *Clin J Am Soc Nephrol,* Vol.4, No.4, 755-762.

[3] Chung, S., et al. (2012). Relationship between erythropoietin resistance index and left ventricular mass and function and cardiovascular events in patients on chronic hemodialysis. *Hemodial Int,* Vol.16, No.2, 181-187.

[4] Ribeiro, S., et al. (2013), 'rhEPO for the Treatment of Erythropoietin Resistant Anemia in Hemodialysis Patients–Risks and Benefits', in H. Suzuki (ed.), *Hemodialysis* (Rijeka, Croatia: InTech), 291-314..

[5] Valderrabano, F. (1996). Erythropoietin in chronic renal failure. *Kidney Int,* Vol.50, No.4, 1373-1391.

[6] Foley, R. N., et al. (1996). The impact of anemia on cardiomyopathy, morbidity, and and mortality in end-stage renal disease. *Am J Kidney Dis,* Vol.28, No.1, 53-61.

[7] Astor, B. C., et al. (2002). Association of kidney function with anemia: the Third National Health and Nutrition Examination Survey (1988-1994). *Arch Intern Med,* Vol.162, No.12, 1401-1408.

[8] McMahon, L. P. & Macginley, R. (2012). KHA-CARI guideline: Biochemical and haematological targets: Haemoglobin concentrations in patients using erythropoietin-stimulating agents. *Nephrology (Carlton),* Vol.17, No.1, 17-19.

[9] Priyadarshi, A. & Shapiro, J. I. (2006). Erythropoietin resistance in the treatment of the anemia of chronic renal failure. *Semin Dial,* Vol.19, No.4, 273-278.

[10] Spivak, J. L. (1986). The mechanism of action of erythropoietin. *Int J Cell Cloning,* Vol.4, No.3, 139-166.

[11] Badve, S. V., et al. (2013). Interventions for erythropoietin-resistant anaemia in dialysis patients. *Cochrane Database Syst Rev,* Vol.8, CD006861.

[12] Badve, S. V., et al. (2011). Is the problem with the vehicle or the destination? Does high-dose ESA or high haemoglobin contribute to poor outcomes in CKD? *Nephrology (Carlton),* Vol.16, No.2, 144-153.

[13] Palmer, S. C., et al. (2010). Meta-analysis: erythropoiesis-stimulating agents in patients with chronic kidney disease. *Ann Intern Med,* Vol.153, No.1, 23-33.

[14] Anonymous (2012). Chapter 4: Red cell transfusion to treat anemia in CKD. *Kidney Int,* Vol.2, No.4, 311-316.

[15] Anonymous (2006). Clinical Practice Recommendations 3.5. Evaluating and Correcting Persistent Failure to Reach or Maintain Intended Hb. *Am J Kidney Dis,* Vol.47, S81-S85.

[16] Locatelli, F., et al. (2004). Revised European best practice guidelines for the management of anaemia in patients with chronic renal failure. *Nephrol Dial Transplant,* Vol.19 Suppl 2, ii1-47.

[17] Lopez-Gomez, Juan M., et al. (2008). Factors that condition the response to erythropoietin in patients on hemodialysis and their relation to mortality. *Kidney Int,* Vol.74, No.S111, S75-S81.

[18] Mitka, M. (2013). HIgh-cost drugs account for most of medicare part b spending. *JAMA,* Vol.310, No.6, 572-572.

[19] Naci, H., et al. (2012). Historical clinical and economic consequences of anemia management in patients with end-stage renal disease on dialysis using erythropoietin stimulating agents versus routine blood transfusions: a retrospective cost-effectiveness analysis. *J Med Econ,* Vol.15, No.2, 293-304.

[20] Clement, F. M., et al. (2010). An economic evaluation of erythropoiesis-stimulating agents in CKD. *Am J Kidney Dis,* Vol.56, No.6, 1050-1061.

[21] Singh, A. K., et al. (2006). Correction of anemia with epoetin alfa in chronic kidney disease. *N Engl J Med,* Vol.355, No.20, 2085-2098.

[22] Singh, A. K., et al. (2006). Correction of anemia with epoetin alfa in chronic kidney disease. *N Engl J Med,* Vol.355, No.20, 2085-2098.

[23] Szczech, L. A., et al. (2008). Secondary analysis of the CHOIR trial epoetin-alpha dose and achieved hemoglobin outcomes. *Kidney Int,* Vol.74, No.6, 791-798.

[24] Besarab, A., et al. (1998). The effects of normal as compared with low hematocrit values in patients with cardiac disease who are receiving hemodialysis and epoetin. *N Engl J Med,* Vol.339, No.9, 584-590.

[25] Pfeffer, M. A., et al. (2009). A trial of darbepoetin alfa in type 2 diabetes and chronic kidney disease. *N Engl J Med,* Vol.361, No.21, 2019-2032.

[26] Phrommintikul, A., et al. (2007). Mortality and target haemoglobin concentrations in anaemic patients with chronic kidney disease treated with erythropoietin: a meta-analysis. *Lancet,* Vol.369, No.9559, 381-388.

[27] Kilpatrick, R. D., et al. (2008). Greater epoetin alfa responsiveness is associated with improved survival in hemodialysis patients. *Clin J Am Soc Nephrol,* Vol.3, No.4, 1077-1083.

[28] Messana, J. M., et al. (2009). Association of quarterly average achieved hematocrit with mortality in dialysis patients: a time-dependent comorbidity-adjusted model. *Am J Kidney Dis,* Vol.53, No.3, 503-512.

[29] Regidor, D. L., et al. (2006). Associations between changes in hemoglobin and administered erythropoiesis-stimulating agent and survival in hemodialysis patients. *J Am Soc Nephrol,* Vol.17, No.4, 1181-1191.

[30] Solomon, Scott D., et al. (2010). Erythropoietic Response and Outcomes in Kidney Disease and Type 2 Diabetes. *N Engl J Med,* Vol.363, No.12, 1146-1155.

[31] Campise, M., et al. (2005). Impact of pre-transplant anaemia correction and erythropoietin resistance on long-term graft survival. *Nephrol Dial Transplant,* Vol.20 Suppl 8, viii8-12.

[32] Gomez-Alamillo, C., et al. (2010). Erythropoietin resistance as surrogate marker of graft and patient survival in renal transplantation: 3-year prospective multicenter study. *Transplant Proc,* Vol.42, No.8, 2935-2937.

[33] Coyne, D. (2006). Iron indices: what do they really mean? *Kidney Int Suppl,* No.101, S4-8.

[34] Coyne, D. (2006). Challenging the boundaries of anemia management: a balanced approach to i.v. iron and EPO therapy. *Kidney Int Suppl,* No.101, S1-3.

[35] Coyne, D. W. (2010). It's time to compare anemia management strategies in hemodialysis. *Clin J Am Soc Nephrol,* Vol.5, No.4, 740-742.

[36] Malyszko, J. & Mysliwiec, M. (2007). Hepcidin in anemia and inflammation in chronic kidney disease. *Kidney Blood Press Res,* Vol.30, No.1, 15-30.

[37] Auerbach, M., et al. (2008). Intravenous iron: from anathema to standard of care. *Am J Hematol,* Vol.83, No.7, 580-588.

[38] Wong, G., et al. (2013). An economic evaluation of intravenous versus oral iron supplementation in people on haemodialysis. *Nephrol Dial Transplant,* Vol.28, No.2, 413-420.

[39] Coyne, D. W., et al. (2007). Ferric gluconate is highly efficacious in anemic hemodialysis patients with high serum ferritin and low transferrin saturation: results of the Dialysis Patients' Response to IV Iron with Elevated Ferritin (DRIVE) Study. *J Am Soc Nephrol,* Vol.18, No.3, 975-984.

[40] Kapoian, T., et al. (2008). Ferric gluconate reduces epoetin requirements in hemodialysis patients with elevated ferritin. *J Am Soc Nephrol,* Vol.19, No.2, 372-379.

[41] Ferrari, P., et al. (2011). Serum iron markers are inadequate for guiding iron repletion in chronic kidney disease. *Clin J Am Soc Nephrol,* Vol.6, No.1, 77-83.

[42] Kalantar-Zadeh, K., et al. (2003). Effect of malnutrition-inflammation complex syndrome on EPO hyporesponsiveness in maintenance hemodialysis patients. *Am J Kidney Dis,* Vol.42, No.4, 761-773.

[43] Coyne, D. W. (2011). Hepcidin: clinical utility as a diagnostic tool and therapeutic target. *Kidney Int,* Vol.80, No.3, 240-244.

[44] Ford, B. A., et al. (2010). Intra-individual variability in serum hepcidin precludes its use as a marker of iron status in hemodialysis patients. *Kidney Int,* Vol.78, No.8, 769-773.

[45] van der Weerd, N. C., et al. (2012). Hepcidin-25 in chronic hemodialysis patients is related to residual kidney function and not to treatment with erythropoiesis stimulating agents. *PLoS One,* Vol.7, No.7, e39783.

[46] Won, H. S., et al. (2012). IL-6 is an independent risk factor for resistance to erythropoiesis-stimulating agents in hemodialysis patients without iron deficiency. *Hemodial Int,* Vol.16, No.1, 31-37.

[47] Kuragano, T., et al. (2010). Determinants of hepcidin in patients on maintenance hemodialysis: role of inflammation. *Am J Nephrol,* Vol.31, No.6, 534-540.

[48] Tessitore, N., et al. (2010). Hepcidin is not useful as a biomarker for iron needs in haemodialysis patients on maintenance erythropoiesis-stimulating agents. *Nephrol Dial Transplant,* Vol.25, No.12, 3996-4002.

[49] Kanbay, M., et al. (2010). Erythropoiesis stimulatory agent- resistant anemia in dialysis patients: review of causes and management. *Blood Purif,* Vol.29, No.1, 1-12.

[50] Panichi, V., et al. (2011). Anaemia and resistance to erythropoiesis-stimulating agents as prognostic factors in haemodialysis patients: results from the RISCAVID study. *Nephrol Dial Transplant,* Vol.26, No.8, 2641-2648.

[51] Khankin, E. V., et al. (2010). Soluble erythropoietin receptor contributes to erythropoietin resistance in end-stage renal disease. *PLoS One,* Vol.5, No.2, e9246.

[52] Kaysen, G. A. (2009). Biochemistry and biomarkers of inflamed patients: why look, what to assess. *Clin J Am Soc Nephrol,* Vol.4 Suppl 1, S56-63.

[53] Battistella, M., et al. (2011). Improved parathyroid hormone control by cinacalcet is associated with reduction in darbepoetin requirement in patients with end-stage renal disease. *Clin Nephrol,* Vol.76, No.2, 99-103.

[54] Kiss, Z., et al. (2011). Serum 25(OH)-cholecalciferol concentration is associated with hemoglobin level and erythropoietin resistance in patients on maintenance hemodialysis. *Nephron Clin Pract,* Vol.117, No.4, c373-378.

[55] Movilli, E., et al. (2003). Epoetin requirement does not depend on dialysis dose when Kt/V > 1.33 in patients on regular dialysis treatment with cellulosic membranes and adequate iron stores. *J Nephrol,* Vol.16, No.4, 546-551.

[56] Locatelli, F., et al. (2012). Predictors of haemoglobin levels and resistance to erythropoiesis-stimulating agents in patients treated with low-flux haemodialysis, haemofiltration and haemodiafiltration: results of a multicentre randomized and controlled trial. *Nephrol Dial Transplant,* Vol.27, No.9, 3594-3600.

[57] Ikee, R., et al. (2012). Potential influence of sevelamer hydrochloride on responsiveness to erythropoiesis-stimulating agents in haemodialysis patients. *Nephrology (Carlton),* Vol.17, No.3, 225-229.

[58] Roger, S. (2006). Iron. *Nephrology (Carlton),* Vol.11, S217-S229.

[59] Johnson, D. W., et al. (2007). Erythropoiesis-stimulating agent hyporesponsiveness. *Nephrology (Carlton),* Vol.12, No.4, 321-330.

[60] Attallah, N., et al. (2006). Effect of intravenous ascorbic acid in hemodialysis patients with EPO-hyporesponsive anemia and hyperferritinemia. *Am J Kidney Dis,* Vol.47, No.4, 644-654.

[61] Ayli, D., et al. (2004). The effect of high-flux hemodialysis on renal anemia. *J Nephrol,* Vol.17, No.5, 701-706.

In: Advances in Drug Resistance Research
Editor: Christudas Morais
ISBN: 978-1-63117-131-4

Chapter 5

Therapeutic Options for Metastatic Castration Resistant Prostate Cancer: Has the Situation Improved?

Varinder Jeet*

Australian Prostate Cancer Research Centre - Queensland,
Institute of Health and Biomedical Innovation,
Queensland University of Technology, Princess Alexandra Hospital,
Translational Research Institute, Brisbane, Australia

Abstract

Limited treatment options for Castration Resistant Prostate Cancer (CRPC) still remain a major challenge. Despite therapeutic advances, most patients with malignant PCa have a poor prognosis. Since the year 2000, we have rapidly expanded our understanding of the molecular mechanisms underlying CRPC and this has led to an unprecedented number of new drug approvals within a short span of time. Recently, four new agents namely Abiraterone Acetate, Enzalutamide, Cabazitaxel, and Radium-223 have been shown to be effective in the post-chemotherapy setting in CRPC. The continued dependency of CRPC on androgen

* Email: varinder.jeet@qut.edu.au.

synthesis has seen the development of a number of new anti-androgen therapies, with abiraterone acetate and Enzalutamide being the most promising discoveries. Immunotherapeutic approaches have also found their niche in PCa with Sipuleucel-T shown to be effective in minimally asymptomatic CRPC. Research focussed on bone-targeting therapies has witnessed the arrival of promising new drugs with Denosumab and Radium-223 displaying improved survival of patients with CRPC. This review briefly discusses the findings and limitations from ongoing and completed clinical trials of novel treatments and regimens. In addition, potential mechanisms of therapy resistance and future challenges are discussed.

Keywords: Prostate cancer, metastatic Castration Resistance Prostate Cancer, therapy resistance, Abiraterone acetate, Enzalutamide, Androgen Receptor

Introduction

Prostate Cancer (PCa) is the most common visceral cancer and the second leading cause of cancer-related death in American men with a total of 238,590 new cases and 29,720 deaths annually [1]. Whilst early stage PCa can be cured with surgery or radiation therapy, the metastatic PCa still remains incurable. For locally advanced and metastatic disease, androgen deprivation therapy (ADT) is the preferred method of treatment. Though effective initially in most patients, the tumours ultimately progress to a stage of Castration Resistant Prostate Cancer (CRPC), which refers to the clinical state at which PCa continues to progress despite castrate levels of testosterone and ADT. In most cases, it takes about 12-24 months for therapy resistance to develop [2].

The growing body of molecular and clinical knowledge gathered in the last two decades provided new insights into the mechanism of therapy resistance in PCa and led to the development of many new agents. The most prominent finding of these studies was that the Androgen Receptor (AR) remains the main driver of tumour growth, spread, and sustenance and therefore the primary therapeutic target. During progression to CRPC, PCa cells may employ different mechanisms to compensate for low androgen level such as amplification or mutation of AR, overexpression of AR coregulators, intracrine production of androgens by PCa cells, generation of AR splice variants, and deregulation of growth factors or cytokines, amongst others [3-7]. The advancement in understanding these molecular mechanisms of therapy resistance paved the way for the screening of novel anti-tumour drugs [8, 9].

The purpose of this chapter is to describe these recent advances including their impact on the quality of life in addition to the ongoing research efforts exploring new agents and future challenges facing medical research in this area.

New Therapies Targeting AR Pathway

Traditionally, ADT is continued in patients with CRPC and is often combined with anti-androgens such as bicalutamide or flutamide as part of the secondary hormonal blockade [10-12]. However, these anti-androgens have a low affinity for the AR and lose their anti-AR ability over time or even become AR agonists in CRPC tumours [13, 14]. Given that AR signalling remains active, the failure of combined androgen blockade suggests that significant levels of androgens are left behind that may be responsible for AR stimulation during progression of CRPC. The knowledge that PCa cells retain the biochemical machinery to synthesize their own androgens and also that several steroid enzymes synthesize androgens from cholesterol led to the discovery of next generation therapeutic agents that target steroidogenesis and more efficient AR inhibition.

Abiraterone Acetate

Abiraterone acetate (AA) is a highly selective irreversible inhibitor of Cytochrome 450 (CYP) 17, which is a key enzyme for the biosynthesis of androgens, estrogens, and glucocorticoids in the adrenal gland [15]. CYP17 inhibition decreases the circulating androgen levels and also reduces androgens within the tumours of CRPC patients [16]. In metastatic CRPC (mCRPC) patients who had progressed after docetaxel treatment, the phase III randomised control trial of AA plus prednisone resulted in an overall median survival benefit of 4.6 months as compared to prednisone plus placebo [17]. Similarly, other studies have also documented a prolonged overall survival (OS) of 14.8 months in the AA arm compared to 10.9 months in mCRPC patients receiving prednisone alone [18]. Furthermore, improvements in the PSA response rates of 29.1% vs. 5.5% and the progression free survival of 5.6 vs. 3.6 months was reported in the AA plus prednisone vs. prednisone alone groups [18]. AA was well tolerated with only mild adverse events. In light of such findings, AA (Zytiga) was approved for the treatment of patients with mCRPC who have received prior docetaxel chemotherapy in 2011. A subsequent study evaluated the effect of AA in CRPC patients who were not treated with chemotherapy before. In these patients, AA in combination with prednisone significantly improved the progression free survival by 8.2 months compared to prednisone alone group [19]. Moreover, delay in cancer-related pain and subsequent chemotherapy besides improved OS was reported in the same study [19]. Based on these results, AA with prednisone has been approved for treating chemotherapy naïve mCRPC in 2013.

Enzalutamide

Enzalutamide (MDV3100) is a potent multilevel second generation AR antagonist that inhibits AR signalling by preventing nuclear translocation and DNA binding, thereby inactivating the AR mediated gene regulation [20]. Enzalutamide offers better AR binding affinity than bicalutamide and in contrast to other anti-androgens has no agonistic activity. Preclinical data show that Enzalutamide induces shrinkage of LNCaP tumour xenografts while other conventional AR antagonists only retard tumour growth [20]. Results from the phase-I and phase-II study showed that Enzalutamide treatment led to substantial anti-tumour activity and also significant PSA decrease in CRPC patients with and without previous chemotherapy [21, 22]. These promising results facilitated the onset of two large phase III trials namely, AFFIRM and PREVAIL. While the PREVAIL trial is still ongoing, results from AFFIRM showed that MDV3100 not only slowed disease progression but also prolonged overall survival and improved the quality of life in mCRPC patients post-docetaxel [23]. Enzalutamide was generally well tolerated with only mild adverse events. As a result, Enzalutamide was approved by the FDA for use in clinic.

Other AR Inhibitors

Apart from AA and Enzalutamide, several promising anti-AR agents are in the pipeline with some of them have entered phase II clinical trials. Of these, three are discussed here briefly.

ARN-509 is a competitive AR inhibitor with a mechanism similar to Enzalutamide. ARN-509 was shown to inhibit tumour growth in a preclinical xenograft model [24]. Phase-I and phase-II trials investigating the efficacy of ARN-509 in three distinct patient populations comprising of high-risk non metastatic CRPC, metastatic treatment naïve CRPC, and progressive disease after Abiraterone Acetate are ongoing.

ODM-201 is another AR antagonist which targets AR nuclear translocation without exerting any agonistic activity. Preliminary results from early stage trials indicate a PSA decline of 50% in 87% of the patients at 12 weeks of treatment. The trials are in progress.

EZN-4176 is a nucleic-acid based antisense oligonucleotide targeting AR mRNA. It was shown to inhibit the growth of both androgen-sensitive and CRPC tumours *in vitro* and *in vivo* [25]. This agent is currently being assessed in a phase I clinical trial.

Immune-Based Therapies

Immune system is body's natural defence mechanism and protects us from multiple ailments. However, in lethal conditions such as cancer this barrier is largely compromised leading to the unchecked expansion of tumour cells. The concept of training immune system to curb cancer induced tolerance was utilised in a number of cancers but PCa was generally ignored due to the common belief that PCa is not immunogenic enough for the success of such approaches. However, recent evidence suggests that PCa has immunogenic potential [26, 27], which spurred the development of immunological anticancer strategies in PCa.

Sipuleucel-T

Sipuleucel-T is a therapeutic cancer vaccine consisting of patients autologous antigen-presenting cells stimulated *ex-vivo* by a recombinant fusion protein called PA2024, which consists of prostatic acid phosphatase (PAP) linked to macrophage colony-stimulating factor (GM-CSF) [28]. Upon stimulation *ex vivo*, the vaccine is intravenously injected into the patient to induce an immune response to PAP expressing PCa cells. The efficacy of Sipuleucel-T was evaluated in a multicentre IMPACT trial. Although this trial did not show significant changes in the PSA response rates and progression free survival (PFS), the overall survival advantage of 4.1 months was reported in addition to 22% relative reduction in the risk of death in the Sipuleucel-T arm as compared with the placebo arm [29]. Influenced by this trial, the FDA approved the use of Sipuleucel-T in asymptomatic or minimally symptomatic CRPC. However, owing to the high therapy costs and limited availability this therapy has not enjoyed widespread reception outside the United States.

Prostvac-VF

Prostvac-VF is a PSA targeting recombinant vaccine that has shown encouraging results in the phase II clinical trials [30, 31]. In a double blinded phase II study involving 125 patients with minimally symptomatic CRPC, Prostvac resulted in a 44% reduction in the mortality rate and also induced an 8.5 month improvement in the overall survival [31]. However, PFS, the primary end point, was unchanged between the control and the treated group. A phase III study is currently ongoing.

Bone-Targeting Agents

Spread of prostate tumours to bone represents the most common type of metastases in PCa. Bone environment serves as the ideal soil for tumours to survive and thrive and therefore considered a key therapeutic target in advanced stage PCa.

Bisphosphonates

Bisphosphonates are a class of drugs that are used to treat osteoporosis and cancer. Bisphosphonates are structurally similar to pyrophosphates, a normal component of bone matrix. Due to this structural similarity, bisphosphonates stably integrate into the bone matrix resulting in the inhibition of osteoclast mediated bone resorption. Studies have shown that bisphosphonates may significantly reduce bone loss in men with non-metastatic PCa [32-34]. Zoledronic acid is the only bisphosphonate which has been approved to treat patients with mCRPC after the success of randomised controlled trials showing favourable outcomes [35, 36]. It produces some adverse events which are easily manageable with medical supervision.

Denosumab

Denosumab is a fully humanised monoclonal antibody that specifically inhibits osteoclast activity by binding to osteoblast-secreted receptor activator of nuclear factor KB ligand (RANK-L), leading to inhibition of bone loss [37]. In a large phase III multicentre study, Denosumab was shown to be superior to Zoledronic acid in terms of the median time to bone metastasis, however, no difference in the overall survival or progression free survival was seen between the two groups [38]. In 2013, Denosumab was approved for the treatment of skeletal related events that are unresectable or where surgical resection is likely to cause severe morbidity.

Radiopharmaceuticals

Radiopharmaceuticals are bone-seeking agents that preferentially deliver radiation to the areas of high bone turnover. Radiopharmaceuticals such as strontium-89 and samarium-153 are recommended for patients with multifocal painful bone metastases [39]. Radium-223 chloride (Alpharadin) belongs to a new class of alpha particle emitting agents that has entered the ongoing phase III trial, ALSYMPCA. Treatment of CRPC patients with bony metastases in this trial resulted in a marked improvement in median overall survival of 3.6 months when compared with placebo. Additionally, significant improvement in time to first skeletal-related event has been reported [40].

Cytotoxic Chemotherapy

In 2004, docetaxel (a taxane that induces polymerization of microtubules and phosphorylation of bcl-2) was approved for use in CRPC patients based largely on the findings of two crucial trials, TAX327 and SWOG 9916 [41, 42]. These trials reported a 2.5 months survival advantage in the docetaxel arm when compared with the mitoxantrone and prednisone treatment groups. In addition, improved quality of life and pain reduction was reported. However, no life-extending second-line treatment options were available once the docetaxel resistance sets upon. FDA has recently approved a new chemotherapeutic agent called Cabazitaxel and new chemotherapies are in advanced clinical development.

Cabazitaxel

Cabazitaxel is a novel taxane that showed anti-tumour activity in docetaxel-resistant cell lines [43] and exerts its cytotoxic activity through mitotic arrest at the metaphase-anaphase transition, thereby causing cell death. However, unlike other taxanes it has a low propensity for multidrug resistance (MDR) proteins such as P-glycoprotein, which makes Cabazitaxel more efficacious in taxane-resistant tumour cells [44]. In the phase III trial TROPIC, cabazitaxel displayed an overall survival benefit of 1.4 months as compared to mitoxantrone in patients previously treated with docetaxel [43, 45]. However, cabazitaxel poses serious side effects which are manageable to some extent but the overall safety profile and its comparative effect on quality of life is still under investigation in multiple clinical studies.

Anti-Angiogenesis Agents

Angiogenesis plays a fundamental role in promoting tumour growth and thereby anti-angiogenesis therapy has been seen as a promising approach for treating patients with CRPC disease. Tumours devise an "angiogenic switch" by perturbing the natural balance of angiogenic inducers and inhibitors in their favour. This angiogenic switch is governed by proangiogenic factors, such as vascular endothelial growth factor-A (VEGF-A) and angiogenin (ANG), allowing the development of malignant tumour phenotype. Multiple therapeutic approaches are under investigation to target steps in the angiogenic cascade, with VEGF inhibitors at the forefront. A number of anti-VEGF therapies have recently been developed e.g. bevacizumab, avastin, sunitib, sorafenib, and SU11248.

Bevacizumab is a monoclonal antibody that specifically targets VEGF signalling through binding and neutralising VEGF-A. Bevacizumab was shown to be effective in metastatic colorectal cancer and breast cancer setting and was approved for these cancer entities. However, addition of bevacizumab to standard docetaxel and prednisone therapy in patients with mCRPC did not improve overall survival and was associated with increased toxicity [46].

Sorafenib is an orally administered multi-tyrosine kinase inhibitor and has inhibitory action against Raf kinase, PDGFR, VEGFR-1, 2 and 3, and c-kit pathways. Currently, sorafenib is approved for the treatment of advanced renal cell carcinoma and hepatocellular carcinoma. Phase II studies in CRPC observed a low rate of PSA responses and a median progression-free survival of 2 to 4 months [47]. Another phase II study investigating the combination of sorafenib with anti-androgen bicalutamide reported a positive PSA response and delay in the onset of treatment failure [48]. Currently, evaluation of sorafenib as a single agent therapy is underway in a phase III study of docetaxel-resistant PCa patients.

Apart from the above mentioned angiogenic targets, testing of many new drugs is currently underway. These include compounds like Sunitinib, Endoglin/CD105, Cedaranib, Aflibercept (VEGF Trap), and many more. These compounds are either being tested alone or in combination with other therapies. They are discussed elsewhere in detail [49].

Targeting Growth Factor Receptor Pathways

Since growth factors supply the cells with necessary armamentarium to grow and proliferate, targeting these pathways has garnered particular interest. Growth factors bind to a wide diversity of receptors on the cell surface, which in-turn trigger the intracellular signalling cascades.

In PCa, abnormalities in epidermal, fibroblast, PDGF, and IGF growth factor families have been reported and agents targeting these signalling cascades have been developed. Epidermal growth factor targeting agent, *Gefitinib*, was trialled in CRPC patients as a monotherapy however with limited success as PSA declines and other clinical parameters were not affected [50]. Similarly, combination of Gefitinib with docetaxel did not yield tangible results either.

Insulin like Growth Factor-1 Receptor (IGF1-R)

Composed of 2 peptide growth factors (IGF-I and -II), 2 transmembrane receptors (IGF-IR and -IIR), and 6 IGF binding proteins (IGFBP-1 to -6), insulin growth factor receptor axis has been investigated in a number of different cancers including PCa. A humanised monoclonal anti-IGF1-R antibody, Figitumumab (CP-751,871), when administered in combination with docetaxel showed radiographic responses and stable disease in CRPC patients [51]. Further studies investigating Figitumumab in different clinical settings are underway.

Phosphatidylinositol-3-Kinase (PI3k)-Akt Signalling Pathway

Situated downstream of the growth factor receptors, PI3K signalling pathway is one of the very well-studied kinase pathways. Upon activation by receptor tyrosine kinases, PI3K/AKT interact with other signalling molecules to regulate multiple cellular functions entailing growth, proliferation, apoptosis, and glucose metabolism amongst other functions. PI3K/AKT axis is frequently deregulated in a broad spectrum of cancers including PCa, thus becoming an important target for anti-cancer therapy. Pan-PI3K inhibitors, GDC-0941 and BKM120, have shown anti-proliferative and anti-tumour effects in preclinical studies [52, 53] and the phase I study of BKM120 showed a partial response with 52% of patients presenting a stable disease for 6 weeks [54].

Clinical trials investigating PI3K/Akt/mTOR pathway inhibitors as single agents and in combination are ongoing in CRPC and are detailed elsewhere [55, 56].

Mechanisms of Resistance and Future Challenges

Over the past decade, a plethora of treatment options have been made available for men with metastatic prostate cancer. Due to the advent of drugs like Abiraterone Acetate and Enzalutamide, those patients who show weak responses to therapies beyond castration can now receive better care. However, as is the case with any new therapy, drug resistance inevitably occurs. Clearly, a better understanding of the biologic underpinnings of these resistance mechanisms has been the focus of ongoing research.

Overcoming Resistance

Mechanisms of resistance to AA are poorly understood at present. However, many putative mechanisms have been proposed including the upregulation of intratumoral CYP17A expression as a result of the selective treatment pressure [57]. This may induce steroidogenesis and upregulation of AR splice variants that confer ligand-independent AR transactivation [58]. Recently, the authors of a follow-up study proposed that resistance to AA could potentially be overcome by dose escalation or simply by administration with food to increase drug exposure [59]. Additionally, an in vitro study in PCa cell lines demonstrated that higher dose or longer exposure of abiraterone could reverse resistance secondary to activation of AR by residual ligands [60]. This study also concluded that combination of AA with AR antagonists such as Enzalutamide may yield better results.

Studies into the mechanisms of resistance to Enzalutamide are also obscure. Resistance to conventional anti-androgens indicate that AR mutations alongside AR splice variants and aberrations in PTEN/PI3K pathways may be responsible for PCa progression to castration resistance. Indeed, a clinically relevant AR mutation, AR F876L, was shown to mediate the resistance to second generation anti-androgens, Enzalutamide and ARN-509 [61]. AR splice variants were also found to be key mediators of persistent AR signalling and resistance to Enzalutamide [62]. Associative evidence was also provided by the studies showing that CRPC cell line, CWR-R1, displays upregulation of AR variant 7 (AR-V7), which may be responsible for resistance to enzalutamide [62-65]. In addition, a very recent study demonstrated that AR gene rearrangements are a unique resistance mechanism by which AR transcriptional program contributes to CRPC growth phenotype independent of full-length AR or androgens [66]. The authors reported that the full length AR and the splice variant, ARv567es, remain constitutively active in CRPC and potentiate a true androgen independent phenotype via switching AR expression from full-length AR to ARv567es [66]. The authors of this study further proposed that AR splice variant mediated therapies must be developed to overcome the resistance to anti-AR therapies and also that AR gene rearrangements may be utilized as biomarkers of resistance to endocrine-targeting therapies for PCa.

In light of these observations, it can be concluded that there is an urgent need to dissect the underlying mechanisms of resistance to the second generation anti-AR drugs like enzalutamide.

Adaptive and Selective Models of Castration Resistant Prostate Cancer

The ability of PCa cells to grow in the absence of androgens is critical in the progression of PCa to CRPC. The adaptation model states that androgen dependent cells undergo a series of genetic or epigenetic events to adapt to androgen-depleted environment, which ultimately leads to therapy resistance and therefore cancer relapse. In contrast, the selection model proposes that PCa contains a spectrum of cells with varying androgen sensitivities even before the androgen therapy is started [67] and the clonal selection under androgen deprivation may be responsible for the development of CRPC. The adaptive and selective models provide crucial mechanistic insights into the onset of CRPC and are not mutually exclusive. These models have been the basis of many new therapeutic approaches and are also suggestive of the fact that PCa is a highly heterogenous disease and therefore strategies other than the development of potent anti-androgens are also of crucial importance. Further studies focussing on understanding the molecular basis and underlying mechanisms of CRPC will significantly aid in the management of the resistant phase of this lethal disease.

Defining the Correct Sequence of Drugs

The expanded arsenal of drugs now available for the treatment of CRPC poses challenging questions about the correct sequence of administration of such therapies. Although the approval of AA and Enzalutamide has brought great hope for patients in the pre- and post-chemotherapy setting, the order of preference of these two drugs is currently ambiguous. Several trials are ongoing to validate the safety of these agents in combination with other existing therapies and their introduction into the earlier stages of disease is also being investigated.

Conclusion

In the last few years, the treatment options for men suffering from CRPC have increased markedly leading to improved quality of life and prolongation of life span. In comparison to the previous decade, androgen targeted therapies such as Abiraterone and Enzalutamide have made a huge contribution in extending the overall survival of mCRPC patients and their impact on the quality of life improvements is also obvious. Sipuleucel-T has come forward as an exciting choice for patients with asymptomatic to minimally symptomatic bone or lymph node metastasis. Novel bone-targeting agents such as Zoledronic acid and Denosumab have shown efficacy in reducing osseous metastasis and associated stress-related bone fractures. In fact, Denosumab was the first agent to significantly delay the onset of bone metastasis in patients with non-metastatic CRPC. A new wave of treatments based on radionuclides has also contributed significantly in alleviating skeleton related events in mCRPC. Ever since its introduction into the clinic in 2004, Docetaxel has been the gold-standard first-line chemotherapeutic option for the treatment of mCRPC and now with the availability of cabazitaxel as a second-line treatment regimen the situation has improved further. Whilst the new range of approved therapies has shown objective clinical benefit, there are a number of new drugs which are either in clinical trials or have shown promising results in the preclinical models. The rate at which these new therapies are successfully extrapolated into the clinic remains to be seen however. Overall, the advancement in the development of novel therapies for various stages of PCa has certainly changed the treatment landscape (Figure 1). However, it has also opened up new questions for clinicians to pick the most relevant drug for the right patient at the right time. It is becoming increasingly evident that personalised approaches for making such complex decisions are the need of the hour. There is also an unmet need for appropriate biomarkers to define the patient populations which will benefit the most from a particular type of therapy. Nonetheless, with all these new drugs and better disease management, there is renewed optimism for patients suffering from the advanced stages of PCa.

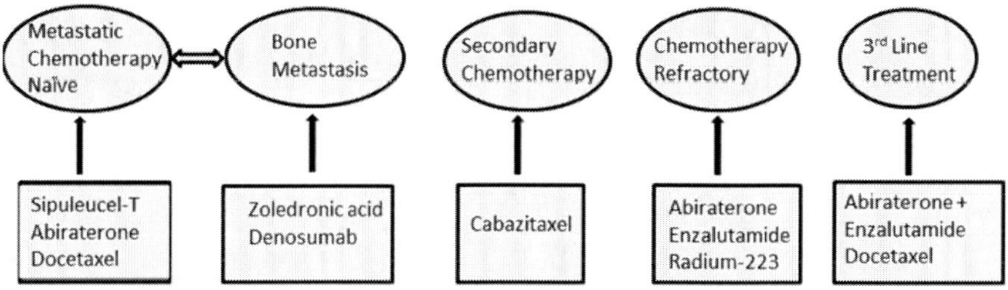

Figure 1. The current treatment landscape of Castration Resistant Prostate Cancer.

References

[1] Siegel, R., D. Naishadham, and A. Jemal, Cancer statistics, 2013. *CA Cancer J Clin*, 2013. 63(1): p. 11-30.

[2] Pagliarulo, V., et al., Contemporary role of androgen deprivation therapy for prostate cancer. *Eur Urol*, 2012. 61(1): p. 11-25.

[3] Steinkamp, M.P., et al., Treatment-dependent androgen receptor mutations in prostate cancer exploit multiple mechanisms to evade therapy. *Cancer Res*, 2009. 69(10): p. 4434-42.

[4] Chen, G., et al., Androgen receptor mutants detected in recurrent prostate cancer exhibit diverse functional characteristics. *Prostate*, 2005. 63(4): p. 395-406.

[5] Buchanan, G., et al., Contribution of the androgen receptor to prostate cancer predisposition and progression. *Cancer Metastasis Rev*, 2001. 20(3-4): p. 207-23.

[6] Locke, J.A., et al., Androgen levels increase by intratumoral de novo steroidogenesis during progression of castration-resistant prostate cancer. *Cancer Res*, 2008. 68(15): p. 6407-15.

[7] Mostaghel, E.A., B. Montgomery, and P.S. Nelson, Castration-resistant prostate cancer: targeting androgen metabolic pathways in recurrent disease. *Urol Oncol*, 2009. 27(3): p. 251-7.

[8] Attard, G. and J.S. de Bono, Translating scientific advancement into clinical benefit for castration-resistant prostate cancer patients. *Clin Cancer Res*, 2011. 17(12): p. 3867-75.

[9] Attard, G., J. Richards, and J.S. de Bono, New strategies in metastatic prostate cancer: targeting the androgen receptor signaling pathway. *Clin Cancer Res*, 2011. 17(7): p. 1649-57.

[10] Culig, Z., G. Bartsch, and A. Hobisch, Antiandrogens in prostate cancer endocrine therapy. *Curr Cancer Drug Targets*, 2004. 4(5): p. 455-61.

[11] Moul, J.W. and G. Chodak, Combination hormonal therapy: a reassessment within advanced prostate cancer. *Prostate Cancer Prostatic Dis*, 2004. 7 Suppl 1: p. S2-7.

[12] Levinson, A., E.A. Nagler, and F.C. Lowe, Approach to management of clinically localized prostate cancer in patients with human immunodeficiency virus. *Urology*, 2005. 65(1): p. 91-4.

[13] Bohl, C.E., et al., Structural basis for antagonism and resistance of bicalutamide in prostate cancer. *Proc Natl Acad Sci U S A*, 2005. 102(17): p. 6201-6.

[14] Lau, Y.K., et al., A dramatic, objective antiandrogen withdrawal response: case report and review of the literature. *J Hematol Oncol*, 2008. 1: p. 21.

[15] Potter, G.A., et al., Novel steroidal inhibitors of human cytochrome P45017 alpha (17 alpha-hydroxylase-C17,20-lyase): potential agents for the treatment of prostatic cancer. *J Med Chem*, 1995. 38(13): p. 2463-71.

[16] Reid, A.H.M., et al., CYP17 inhibition as a hormonal strategy for prostate cancer. *Nature Clinical Practice Urology*, 2008. 5(11): p. 610-620.

[17] Fizazi, K., et al., Abiraterone acetate for treatment of metastatic castration-resistant prostate cancer: final overall survival analysis of the COU-AA-301 randomised, double-blind, placebo-controlled phase 3 study (vol 13, pg 983, 2012). *Lancet Oncology*, 2012. 13(11): p. E464-E464.

[18] De Bono, J.S., et al., Abiraterone and Increased Survival in Metastatic Prostate Cancer. *New England Journal of Medicine,* 2011. 364(21): p. 1995-2005.

[19] Ryan, C.J., et al., Abiraterone in Metastatic Prostate Cancer without Previous Chemotherapy. *New England Journal of Medicine*, 2013. 368(2): p. 138-148.

[20] Tran, C., et al., Development of a second-generation antiandrogen for treatment of advanced prostate cancer. *Science*, 2009. 324(5928): p. 787-90.

[21] Mukherji, D., C.J. Pezaro, and J.S. De-Bono, MDV3100 for the treatment of prostate cancer. *Expert Opin Investig Drugs*, 2012. 21(2): p. 227-33.

[22] Scher, H.I., et al., Antitumour activity of MDV3100 in castration-resistant prostate cancer: a phase 1-2 study. *Lancet,* 2010. 375(9724): p. 1437-46.

[23] Scher, H.I., et al., Increased survival with enzalutamide in prostate cancer after chemotherapy. *N Engl J Med*, 2012. 367(13): p. 1187-97.

[24] Clegg, N.J., et al., ARN-509: a novel antiandrogen for prostate cancer treatment. *Cancer Res*, 2012. 72(6): p. 1494-503.

[25] Zhang, Y.X., et al., Reduced Expression of the Androgen Receptor by Third Generation of Antisense Shows Antitumor Activity in Models of Prostate Cancer. *Molecular Cancer Therapeutics*, 2011. 10(12): p. 2309-2319.

[26] Fong, L. and E.J. Small, Immunotherapy for prostate cancer. *Curr Urol Rep*, 2006. 7(3): p. 239-46.

[27] Cha, E. and L. Fong, Immunotherapy for prostate cancer: biology and therapeutic approaches. *J Clin Oncol*, 2011. 29(27): p. 3677-85.

[28] Small, E.J., et al., Immunotherapy of hormone-refractory prostate cancer with antigen-loaded dendritic cells. *J Clin Oncol*, 2000. 18(23): p. 3894-903.

[29] Kantoff, P.W., et al., Sipuleucel-T Immunotherapy for Castration-Resistant Prostate Cancer. *New England Journal of Medicine*, 2010. 363(5): p. 411-422.

[30] Kaufman, H.L., et al., Phase II randomized study of vaccine treatment of advanced prostate cancer (E7897): A trial of the Eastern Cooperative Oncology group. *Journal of Clinical Oncology*, 2004. 22(11): p. 2122-2132.

[31] Kantoff, P.W., et al., Overall Survival Analysis of a Phase II Randomized Controlled Trial of a Poxviral-Based PSA-Targeted Immunotherapy in Metastatic Castration-Resistant Prostate Cancer. *Journal of Clinical Oncology*, 2010. 28(7): p. 1099-1105.

[32] Smith, M.R., et al., Randomized controlled trial of zoledronic acid to prevent bone loss in men receiving androgen deprivation therapy for nonmetastatic prostate cancer. *J Urol*, 2003. 169(6): p. 2008-12.

[33] Smith, M.R., et al., Pamidronate to prevent bone loss during androgen-deprivation therapy for prostate cancer. *N Engl J Med*, 2001. 345(13): p. 948-55.

[34] Michaelson, M.D., et al., Randomized controlled trial of annual zoledronic acid to prevent gonadotropin-releasing hormone agonist-induced bone loss in men with prostate cancer. *J Clin Oncol*, 2007. 25(9): p. 1038-42.

[35] Saad, F., et al., A randomized, placebo-controlled trial of zoledronic acid in patients with hormone-refractory metastatic prostate carcinoma. *J Natl Cancer Inst*, 2002. 94(19): p. 1458-68.

[36] Saad, F., et al., Long-term efficacy of zoledronic acid for the prevention of skeletal complications in patients with metastatic hormone-refractory prostate cancer. *J Natl Cancer Inst*, 2004. 96(11): p. 879-82.

[37] Boyle, W.J., W.S. Simonet, and D.L. Lacey, Osteoclast differentiation and activation. *Nature,* 2003. 423(6937): p. 337-42.

[38] Fizazi, K., et al., Denosumab versus zoledronic acid for treatment of bone metastases in men with castration-resistant prostate cancer: a randomised, double-blind study. *Lancet*, 2011. 377(9768): p. 813-22.

[39] Paes, F.M. and A.N. Serafini, Systemic metabolic radiopharmaceutical therapy in the treatment of metastatic bone pain. *Semin Nucl Med*, 2010. 40(2): p. 89-104.

[40] Sartor, A.O.e.a., Radium-223 chloride impact on skeletal-related events in patients with castration-resistant prostate cancer (CRPC) with bone metastases: A phase III randomized trial (ALSYMPCA). *J. Clin. Oncol.*, 2012. 30 (Suppl. 5), a4551.

[41] Petrylak, D.P., et al., Docetaxel and estramustine compared with mitoxantrone and prednisone for advanced refractory prostate cancer. *N Engl J Med*, 2004. 351(15): p. 1513-20.

[42] Tannock, I.F., et al., Docetaxel plus prednisone or mitoxantrone plus prednisone for advanced prostate cancer. *N Engl J Med*, 2004. 351(15): p. 1502-12.

[43] de Bono, J.S., et al., Prednisone plus cabazitaxel or mitoxantrone for metastatic castration-resistant prostate cancer progressing after docetaxel treatment: a randomised open-label trial. *Lancet*, 2010. 376(9747): p. 1147-54.

[44] Paller, C.J. and E.S. Antonarakis, Cabazitaxel: a novel second-line treatment for metastatic castration-resistant prostate cancer. *Drug Des Devel Ther*, 2011. 5: p. 117-24.

[45] Oudard, S., TROPIC: Phase III trial of cabazitaxel for the treatment of metastatic castration-resistant prostate cancer. *Future Oncol*, 2011. 7(4): p. 497-506.

[46] Kelly, W.K., et al., Randomized, double-blind, placebo-controlled phase III trial comparing docetaxel and prednisone with or without bevacizumab in men with metastatic castration-resistant prostate cancer: CALGB 90401. *J Clin Oncol*, 2012. 30(13): p. 1534-40.

[47] Aragon-Ching, J.B., et al., Final analysis of a phase II trial using sorafenib for metastatic castration-resistant prostate cancer. *BJU International*, 2009. 103(12): p. 1636-1640.

[48] Beardsley, E.K., et al., A phase II study of sorafenib in combination with bicalutamide in patients with chemotherapy-naive castration resistant prostate cancer. *Investigational New Drugs*, 2012. 30(4): p. 1652-1659.

[49] Mukherji, D., et al., Angiogenesis and anti-angiogenic therapy in prostate cancer. *Critical Reviews in Oncology Hematology*, 2013. 87(2): p. 122-131.

[50] Pezaro, C., et al., An Open-Label, Single-Arm Phase Two Trial of Gefitinib in Patients With Advanced or Metastatic Castration-Resistant Prostate Cancer. *American Journal of Clinical Oncology-Cancer Clinical Trials*, 2009. 32(4): p. 338-341.

[51] Kurzrock, R., et al., Activity of XL184 (Cabozantinib), an Oral Tyrosine Kinase Inhibitor, in Patients With Medullary Thyroid *Cancer. Journal of Clinical Oncology,* 2011. 29(19): p. 2660-2666.

[52] Raynaud, F.I., et al., Biological properties of potent inhibitors of class I phosphatidylinositide 3-kinases: from PI-103 through PI-540, PI-620 to the oral agent GDC-0941. *Molecular Cancer Therapeutics*, 2009. 8(7): p. 1725-1738.

[53] Maira, S.M., et al., Identification and Characterization of NVP-BKM120, an Orally Available Pan-Class I PI3-Kinase Inhibitor. *Molecular Cancer Therapeutics*, 2012. 11(2): p. 317-328.

[54] Bendell, J.C., et al., Phase I, Dose-Escalation Study of BKM120, an Oral Pan-Class I PI3K Inhibitor, in Patients With Advanced Solid Tumors. *Journal of Clinical Oncology,* 2012. 30(3): p. 282-290.

[55] Sarker, D., et al., Targeting the PI3K/AKT Pathway for the Treatment of Prostate Cancer. *Clinical Cancer Research*, 2009. 15(15): p. 4799-4805.

[56] Morgan, T.M., T.D. Koreckij, and E. Corey, Targeted Therapy for Advanced Prostate Cancer: Inhibition of the PI3K/Akt/mTOR Pathway. *Current Cancer Drug Targets*, 2009. 9(2): p. 237-249.

[57] Cai, C.M., et al., Intratumoral De Novo Steroid Synthesis Activates Androgen Receptor in Castration-Resistant Prostate Cancer and Is Upregulated by Treatment with CYP17A1 Inhibitors. *Cancer Research*, 2011. 71(20): p. 6503-6513.

[58] Mostaghel, E.A., et al., Resistance to CYP17A1 Inhibition with Abiraterone in Castration-Resistant Prostate Cancer: Induction of Steroidogenesis and Androgen Receptor Splice Variants. *Clinical Cancer Research*, 2011. 17(18): p. 5913-5925.

[59] Li, R., et al., Abiraterone Inhibits 3 beta-Hydroxysteroid Dehydrogenase: A Rationale for Increasing Drug Exposure in Castration-Resistant Prostate Cancer. *Clinical Cancer Research*, 2012. 18(13): p. 3571-3579.

[60] Richards, J., et al., Interactions of Abiraterone, Eplerenone, and Prednisolone with Wild-type and Mutant Androgen Receptor: A Rationale for Increasing Abiraterone Exposure or Combining with MDV3100. *Cancer Research*, 2012. 72(9): p. 2176-2182.

[61] Joseph, J.D., et al., A Clinically Relevant Androgen Receptor Mutation Confers Resistance to Second-Generation Antiandrogens Enzalutamide and ARN-509. *Cancer Discov*, 2013. 3(9): p. 1020-9.

[62] Li, Y., et al., Androgen receptor splice variants mediate enzalutamide resistance in castration-resistant prostate cancer cell lines. *Cancer Res*, 2013. 73(2): p. 483-9.

[63] Guo, Z., et al., A novel androgen receptor splice variant is up-regulated during prostate cancer progression and promotes androgen depletion-resistant growth. *Cancer Res*, 2009. 69(6): p. 2305-13.

[64] Hu, R., et al., Ligand-independent androgen receptor variants derived from splicing of cryptic exons signify hormone-refractory prostate cancer. *Cancer Res*, 2009. 69(1): p. 16-22.

[65] Li, Y., et al., AR intragenic deletions linked to androgen receptor splice variant expression and activity in models of prostate cancer progression. *Oncogene*, 2012. 31(45): p. 4759-67.

[66] Nyquist, M.D., et al., TALEN-engineered AR gene rearrangements reveal endocrine uncoupling of androgen receptor in prostate cancer. *Proc Natl Acad Sci U S A*, 2013.

[67] Bostwick, D.G., et al., Independent origin of multiple foci of prostatic intraepithelial neoplasia: comparison with matched foci of prostate carcinoma. *Cancer,* 1998. 83(9): p. 1995-2002.

In: Advances in Drug Resistance Research ISBN: 978-1-63117-131-4
Editor: Christudas Morais

Chapter 6

Current Trends in Prostate Cancer Treatment and Drug Resistance

***Raja S. Vasireddy*[1,2,3,*] *and Colleen C. Nelson*[1,2,3]**

[1]Australian Prostate Cancer Research Centre - Queensland, Brisbane, Queensland, Australia

[2]Institute of Health and Biomedical Innovation (IHBI), Queensland University of Technology, Brisbane, Queensland, Australia

[3]Translational Research Institute, Brisbane, Queensland, Australia

Abstract

Prostate cancer is the second most common cancer in men with approximately 256,000 deaths reported worldwide. Active surveillance which involves careful monitoring of the tumour over time is often considered in patients with low risk and slow progressing tumours. Surgery and radiation therapy are also used to treat patients with localised tumours. However, for patients with aggressive tumours or patients who fail localised treatment androgen-deprivation therapy (ADT) is the mainstay of treatment. Despite initial tumour regression and prostate-

* E-mail: raja.vasireddy@qut.edu.au.

specific antigen (PSA) decline in about 90% of patients treated with ADT, relapse occurs in many patients after a mean of 2 to 3 years leading to the development of more aggressive castration-resistant prostate cancer (CRPC). CRPC is often metastatic, associated with poor prognosis, and patients die within 2 years. Currently available chemotherapeutics to treat metastatic tumours extend the life span of patients by only a few months. Majority of prostate cancer drugs target either androgen signalling or cell division in prostate cancer cells. Novel immunotherapeutic and natural compound approaches are currently being tested to treat prostate cancer. However, resistance to therapy continues to be one of the major hurdles for the successful treatment of CRPC. To overcome drug resistance multiple approaches have been employed. For example, prostate cancer cells depend on androgens and its cognate receptor androgen-receptor (AR) for their growth and survival. Therefore, targeting androgen synthesis and AR provides a main avenue for drug discovery research. Drugs that target tumour cell survival also offer therapeutic benefit and are used either alone or in combination therapy.

Keywords: Prostate cancer, drug resistance, androgen signaling

Introduction

Prostate cancer (PCa) is the carcinoma of the prostate gland which is a part of the male reproductive system. PCa is the leading cause of death in men in majority of developed countries. Prostate cancer predominantly occurs in older men at a frequency of 1 in 10,000 at the age below 40 and 1 in 7 above 60 years [1]. Besides aging other risk factors include ethnicity, familial history and genetic susceptibility [1].

Conventional therapies to treat primary PCa include active surveillance, surgery and radiation therapy [2, 3]. Active surveillance is often considered during early stages of disease, when the disease is localised and slow progressing.

This involves repeated PSA testing, physical examination and or repeated biopsies. Surgery and radiation treatment are typically used to treat pre-metastatic stage of the disease and are often associated with the loss of libido and impotence.

These treatments are used either alone or in combination and are decided based on factors such as disease stage, Gleason grade of the tumour, patient's age and potential benefits of the treatment. Patients who fail either localised treatment or at the risk of relapse, are treated with multiple lines of treatment regimens depending on the factors that contribute to the progression of the disease. These treatment regimens can be categorised based on their mode of action or the target and are discussed below.

Drugs That Target Androgen-Signalling

Similar to the normal prostate tissue, tumours of the prostate depend on androgens for their growthand development. Androgens signal through the androgen-receptor (AR) and AR plays an important role in PCa initiation and progression. In patients who fail surgery and radiation therapy the first line of treatment involves Androgen-Deprivation Therapy (ADT). ADT may be used either alone or in combination with surgical castration. Therefore,androgen-deprivation therapy (ADT) has been explored as a first line of systemic treatment to control the progression of disease to the more aggressive and lethal Castration-Resistant prostate cancer (CRPC). During the earlier stages of the disease most primary tumours are androgen-dependent and many patients respond favourably to ADT and tumours regress. However failure of ADT occurs in majority of the cases and progress to CRPC and 50 to 70% of the CRPC patients develop metastasis and tumours spread to bone and axial skeleton. Metastatic PCa is a fatal disease and currently there are no treatments available to treat the patients with terminal metastatic disease. Drugs that are used in ADT can be categorised into two classes:drugs that target AR activity and drugs that target androgen synthesis.

Drugs That Target AR Activity

Failure of ADT occurs due to factors such as intratumoural androgen synthesis, amplification of AR and adaptive cell survival. Despite of castrate levels of serum androgens, PCa cells manage to restore AR-signalling. This abnormal restoration of AR-signalling can be because of AR amplification, gain of function mutations in AR making it more promiscuous. AR becomes active upon its ligand binding and translocates to nucleus to initiate transcriptional regulation of its target genes. Therefore drugs have been developed that inhibit its nuclear translocation or binding to its ligand.

Bicalutamide: Bicalutamide (Casodex) is a non-steroidal anti-androgen and inhibits the AR-mediated prostate cancer cell growth [4]. It's a competitive AR antagonist and is given orally as a single 150 mg dose/day [5].

Bicalutamide is used either alone or in combination with surgical or medical castration in pre-metastatic stage of the disease. Patients with locally advanced PCa showed disease-free survival benefits compared to men who received standard care. Bicalutamide also improved the overall survival of patients when used in combination with radiation therapy [6]. Unlike surgical castration non-steroidal antiandorgens such as bicalutamide have the benefit of inhibiting AR-signalling and not affecting testosterone production. Bicalutamide acts as an AR antagonist, however it is also reported to act as an AR agonist. Although patients treated with bicalutamide show survival benefit some patients fail the therapy and progress to fatal disease [7-9].

Several mechanisms have been explained for the failure of bicalutamide therapy in CRPC patients. These include over-expression [10], gain of function mutations altering the AR protein structure and converting bicalutamide to an AR agonist [11] and up-regulation of multidrug resistance proteins [12].

Enzalutamide: Resistance to bicalutamide can be conferred by overexpression of AR, novel mutations in AR or due to multi-drug resistance proteins [7, 12, 13]. Therefore search for new AR-antagonists has continued. Enzalutamide, formerly known as MDV3100 is a new FDA approved AR antagonist that is currently under clinical development. Compared to bicalutamide, enzalutamide is more effective in prostate cancer models with androgen-receptor overexpression and with no reported agonist activity [14, 15]. Enzalutamide inhibits AR-signalling by preventing its nuclear translocation, DNA binding and recruitment of co-activators. In a large international, randomised, double-blinded, placebo-controlled phase-III clinical trial patients treated with enzalutamide at a dose of 160mg per day showed better response with respect to multiple secondary end points such as PSA decline, progression-free survival, soft-tissue response rate and quality of life. The results from this study also show that enzalutamide prolonged the survival of patients with metastatic CRPC [16].

Despite clinical trials reporting an increased overall survival in response to enzalutamidein CRPC patients, there are several views predicting the resistance to enzalutamide in a manner similar to Bicalutamide [17]. These include adaptive survival by shifting towards AR-splice variant signalling, Fas-mediated drug resistance leading to increased cell survival, and mutations in AR.But this cannot be conformed until the results from the current clinical trials are released.

Peptidomimeticdrugs: AR is a ligand dependent transcriptional factor and predominantly activated upon binding to its ligand for instance DHT or testosterone. Once bound to ligand AR-translocates to nucleus and binds to androgen-responsiveelements (ARE) present in the targetgenes. Transcriptional co-regulators play an important role in activation of AR-target genes, one such example is PELP1that serves as scaffold between AR and coactivators [18]. PELP1 is overexpressed in high-grade prostate tumours and shown to play a critical role in AR-signalling [19, 20]. PELP1 interacts with AR through its conserved LXXLL motif where L is leucine and X is any amino acid including leucine. This short consensus sequence is shown to be critical for interactions between AR and its co-regulators. Peptide molecules that mimic LXXLL motif have been tested for their efficacy in inhibiting AR-signalling. Results show that peptidomimetic D2 being effective in blocking the AR nuclear translocation and attenuating the interaction between AR and its co-regulators.

Drugs That Target Androgen Synthesis

Ketaconazole: Ketoconazole is a synthetic broad-spectrum antifungal agent. Ketaconazole was first used in 1977 to treat patients with systemic fungal infections who later developed gynaecomastia because of inhibitory effect of ketoconazole on steroidogenesis [21]. This led to the idea of using this drug as an antiandrogen in patients with advanced prostate cancer. Initial studies with ketoconazole showed a greater response rate which however showed a modest response in subsequent studies [22, 23]. Some studies have also reported the ketoconazole induced cytotoxicity including liver damage and adrenal suppression [24]. Interest in the use of ketoconazole was further subsided with the development of new therapies such as LHRS agonists and abiraterone. However, ketoconazole is still considered as a valuable second line hormonal treatment.

Abiraterone: As mentioned before majority of patients who receive first line treatment (surgical or medical castration) for advanced PCa progress to more aggressive CRPC. One potential reason for the failure of ADT can be due to intratumoural androgen synthesis using back-door pathways, for example by conversion of androstanedioldirectly to DHT [25]. Therefore, drugs that target intratumoural androgen synthesis would benefit patients with advanced CRPC.

Abiraterone acetate is an oral antiandrogen that inhibits androgen synthesis by blocking the enzymatic activity of CYP17a [26]. CYP17a is member of the cytochrome p450 family and plays a critical role in converting cholesterol into DHT [27]. In a phase III, randomised, placebo controlled trial men who failed docetaxel therapy showed overall survival benefit upon receiving aberaterone in combination with prednisone [28]. Testing the efficacy of abiraterone acetate in chemotherapy naïve CRPC patients is currently ongoing and results are awaiting from phase III clinical trials (NCT00887198).

Patients treated with abiraterone alone may develop resistance and possible mechanisms include mutations in AR or CYP17a, synthesis of androgens by CYP17 independent pathways [29]. Therefore, combination treatment of abiraterone with other antiandrogens such as enzalutamide is currently under investigation and pre-clinical studies showed the better outcome when used in combination.

Drugs That Target Cell Survival and Cell Proliferation

Adaptive upregulation of cell survival pathways is one of the mechanisms by which prostate cancer cells develop resistance to anticancer therapies such as ADT. Drugs that target tumour cell survival offer a benefit of reducing tumour burden and prolonged survival. Currently there are several chemotherapeutic drugs that are approved to treat prostate cancer patients with advanced disease.

Docetaxel: Docetaxel belongs to the class of taxanes and acts as an anti-mitotic agent. Docetaxel was first approved in 2004 for the treatment of metastatic CRPC (mCRPC) after it was shown to be effective in increasing the overall survival in patents with mCRPC [30]. Docetaxel in combination with prednisone or estramusine was approved as a first line treatment. Docetaxel acts as a microtubule stabilising agent and leads to mitotic arrest and cell death.In addition to prostate cancer, docetaxel also shown to be effective in other cancers such as breast, head and neck, lung and ovarian cancers [30]. A meta-analysis of 2244 patients from 12 randomized clinical trials showed a higher benefit of PSA decline in patients treated with docetaxel based combination therapies [31]. Although docetaxel is effective in improving the quality of life, the overall-survival for patients with mCRPC is <20 months [32].

Despite its effectiveness in targeting cancer cell survival and reducing the tumour burden, cancer cells develop resistance to docetaxel leading to the failure of therapy. Development of cellular resistance to taxanes represents a major limitation in using taxane based therapy. Resistance to docetaxel can be acquired by multiple mechanisms including expression of multidrug resistance phenotype (MDR), alterations in the structure of tubulin/microtubule system, by pass mechanisms of cell cycle and apoptosis [33, 34]. Development of resistance to docetaxel leads to failure of treatment and only a quarter of patients experience improvement in quality of life. This led to a search for the second line post-docetaxel treatment regimes in patients who fail docetaxel therapy.

Carbazitaxel: Until 2010 there were no second-line treatment options or drugs available to treat patients who fail docetaxel therapy. On June 17, 2010, the US Food and Drug Administration (FDA) approved cabazitaxel as asecond-line drugfor the treatment ofpatients with mCRPC who were previously treated with a docetaxel-containing regimen [35].

The clinical benefit and safety of carbazitaxel was first evaluated in 2008 in a large multi-centre phase-III clinical trial [36]. This phase-III trial known as TROPIC (treatment of hormonerefractorymetastatic prostate cancer previously treated with a docetaxel-containing regimen) recruited 755 men who developed mCRPC and failed first line docetaxel therapy. Results from this trial showed a benefit of increase in median overall survival by 2.4 months in patients who received carbazitaxel compared to those who received mitoxantrone [36]. In addition, carbazitaxel showed a decline in risk of all-cause mortality by 30% in patients who received carbazitaxel compared to men on mitoxantrone. At present carbazitaxel is confined to post-docetaxel space however its use as a first line treatment in comparison to docetaxel is forecasted.

Radium-223: Majority of castration-resistant prostate cancer patients die because of the spread of the disease to other parts of the body particularly to the bone [37]. Currently there are no treatments available that can effectively target metastatic tumours, particularly tumours in the bone. This can be attributed to its environment which is hard to reach for many drugs. Radium-223 dichloride is a targeted alpha emitter and emits high energy alpha particles of short range (<100μm).

Radium-223 is a bone-seeking calciummimeticand selectively binds to the areas of high bone turnover that commonly occurs in metastatic sites of the tumours [38]. Radium-223 binds to the newly formedbone stroma, especially within the microenvironment that is rich in osteoblasts or osteoclasts [39]. As Radium-223 emits high energy alpha particles it induces lethal DNAdouble-strand break damage in target cells [38]. Another advantage of Radium-223 is its less cytotoxic effect on normal tissue as it emits short range alpha particles that target tumour cells. This was shown to be true in phase-I and phase-II clinical trials in men with bone metastasis. Radium-223 was shown to reduce pain and improve the prognosis of the patients with mCRPC [40]. This was followed by a large (921 patients), prospective, randomised, double-blinded, placebo-controlled, phase-III clinical trial, Alpharadinin Symptomatic Prostate Cancer Patients (ALSYMPCA) and radium-223 was shown to extend the median survival by 3.6 months and reduce the risk of death by 30% in men with mCRPC [41]. Because of its distinct non-overlapping mechanism of action and safety profile radium-223 is currently being investigated in phase-I and II clinical trials as a combination drug with taxanes (ClinicalTrials.gov number, NCT01106352).

Drugs That Target Metabolic Activity

Metformin: ADT is the main mode of treatment in majority of prostate cancer patients with advanced disease. Although ADT leads to tumour regression in majority of PCa patients, the main side effect of ADT is the development of metabolic syndrome characterised by insulin resistance, obesity, gynecomastia, osteoporosis and loss of libido [42]. More than 50% of PCa patients undergoing long-term ADT develop metabolic syndrome. Metabolic syndrome is shown to increase the fatality rate in PCa patients for example by increasing the risk of cardio-vascular diseases [43].Recent studies have shown that prostate cancer cells can use lipids to synthesise androgens via back-door pathways [44, 45]. Therefore, drugs that target intra-tumoural androgen synthesis offer a novel approach of targeting PCa.

Metformin is an oral biguanide and is mainly used to treat type-2 diabetes-mellitus. Metformin is used as a first-line hypoglycemic drug in diabetic patients and helps to reduce the levels of LDL cholesterol and triglycerides. Metformin reduces glucose levels and also regulates insulin levels through activation of AMPK [46]. In many studies, it was observed that diabetic patients treated with metformin showed lower risk of cancer compared to patients who received non-metformin drugs [47, 48]. This has led to the hypothesis that metformin acts as an anti-cancer drug. Metformin has been shown to inhibit the growth of various cancer cell lines such as colon, glial, pancreatic, breast and prostate [49]. Prostate cancer cells treated with metformin showed approximately 50% decrease in cell viability compared to prostate epithelial cells, indicating that metformin specifically targets the proliferation of cancer cells [50]. In addition, metformin has also shown to exert selective toxicity towards cancer stem cells both in vitro and in in vivo using xenograft models.

The exact mechanism action of anti-neoplastic activity of metformin is still not clear but several mechanisms have been proposed. These include but not limited to the effect of metformin on AMPK, c-MYC, Akt and cyclinD1 and other cell cycle proteins [49]. AMPK acts as a sensor of starvation and is activated in nutrient deprived conditions. Activated AMPK halts the translation machinery of cells by inhibiting the mammalian target of rapamycin (mTOR) pathway [46]. This leads decreased cell proliferation and ultimately cell death. In addition, metformin also shown to induce the activation of tumour suppressor gene liver kinase B1 (LKB1) [51]. Results from the pre-clinical studies were further supported by clinical trials where metformin was shown to reduce the risk of PCa by 44% in Caucasians [52]. However, two recent retrospective studies showed no significant difference in biochemical recurrence between metformin treated and non-metformin treated groups [53]. This difference in the data can be due to the nature and method of analysis and therefore further studies are warranted.

Selenium: selenium is a nutritionally essential micronutrient. Selenium is incorporated into amino acids for example selenocysteine and is essential for the synthesis of selenoproteins. The amount of selenium intake varies significantly across the world and depends on the selenium content in soil and the type of food consumed. For instance, the average selenium intake is high in US where as it is low in Europe [54]. The evidence for the role of selenium in preventing cancer came from an ecological study that suggested an inverse correlation between selenium intake and cancer incidence [55]. Since then results from several case-controlled studies showed the negative effect of selenium on cancer incidence. The same is reported in terms of prostate cancer incidence and selenium levels [56]. For example, in a matched case controlled prospective study conducted in late nineties the amount of selenium in toe nails is shown to be associated with decreased risk in development of advance prostate cancer [57]. However, further prospective studies including the results from SELECT trial done on large patient cohort showed no such a correlation. Results from SELECT trail showed that neither selenium nor vitamin E alone or in combination reduce the risk of prostate cancer incidence [54]. But a recent report from Netherlands where the levels of selenium in toe nails were compared to risk of advance PCa in a large patient cohort invoked the interest in using selenium as dietary supplement to reduce the risk of PCa [58].

Vitamin E and Gamma tocotrienol: Vitamin-E refers to a group of fat-soluble tocopherols and tocotrienols. Based on the position of methyl groups on their chromonal ring tocopherols and tocotrienols can be categorised into four isomeric forms; alpha (α), beta (β), gamma (γ) and delta (δ) [59]. α-tocopherol is the most biologically active form of vitamin-E. Vitamin-E acts as a potent anti-oxidant by reducing the free-radical formation such as reactive-oxygen species. Besides their antioxidant, anti-inflammatory, antiangiogenic and antimicrobial properties recent studies showed the evidencc for the anticancer activity of tocotrienols on numerous cancer cell lines including breast, colon, liver and prostate [60]. Plasma levels of α-tocopherols were shown to be associated with the decreased risk of prostate cancer [60]. However this is questioned by a population based study were plasma levels of γ-tocopherol were shown to reduce the risk [61, 62].Among various isoforms of vitamin-E γ-tocotrienol (γTE) was shown to supress prostate cancer cell growth.

One of the reasons explained for the failure of current treatment regimens in targeting prostate cancer includes their inability to target cancer stem cells (CSCs). Cancer stem cells share some of the characteristics of normal stem cell such as being quiescent and resistant to chemotherapeutic drugs. Chemotherapeutic drugs mainly target actively diving cells. In addition (CSCs) can also develop acquired drug resistance by expressing multidrug resistance proteins. γTE was shown to increase the sensitivity of (CSCs) to chemotherapeutic drugs by down regulation of CSC markers such as CD44 and CD133 in prostate cancer cells [63]. In addition, γTE was also shown to compromise the tumourogenesis as demonstrated by suppressed spheroid and tumour formation in both *in vitro* and *in vivo* experiments. The exact mechanism of action of γTE is still not clear but various mechanisms have been proposed. For example γTE was shown to induce apoptosis by activation p53 and JNK [64]. γTE was also shown to down-regulate pro-survival signalling such as NF-kB, EFG-R and pAKT pathway.

Immunotherapeutic Targets

Targeting cancer using immunotherapeutic approaches has been considered for more than a century [65]. Although there are several studies that proved the benefit of these drugs in pre-clinical investigations none demonstrated the clinical benefit of improving the survival of patients. However, recent studies proved the efficacy of immunotherapeutic drugs in targeting cancers such as melanoma and prostate cancer. These drugs harness the patient's immune system in targeting cancer cells.

Sipuleucel-T: Sipuleucel-Tis the first autologous immunotherapeutic agent approved by FDA on 29th April, 2010 to treat asymptomatic and minimally symptomatic CRPC patients [66]. There are several other immunotherapeutic agents that are in late-phase development for prostate cancer and include prostate-specific antigen (PSA)-TRICOM vaccine (a poxviral-based vaccine directed against PSA) and ipilimumab (an anticytotoxic T-lymphpcyte antigen [CTLA-4] monoclonal antibody) that is currently approved for melanoma [67, 68].

Sipuleucel-T is the first immunotherapeutic agent demonstrated to offer the overall survival benefit for asymptomatic and minimally symptomatic PCa patients [66]. Sipuleucel-T is designed to prime the immune response against prostate cancer cells. Sipuleucel-T is a cellular product and contains peripheral blood mononuclear cells (PBMCs), including antigen-presenting cells (APCs) that express CD54, B and T lymphocytes that are activated *ex-vivo* to activate APCs [69]. Sipuleucel-T is manufactured from the patient's immune cells and is designed for an individualised treatment. A standard course of Sipuleucel-T consists of 3 doses and each dose is manufactured from standard leukapheresis procedure using patient's PBMCs [70]. These cells are then incubated with a recombinant fusion protein comprising the prostate protein prostatic acid phosphatase (PAP) fused to cytokine, granulocyte-macrophage colony-stimulating factor (GM-CSF). This design was based on pre-clinical observation that rat APCs activated ex vivo with fusion protein containing PAP and GM-CSF induced autoimmune prostatitis [71].

Use of Sipuleucel-T in treating prostate cancer patients is supported by data from various clinical trials. Results from three randomized, double-blinded, placebo-controlled phase-III clinical trials that used Sipuleucel-Tin patients with metastatic CRPC were released [72]. The first two trials designated D9901 and D9902A were identically designed, controlled, double-blinded, multicentre studies and patients were randomized in a 2:1 ratio to receive Sipuleucel-T or control infusions at weeks 0, 2 and 4. Time to disease progression (TTP) was chosen as the primary end point and both studies have pre-specified protocols for analysis of overall survival after patients were followed for 36 months or until death of the patients [72]. Both studies demonstrated a benefit of statistically significant prolongation of median overall survival (OS) in patients receiving Sipuleucel-T [72].

In study D9901 patients treated with Sipuleucel-Tshowed a statistically significant 4.5 month prolongation in median OS compared to controls. Results from these two studies were supported by a much larger pivotal phase-III IMPACT clinical trial [66]. A total of 512 men with asymptomatic or minimally symptomatic metastatic CRPC were randomized in a 2:1 ratio to receive Sipuleucel-T.

The primary and secondary end points were OS and time to objective disease progression. Patients treated with Sipuleucel-T showed a 22% reduction in the risk of death and a 4.1-month prolongation of median OS. The safety of Sipuleucel-T was evaluated in four randomized phase-III studies and adverse events were reported in more than 15% of patients, which included chills, fatigue, back pain, arthralgia and pyrexia. The incidence of cerebrovascular events was 3.5 in Sipuleucel-T treated group and 2.6% in control group [73]. The risk of developing cerebrovascular events from using Sipuleucel-T is currently being re-assessed by a phase-IV prospective study (PROCEED, trail NCT01306890) and is currently enrolling patients.

Effect of sipuleucel-T in increasing the overall survival in PCa patients has been called into question by a report showing the lack of demonstrable anti-tumour activity of sipuleucel-T. This study argues that the overall survival benefit observed in clinical trials can be due to the harmful effect of placebo on older patients with PCa [74].

Denosumab: Denosumab is a fully humanised monoclonal antibody of IgG2 subtype that selectively binds to Receptor Activator of NF Kappa B Ligand (RANKL) with high affinity [75]. Binding of Denosumab to RANKL prevents its binding to RANK on the surface of osteoclast precursors and osteoclasts. RANKL is a membrane-bound protein and plays a critical role in differentiation, activation and survival of osteoclasts [76]. Denosumab is licenced for the treatment of bone loss as it inhibits the differentiation, activation and survival of osteoclasts. Bone loss is usually seen in conditions such as postmenopausal period or in men with prostate cancer undergoing hormone ablation therapy. Hormones such as estrogen and testosterone play an important role in maintaining bone density. ADT was shown to increase the bone resorption by approximately 2-4% per year irrespective of dietary supplementation.

Bone homeostasis is maintained by the bone turnover and is a fine balance between the formation of new bone and bone resorption. Osteoclast mediated bone resorption is regulated by a cytokine pathway that belongs to tumour necrosis factor family and comprised of RANK, RANKL and osteoprotegerin (OPG) which is a decoy receptor [77]. OPG inhibits the binding of RANK and its ligand RANKL on the surface of osteoclasts and inhibits osteoclastogenesis. OPG is a soluble protein secreted by osteoblasts and stromal cell in the bone [77].

Prostate cancer has a high tropism for bone tissue and approximately 80% of CRPC patients develop bone metastasis. Metastatic lesions in the bone induce skeletal-related events (SREs).

Examples of SREs include pathological fractures, radiculopathy, cytopenias and spinal cord compression. Osteoclast mediated bone resorption is high in areas of bone metastasis leading to SREs. It was hypothesised that inhibition of osteoclasts using RANKL antagonists would have a therapeutic value and preclinical models demonstrated the benefit of using RANKL inhibitors in reducing the SREs. Denosumab inhibits the activity of RANKL using the mechanism similar to OPG [76]. When given subcutaneously to prostate cancer patients Denosumab resulted in decreased bone turnover in phase-II and III clinical trials and patients treated with Denosumab showed approximately 5.6% increase in bone density compared to controls [75].Currently Denosumab is used to treat SREs in patients with non-metastatic prostate cancer who is on ADT as well as patients with bone metastasis from solid tumours.

Drugs That Target Tumour Microenvironment

Tasquinimod: Tasquinimod is an anti-angiogenic agent used in the treatment of advanced prostate cancer [78]. Angiogenesis plays an important role in tumour growth and differentiation. Therefore drugs that inhibit molecular pathways involved in angiogenesis offers an advantage of treating prostate cancer patients. Tumours are high in cell density because of their uncontrolled cell division and require higher levels of oxygen for their metabolic activity. Because oxygen cannot diffuse into tissues thicker than 200μm, cancer cells secrete angiogenic factors such as vascular endothelial growth factor (VEGF) and hypoxia-inducible factor-1 alpha (HIF-1α) that switch on the neovascularising state referred to as "angiogenic switch". This angiogenic switch initiates the formation of new vessels and promotes exponential tumour growth. Neovascularisation or tumour angiogenesis provides a new avenue for the tumour cells to spread to other parts of the body. As a result tumour angiogenesis plays an important role in disease progression and is an area of therapeutic research.

Tasquinimod is a second generation quinolone-3-carboxamide developed from its first generation agent linomide. Linomide was shown to inhibit prostate cancer growth in vivo.

However clinical use of linomide is limited by its cytotoxicity and led to the development of less toxic second generation agents. Tasquinimod suppresses tumour growth by acting as aantiangiogenic agent by down regulation of angiogenic factors for example VEGF and HIF-1α [79]. Tasquinimod exerts this by regulating acetylation of target gene promoters [79].

When used in combination with ADT, tasquinimod demonstrated a synergistic action resulting in suppression of tumour growth by significantly reducing the tumour vasculature [79]. Tasquinimod showed a similar synergistic action when used in combination with docetaxel and ADT in metastatic CRPC patients. In phase-I and II clinical studies tasquinimod showed a greater tolerability and improved the progression-free survival by a median of 4.3 months in minimally symptomatic and chemotherapy naive CRPCpatients [79]. Based on the promising results from phase-II trials, a randomized, double-blinded, placebo-controlled phase-III trial has now begun and is currently recruiting patients (NCT01234311).

Conclusion

Prostate cancer causes a significant morbidity and mortality in men and is a major economic burden in many developed countries. For many decades ADT has been the main stay of treating prostate cancer patients with advanced disease.

Despite initial tumour regression many patients fail ADT and develop more aggressive castration-resistant phenotype. Docetaxel is available to treat patients who fail ADT and eventually develop fatal metastatic phenotype. Reasons for the failure of ADT include intratumoural androgen synthesis and AR mutations, which leads to adaptive cell survival through the restoration of AR signalling. Bicalutamide was the first anti-androgen agent developed to inhibit AR-signalling. Bicalutamide acts as an AR-antagonist and is still used to treat CRPC patients. Despite its effectiveness in increasing overall survival bicalutamide treatment fails in many patients. Resistance to bicalutamide is due to mutations in AR where bicalutamide is used as AR-agonist. Intensive research to overcome resistance has led to the development of at least six drugs are either in phase-III clinical trials or clinically available. These include abiraterone, carbazitaxel, radium-223, denosumab, metformin and enzalutamide.

Another exciting area of research in drug development against prostate cancer includes immunotherapeutic targeting of tumour cells. Sipuleucel-T is the immunotherapeutic agent that is currently under phase-III clinical trials. [74] Results from studies that tested these new drugs show a promising clinical benefit in increasing the overall survival and quality of life in patients with advanced prostate cancer and future looks optimistic in treating patients with prostate cancer.

References

[1] Baade P. D., Youlden D. R., Krnjacki L. J. International epidemiology of prostate cancer; geographical distribution and secular trends (2009). *Molecular nutrition and food research,* 53; 171-84.

[2] Klotz L. Active surveillance for prostate cancer; overview and update (2013). *Current treatment options in oncology,* 14; 97-108.

[3] Nguyen P. L., Zietman A. L. High-dose external beam radiation for localized prostate cancer; current status and future challenges (2007). *Cancer journal,* 13; 295-301.

[4] Fradet Y. Bicalutamide (Casodex) in the treatment of prostate cancer (2004). *Expert review of anticancer therapy,* 4; 37-48.

[5] Osguthorpe D. J., Hagler A. T. Mechanism of androgen receptor antagonism by bicalutamide in the treatment of prostate cancer (2011). *Biochemistry,* 50; 4105-13.

[6] Tyrrell C. Immediate Treatment with Bicalutamide, 150 mg/d, Following Radiotherapy in Localized or Locally Advanced Prostate Cancer (2004). *Reviews in urology,* 6 Suppl., 2; S29-36.

[7] Hara T., Miyazaki J., Araki H., Yamaoka M., Kanzaki N., et al. Novel mutations of androgen receptor; a possible mechanism of bicalutamide withdrawal syndrome 2003. *Cancer research,* 63; 149-53.

[8] Schellhammer P. F., Sharifi R., Block N. L., Soloway M. S., Venner P. M., et al. A controlled trial of bicalutamide versus flutamide, each in combination with luteinizing hormone-releasing hormone analogue therapy, in patients with advanced prostate carcinoma. Analysis of time to progression. CASODEX Combination Study Group (1996). *Cancer,* 78; 2164-9.

[9] Soloway M. S., Schellhammer P. F., Smith J. A., Chodak G. W., Kennealey G. T. Bicalutamide in the treatment of advanced prostatic

carcinoma; a phase II multicenter trial (1996). *Urology,* 47; 33-7; discussion 48-53.

[10] Chen Y., Clegg N. J., Scher H. I. Anti-androgens and androgen-depleting therapies in prostate cancer; new agents for an established target (2009). *The lancet oncology,* 10; 981-91.

[11] Bohl C. E., Gao W., Miller D. D., Bell C. E., Dalton J. T. Structural basis for antagonism and resistance of bicalutamide in prostate cancer (2005). *Proceedings of the National Academy of Sciences of the United States of America,* 102; 6201-6.

[12] Colabufo N. A., Pagliarulo V., Berardi F., Contino M., Inglese C., et al. Bicalutamide failure in prostate cancer treatment; involvement of Multi Drug Resistance proteins (2008). *European journal of pharmacology,* 601; 38-42.

[13] Chen C. D., Welsbie D. S., Tran C., Baek S. H., Chen R., et al. Molecular determinants of resistance to antiandrogen therapy (2004). *Nature medicine,* 10; 33-9.

[14] Jung M. E., Ouk S., Yoo D., Sawyers C. L., Chen C., et al. Structure-activity relationship for thiohydantoin androgen receptor antagonists for castration-resistant prostate cancer (CRPC) (2010). *Journal of medicinal chemistry,* 53; 2779-96.

[15] Tran C., Ouk S., Clegg N. J., Chen Y., Watson P. A., et al. Development of a second-generation antiandrogen for treatment of advanced prostate cancer (2009). *Science,* 324; 787-90.

[16] Scher H. I., Fizazi K., Saad F., Taplin M. E., Sternberg C. N., et al. Increased survival with enzalutamide in prostate cancer after chemotherapy (2012). *The New England journal of medicine,* 367; 1187-97.

[17] El-Amm J., Patel N., Freeman A., Aragon-Ching J. B. Metastatic Castration-Resistant Prostate Cancer; Critical Review of Enzalutamide (2013). *Clinical Medicine Insights. Oncology,* 7; 235-45.

[18] Ravindranathan P., Lee T. K., Yang L., Centenera M. M., Butler L., et al. Peptidomimetic targeting of critical androgen receptor-coregulator interactions in prostate cancer (2013). *Nature communications,* 4; 1923.

[19] Yang L., Ravindranathan P., Ramanan M., Kapur P., Hammes S. R., et al. Central role for PELP1 in nonandrogenic activation of the androgen receptor in prostate cancer (2012). *Molecular endocrinology,* 26; 550-61.

[20] Chakravarty D., Tekmal R. R., Vadlamudi R. K. PELP1; A novel therapeutic target for hormonal cancers (2010). *IUBMB life,* 62; 162-9.

[21] Pont A., Goldman E. S., Sugar A. M., Siiteri P. K., Stevens D. A. Ketoconazole-induced increase in estradiol-testosterone ratio. Probable explanation for gynecomastia 1985. *Archives of internal medicine,* 145; 1429-31.

[22] Trachtenberg J., Pont A. Ketoconazole therapy for advanced prostate cancer 1984. *Lancet,* 2; 433-5.

[23] Mahler C., Verhelst J., Denis L. Ketoconazole and liarozole in the treatment of advanced prostatic cancer 1993. *Cancer,* 71; 1068-73.

[24] Bok R. A., Small E. J. The treatment of advanced prostate cancer with ketoconazole; safety issues 1999. *Drug safety ; an international journal of medical toxicology and drug experience,* 20; 451-8.

[25] Mohler J. L., Titus M. A., Wilson E. M. Potential prostate cancer drug target; bioactivation of androstanediol by conversion to dihydrotestosterone (2011). *Clinical cancer research; an official journal of the American Association for Cancer Research,* 17; 5844-9.

[26] Stein M. N., Goodin S., Dipaola R. S. Abiraterone in prostate cancer; a new angle to an old problem (2012). *Clinical cancer research ; an official journal of the American Association for Cancer Research,* 18; 1848-54.

[27] Hakki T., Bernhardt R. CYP17- and CYP11B-dependent steroid hydroxylases as drug development targets (2006). *Pharmacology and therapeutics,* 111; 27-52.

[28] de Bono J. S., Logothetis C. J., Molina A., Fizazi K., North S., et al. Abiraterone and increased survival in metastatic prostate cancer (2011). *The New England journal of medicine,* 364; 1995-(2005).

[29] Attard G., Cooper C. S., de Bono J. S. Steroid hormone receptors in prostate cancer; a hard habit to break? (2009). *Cancer cell,* 16; 458-62.

[30] De Dosso S., Berthold D. R. Docetaxel in the management of prostate cancer; current standard of care and future directions (2008). *Expert opinion on pharmacotherapy,* 9; 1969-79.

[31] Serpa Neto A., Tobias-Machado M., Kaliks R., Wroclawski M. L., Pompeo A. C., Del Giglio A. Ten years of docetaxel-based therapies in prostate adenocarcinoma; a systematic review and meta-analysis of 2244 patients in 12 randomized clinical trials (2011). *Clinical genitourinary cancer,* 9; 115-23.

[32] Altavilla A., Iacovelli R., Procopio G., Alesini D., Risi E., et al. Medical strategies for treatment of castration resistant prostate cancer (CRPC) docetaxel resistant (2012). *Cancer Biol. Ther.,* 13; 1001-8.

[33] Krishna R., Mayer L. D. Multidrug resistance (MDR) in cancer. Mechanisms, reversal using modulators of MDR and the role of MDR modulators in influencing the pharmacokinetics of anticancer drugs 2000. *European journal of pharmaceutical sciences ; official journal of the European Federation for Pharmaceutical Sciences,* 11; 265-83.

[34] Luqmani Y. A. (2005). Mechanisms of drug resistance in cancer chemotherapy. *Medical principles and practice ; international journal of the Kuwait University, Health Science Centre,* 14 Suppl 1; 35-48.

[35] FDA Center for Drug Evaluation and Research. Approval Package for; Jevtana. June 17, (2010). Available from;http;//www.accessdata.fda.gov/ drugsatfda_docs/nda/(2010)/(2010)23s000Approv.pdf. Accessed Feb. 2, (2011).

[36] de Bono J. S., Oudard S., Ozguroglu M., Hansen S., Machiels J. P., et al. Prednisone plus cabazitaxel or mitoxantrone for metastatic castration-resistant prostate cancer progressing after docetaxel treatment; a randomised open-label trial (2010). *Lancet,* 376; 1147-54.

[37] Lange P. H., Vessella R. L. Mechanisms, hypotheses and questions regarding prostate cancer micrometastases to bone 1998. *Cancer metastasis reviews,* 17; 331-6.

[38] Parker C., Sartor O. Radium-223 in prostate cancer (2013). *The New England journal of medicine,* 369; 1659-60.

[39] Harrison M. R., Wong T. Z., Armstrong A. J., George D. J. Radium-223 chloride; a potential new treatment for castration-resistant prostate cancer patients with metastatic bone disease (2013). *Cancer management and research,* 5; 1-14.

[40] Nilsson S., Larsen R. H., Fossa S. D., Balteskard L., Borch K. W., et al. First clinical experience with alpha-emitting radium-223 in the treatment of skeletal metastases (2005). *Clinical cancer research ; an official journal of the American Association for Cancer Research,* 11; 4451-9.

[41] Parker C., Nilsson S., Heinrich D., Helle S. I., O'Sullivan J. M., et al. Alpha emitter radium-223 and survival in metastatic prostate cancer (2013). *The New England journal of medicine,* 369; 213-23.

[42] Morote J., Ropero J., Planas J., Bastaros J. M., Delgado G., et al. Metabolic syndrome increases the risk of aggressive prostate cancer detection (2013). *BJU international,* 111; 1031-6.

[43] Lu-Yao G., Stukel T. A., Yao S. L. Changing patterns in competing causes of death in men with prostate cancer; a population based study (2004). *The Journal of urology,* 171; 2285-90.

[44] Locke J. A., Guns E. S., Lubik A. A., Adomat H. H., Hendy S. C., et al. Androgen levels increase by intratumoral de novo steroidogenesis during progression of castration-resistant prostate cancer (2008). *Cancer research,* 68; 6407-15.

[45] Lubik A. A., Gunter J. H., Hendy S. C., Locke J. A., Adomat H. H., et al. Insulin increases de novo steroidogenesis in prostate cancer cells (2011). *Cancer research,* 71; 5754-64.

[46] Zhou G., Myers R., Li Y., Chen Y., Shen X., et al. Role of AMP-activated protein kinase in mechanism of metformin action 2001. *The Journal of clinical investigation,* 108; 1167-74.

[47] Sadeghi N., Abbruzzese J. L., Yeung S. C., Hassan M., Li D. Metformin use is associated with better survival of diabetic patients with pancreatic cancer (2012). *Clinical cancer research ; an official journal of the American Association for Cancer Research,* 18; 2905-12.

[48] Evans J. M., Donnelly L. A., Emslie-Smith A. M., Alessi D. R., Morris A. D. Metformin and reduced risk of cancer in diabetic patients (2005). *Bmj,* 330; 1304-5.

[49] Ben Sahra I., Laurent K., Loubat A., Giorgetti-Peraldi S., Colosetti P., et al. The antidiabetic drug metformin exerts an antitumoral effect in vitro and in vivo through a decrease of cyclin D1 level (2008). *Oncogene,* 27; 3576-86.

[50] Zakikhani M., Dowling R. J., Sonenberg N., Pollak M. N. The effects of adiponectin and metformin on prostate and colon neoplasia involve activation of AMP-activated protein kinase (2008). *Cancer prevention research,* 1; 369-75.

[51] Shaw R. J., Bardeesy N., Manning B. D., Lopez L., Kosmatka M., et al. The LKB1 tumor suppressor negatively regulates mTOR signaling (2004). *Cancer cell,* 6; 91-9.

[52] Wright J. L., Stanford J. L. Metformin use and prostate cancer in Caucasian men; results from a population-based case-control study (2009). *Cancer causes and control, CCC* 20; 1617-22.

[53] Patel T., Hruby G., Badani K., Abate-Shen C., McKiernan J. M. Clinical outcomes after radical prostatectomy in diabetic patients treated with metformin (2010). *Urology,* 76; 1240-4.

[54] Nicastro H. L., Dunn B. K. Selenium and prostate cancer prevention; insights from the selenium and vitamin E cancer prevention trial (SELECT) (2013). *Nutrients,* 5; 1122-48.

[55] Shamberger R. J., Frost D. V. Possible protective effect of selenium against human cancer 1969. *Canadian Medical Association journal,* 100; 682.

[56] Etminan M., FitzGerald J. M., Gleave M., Chambers K. Intake of selenium in the prevention of prostate cancer; a systematic review and meta-analysis (2005). *Cancer causes and control, CCC* 16; 1125-31.

[57] Yoshizawa K., Willett W. C., Morris S. J., Stampfer M. J., Spiegelman D., et al. Study of prediagnostic selenium level in toenails and the risk of advanced prostate cancer 1998. *Journal of the National Cancer Institute,* 90; 1219-24.

[58] Geybels M. S., Verhage B. A., van Schooten F. J., Goldbohm R. A., van den Brandt P. A. Advanced prostate cancer risk in relation to toenail selenium levels (2013). *Journal of the National Cancer Institute,* 105; 1394-401.

[59] Monsen E. R. Dietary reference intakes for the antioxidant nutrients; vitamin C, vitamin E, selenium, and carotenoids 2000. *Journal of the American Dietetic Association,* 100; 637-40.

[60] Heinonen O. P., Albanes D., Virtamo J., Taylor P. R., Huttunen J. K., et al. Prostate cancer and supplementation with alpha-tocopherol and beta-carotene; incidence and mortality in a controlled trial 1998. *Journal of the National Cancer Institute,* 90; 440-6.

[61] Walsh P. C. Vitamin E supplements and risk of prostate cancer in U.S. men (2005). *The Journal of urology,* 173; 87-8.

[62] Rodriguez C., Jacobs E. J., Mondul A. M., Calle E. E., McCullough M. L., Thun M. J. Vitamin E supplements and risk of prostate cancer in U.S. men (2004). *Cancer epidemiology, biomarkers and prevention; a publication of the American Association for Cancer Research, cosponsored by the American Society of Preventive Oncology.,* 13; 378-82.

[63] Luk S. U., Yap W. N., Chiu Y. T., Lee D. T., Ma S., et al. Gamma-tocotrienol as an effective agent in targeting prostate cancer stem cell-like population (2011). *International journal of cancer. Journal international du cancer,* 128; 2182-91.

[64] Yap W. N., Chang P. N., Han H. Y., Lee D. T., Ling M. T., et al. Gamma-tocotrienol suppresses prostate cancer cell proliferation and invasion through multiple-signalling pathways (2008). *British journal of cancer,* 99; 1832-41.

[65] Kim C. J., Dessureault S., Gabrilovich D., Reintgen D. S., Slingluff C. L. Jr., Immunotherapy for melanoma 2002. *Cancer control; journal of the Moffitt Cancer Center,* 9; 22-30.

[66] Kantoff P. W., Higano C. S., Shore N. D., Berger E. R., Small E. J., et al. Sipuleucel-T immunotherapy for castration-resistant prostate cancer (2010). *The New England journal of medicine,* 363; 411-22.

[67] Kantoff P. W., Schuetz T. J., Blumenstein B. A., Glode L. M., Bilhartz D. L., et al. Overall survival analysis of a phase II randomized controlled trial of a Poxviral-based PSA-targeted immunotherapy in metastatic castration-resistant prostate cancer (2010). *Journal of clinical oncology; official journal of the American Society of Clinical Oncology,* 28; 1099-105.

[68] Hodi F. S., O'Day S. J., McDermott D. F., Weber R. W., Sosman J. A., et al. Improved survival with ipilimumab in patients with metastatic melanoma (2010). *The New England journal of medicine,* 363; 711-23.

[69] Shore N. D., Mantz C. A., Dosoretz D. E., Fernandez E., Myslicki F. A., et al. Building on sipuleucel-T for immunologic treatment of castration-resistant prostate cancer (2013). *Cancer control; journal of the Moffitt Cancer Center,* 20; 7-16.

[70] Frohlich M. W. Sipuleucel-T for the treatment of advanced prostate cancer (2012). *Seminars in oncology,* 39; 245-52.

[71] Valone F. H., Small E., MacKenzie M., Burch P., Lacy M., et al. Dendritic cell-based treatment of cancer; closing in on a cellular therapy 2001. *Cancer journal,* 7 Suppl 2; S53-61.

[72] Higano C. S., Schellhammer P. F., Small E. J., Burch P. A., Nemunaitis J., et al. Integrated data from 2 randomized, double-blind, placebo-controlled, phase 3 trials of active cellular immunotherapy with sipuleucel-T in advanced prostate cancer (2009). *Cancer,* 115; 3670-9.

[73] Hall S. J., Klotz L., Pantuck A. J., George D. J., Whitmore J. B., et al. Integrated safety data from 4 randomized, double-blind, controlled trials of autologous cellular immunotherapy with sipuleucel-T in patients with prostate cancer (2011). *The Journal of urology,* 186; 877-81.

[74] Huber M. L., Haynes L., Parker C., Iversen P. Interdisciplinary critique of sipuleucel-T as immunotherapy in castration-resistant prostate cancer (2012). *Journal of the National Cancer Institute,* 104; 273-9.

[75] Paller C. J., Carducci M. A., Philips G. K. Management of bone metastases in refractory prostate cancer--role of denosumab (2012). *Clinical interventions in aging,* 7; 363-72.

[76] Dellis A., Papatsoris A. G. Denosumab as a promising novel bone-targeted agent in castration resistant prostate cancer (2013). Expert opinion on biological therapy.

[77] Helo S., Manger J. P., Krupski T. L. Role of denosumab in prostate cancer (2012). *Prostate cancer and prostatic diseases,* 15; 231-6.

[78] Williamson S. C., Hartley A. E., Heer R. A review of tasquinimod in the treatment of advanced prostate cancer (2013). *Drug design, development and therapy,* 7; 167-74.

[79] Osanto S., van Poppel H., Burggraaf J. Tasquinimod; a novel drug in advanced prostate cancer (2013). *Future oncology,* 9; 1271-81.

In: Advances in Drug Resistance Research
Editor: Christudas Morais ISBN: 978-1-63117-131-4

Chapter 7

Resistance of Metastatic Renal Cell Carcinomas to Chemo and Immunotherapy: Clinicians' Perspective

Ng Keng Lim[1,2,3,*] *and Simon T. Wood*[2]
[1]Department of Surgery, University Malaya, Kuala Lumpur, Malaysia
[2]Department of Urology, Princess Alexandra Hospital, Brisbane, Australia
[3]Centre for Kidney Disease Research, University of Queensland, Brisbane, Australia

Abstract

Metastatic renal cell carcinoma (mRCC) confers poor prognosis despite remarkable advances in treatment modalities. Traditionally RCC has been known to be refractory to chemotherapy regimen. Immunotherapy had been the mainstay of treatment until the recent explosion of targeted therapies. Patients with mRCC are reported to experience significantly better clinical responses with targeted therapies which have become standard of care. Nevertheless, a sizeable proportion

* Author of correspondence: kenglimng@yahoo.com. This work was supported by Ministry of Science, Technology and Innovation, Malaysia; ID: 02-01-03-SF0919.

of patients do not show response to any form of treatment (intrinsic resistance) and another proportion develop resistance during the course of the treatment despite initial responses (extrinsic resistance). In this chapter, we present an overview of chemotherapy and immunotherapy resistance in mRCC.

Keywords: Metastatic renal cell carcinoma, chemotherapy, immunotherapy

Introduction

The worldwide incidence of renal cancers is on an increasing trend and usually accounts for 2-3% of all adult cancers. Clear cell RCC is the most common subtype originating from proximal tubules (more than 80%), followed by papillary RCC (pRCC) (10-15%) and chromophobe RCC (chRCC). Collecting duct, unclassified, and medullary (occurring almost exclusively in patients with sickle-cell trait) are rare subtypes (about 3-5%) [1]. Sarcomatoid differentiation is not a distinct histological subtype but is a growth pattern that can occur in all subtypes characterized by a spindle-cell appearance, epithelial and mesenchymal differentiation, increased cellularity, and cellular atypia that portend an aggressive disease course [2, 3]. Metastatic non-clear cell RCCs are characterized by resistance to systemic therapy and poor survival, with longer survival for chRCC than for pRCC or collecting duct tumours in historic data (20 vs 5.5 months, respectively) [4].

Surgical Management of Localised RCC

With increasing availability and utilization of cross-sectional imaging techniques, more patients are being diagnosed with incidental renal tumours. This has led to a shift in clinical presentation of renal cancer in the last decade, where renal tumours are increasingly found as asymptomatic small renal masses on imaging studies obtained for other purposes [5, 6]. The treatment paradigm for small localized renal cancers is rapidly evolving. Surgical innovation has focused on minimally invasive nephron-sparing surgery and focal ablative therapies which are replacing radical nephrectomy in many urological centres worldwide. This treatment approach offers good functional renal preservation while maintaining proper oncological outcomes.

Patients with RCC typically present in the sixth and seventh decades of life. While incidental detection of asymptomatic tumors is increasingly common, patients may present with symptomatic disease including localized, constitutional, paraneoplastic and metastatic symptoms. Local symptoms include gross haematuria, flank pain and loin mass, while constitutional symptoms often include loss of apetite, weight loss and cachexia. Occasionally, RCC patients can present with a wide variety of paraneoplastic manifestations including hypercalcaemia (due to secreted parathyroid hormone related protein), hypertension (renin secretion), liver dysfunction (Stauffer's syndrome), erthrocytosis (erythropoietin production), fever and night sweats.

Despite increased detection of early stage disease, around 20-30% of patients with RCC still present with metastatic disease at diagnosis, and about a third of patients undergoing nephrectomy for localized disease eventually develop metastases [7]. Metastatic RCC carries a poor prognosis with overall 5 year survival of less than 5% [8]. Common metastatic sites include lungs, bones, liver and occasionally the brain. Clinical diagnosis and tumour staging is accomplished mainly by four phase computed tomography scans which include control, arterial, nephrographic and excretory phases. Treatment strategy depends on tumor stage. For tumors limited to the kidney surgical excision via complete or partial nephrectomy remains the most effective treatment with robust clinical outcomes. Nephrectomy can be performed via open, laparoscopic and robotic assisted modes depending on surgical expertise and infrastructure.

Treatment options for small renal masses include surgical excision, active surveillance and focal ablative therapies (e. g. cryosurgery and radiofrequency ablation). Nephron sparing approaches are preferred whenever imperative or relative indications exist such as bilateral tumours, solitary kidney status, chronic kidney disease or medical conditions likely to adversely impact renal function in the longer-term [9]. Most therapeutic guidelines currently recommend partial nephrectomy as first line treatment for surgically suitable lesions due to excellent oncological efficacy and the potential benefits of preservation of renal mass. Most surgical series suggest around 20% of masses are benign, 60% are probably indolent variants of renal cell carcinoma, and only 20% are potentially aggressive tumours. [10, 11] In a meta-analysis of almost 300 patients with small kidney masses, who did not receive intervention, the average growth rate of the tumours was only 0·28 cm per year, and only 1% of tumours metastasized [12]. Therefore, active surveillance approach can be used to avoid the morbidity of surgical excision or ablation in select patients such as older persons or those at high risk from surgical intervention.

Focal ablative techniques such as radiofrequency ablation and cryosurgery can also be an option for small renal masses. These have an advantage of lower surgical morbidity, reduced pain, faster recovery and preservation of renal function. However there are several issues of concern, for example, increased rates of local recurrence and difficulties in defining post ablative imaging success. At present, energy ablative therapy is usually offered to selected patients who are elderly or who have multiple comorbidities with high surgical risks [13].

Surgical Management of Advanced RCC

Larger or locally advanced renal tumours are best treated with surgical excision where technically feasible. Medial extent of the tumor to involve major vasculature and regional lymph node metastases are often determinates of resectability. RCC has a propensity for growth within venous spaces and may expand to fill and occlude the inferior vena cava. Cure can still be achieved in these cases if metastatic disease does not exist and complete surgical excision is undertaken.

Selective cases of mRCC can still benefit from surgery and these include cytoreductive nephrectomy and metastatectomy usually for synchronous and metachronous single site lesion. Cytoreductive nephrectomy has been shown to be beneficial by the findings of two phase III studies in which patients with metastatic renal cell carcinoma were randomly assigned to nephrectomy or no surgery followed by interferon alfa. In a combined analysis of these trials, median overall survival was 13·6 months (95% CI 9·7–17·4) for nephrectomy plus interferon versus 7·8 months (5·9-9·7) for interferon alone (hazard ratio 0·69, 0·55–0·87, p=0·002) [14-16]. The exact mechanism that accounts for this beneficial effect is not known. Patients most likely to benefit from cytoreduction include those with a substantial proportion of the total tumour burden (e. g, >75%) in the involved kidney; good performance status with adequate cardiac and pulmonary function; and no CNS or liver metastases (with rare exceptions) [17]. Another beneficial reason for cytoreductive nephrectomy is for palliation of symptoms of pain, haematuria or mass effect caused by the renal tumour mass. Metastatectomy can also be beneficial for the patient with favourable prognostic factors which include complete resectability (e. g., solitary lung metastasis) and a long interval between initial diagnosis and development of metastases, indicating an indolent course and reinforcing the likelihood that the metastasis is truly solitary [18, 19]. Patients with favourable features can achieve a 5 year survival of 30% with metastasectomy, and thus surgical resection of metastases should be considered in highly select patients with renal cell carcinoma [20].

Non-Surgical Management of Metastatic RCC

In regards to non-surgical treatment for mRCCs, the armamentarium in the past included hormonal, chemo, radio and immunotherapies. The most successful treatment modality was immunotherapy. High-dose interleukin-2 (IL-2) and interferon-α (IFN-α) remained the standard of care for patients with mRCC [21]. However, these cytokines had a positive effect in only 10-20% of patients [22]. With the introduction of molecular targeted therapies, the clinical outcomes of these mRCC patients have improved. Before their introduction, the median overall survival for patients with RCC was around 1 year, and only 10% of patients with metastatic disease survived past 5 years [23]. By contrast, the sequential use of targeted therapies can result in a progression-free survival of up to 27 months, and an overall survival of 40 months [24]. However, despite this substantial improvement in clinical responses, treatment with these targeted agents rarely achieves complete responses, some patients do not respond at all and most patients ultimately develop resistance to therapy [25]. Therefore, there is resurgence in the use of newer chemotherapy agents or polychemotherapy, emerging immunotherapies, novel molecular agents and various combinations of chemoimmunotherapies with molecular agents to add further improvements in the clinical outcomes of patients who failed targeted therapies. In the subsequent part of this chapter we discuss resistance of mRCC, with emphasis on radio, hormonal, chemo and immunotherapies, while the issue of molecular targeted therapy is discussed elsewhere in this book.

Resistance to Radiotherapy

Renal cell carcinoma has low radiosensitivity compared to other solid organ tumours [26]. There is also no role of radiotherapy as an adjuvant therapy following nephrectomy as shown by randomized trials [27, 28]. Therefore currently, the use of radiotherapy is largely for palliation of symptoms of metastatic sites, especially in the control of pain from bone metastases and occasionally in the control of mass effect from metastases.

Resistance to Hormonal Therapy

Following the discovery of oestrogen receptors in mRCC in animal models, hormonal therapy has been applied in the clinical setting. Hormonal treatment using progestational agents such as medroxyprogesterone acetate and antioestrogen agents such as tamoxifen have been assessed for use in metastatic renal cell carcinoma [29, 30]. Some tumour regression and symptom reduction, largely applied to patients with very advanced, symptomatic carcinoma were reported. In multicentre randomised trials, uniformly low response rates were reported [31]. In current clinical practice hormonal therapy is sometimes utilized in the palliative care setting but does not seem to have any substantial antitumour effects.

Resistance to Chemotherapy

The first set of conventional chemotherapeutic agents that were used in the treatment of mRCC included fluropyrimidine derivatives (e. g. floxuridine) and vinblastine. The response rate to vinblastine alone was 3% [32]. Keeping in mind the peculiar behaviour of mRCC with a natural course ranging from a few months to several years, and a spontaneous remission rate of 5% [33], vinblastine must be regarded as ineffective.

In the 1990s, the most extensively studied drugs were floxuridine and fluorouracil (5-FU). In one trial, a 20% response rate was reported with continuous infusion of floxuridine administered according to a circadian schedule [34]. A comprehensive review on these regimens by Yagoda et al. in 1995 revealed an overall response rate of 6% among 4,093 patients with advanced mRCC who received adequate treatment, with only a slight improvement (response rate 14.6%) in a subgroup of patients who were treated with an antimetabolite (floxuridine or 5-FU) [35]. Responses were generally short, lasting a few months. Moreover, the addition of fluoruracil modulators, such as calcium folinate did not increase the response rates [36].

In 1993, Yagoda et al. [37] reviewed the role of chemotherapy in RCC and analyzed 72 cytotoxic chemotherapeutic agents used singly or in a limited number of two-drug combinations in 3502 patients, and found reports of objective responses (complete and partial remissions) in only 197 or 5.6% of patients (95% confidence interval, 4.8% to 6.4%). The authors concluded that RCC "must be considered a chemotherapeutically resistant cancer." Another review of over 50 chemotherapy trials for RCC found that no single agent produced a response rate greater than 6% [38]. Most conventional agents have proved ineffective in the treatment of mRCC with a response rate of less than 10% [35].

Molecular Mechanisms of Chemotherapy Resistance

The reasons for such chemoresistance in mRCC have been extensively studied and new knowledge of the pathways and mechanisms have been constantly added to the known old evidences of drug resistance. These pathways and molecules include: multi-drug resistance gene (MDR-1), gene product P-glycoprotein, glutathione S-transferase, topoisomerase II, loss of hypoxia-inducible factor 1α (HIF-1α) regulation, accumulation of hypoxia-inducible factor 2α (HIF-2α), and consequent Hdm2-mediated suppression of p53, expression of PKC-ς and of the L1 cell adhesion molecule (L1-CAM), overexpression of cell survival gene clusterin, of STAT1 and of the antiapoptotic gene bcl-2 have all been proven to be involved in RCC chemoresistance [39-54]. The clinical problem of MDR can be divided into two main types, one acquired during treatment and the other pre-existing at the time of diagnosis [55]. It is important to realise that multiple mechanisms are likely to contribute to clinical MDR.

Multi-Drug Resistance Molecules

Historically, the first significant advance in our understanding of MDR came with the identification of the membrane transporter P-glycoprotein, followed by that of other transporters of the ATP-binding cassette (ABC) family, which could catalyze the efflux of a range of structurally unrelated anticancer drugs. The prototypic transporter protein responsible for this phenomenon is MDR1-P-glycoprotein (MDR1-Pgp), discovered in 1976 by Juliano and Ling [56]. Overexpression of MDR1-Pgp protects kidney cancer cells and normal tissue from penetration by drugs and toxins [54, 57]. P-glycoprotein carries out an ATP-dependent conformational change that moves the substrate to the exterior of the cell [58]. At least 48 structurally related transporters, known collectively as the ABC family, have been reported [59]. Some of these transporters act directly on the drug while others act on conjugates in concert with cellular conjugating enzymes that first link the drug to glutathione, glucuronide or sulphate [55].

Another mechanism of drug resistance is impaired topoisomerase II activity, was applied to a structurally varied class of topoisomerase poisons such as doxorubicin and etoposide [60]. This further form of multidrug resistance, termed 'atypical' multidrug resistance was found to arise either from reduced expression, or from expression in a mutated form, of the enzyme topoisomerase II[alpha] and does not, therefore, involve drug transport/metabolism.

Other factors involved in MDR are lung cancer multidrug resistance protein (LRP), glutathione increase and p53 mutations. The activity of detoxifying enzymes such as glutathione-S-transferase might contribute to cellular MDR in kidney cancer [61]. Glutathione reacts enzymatically (glutathione *S*-transferase family) or non-enzymatically with toxic compounds to form glutathione conjugates. In primary human RCC cell lines, glutathione content was significantly higher and the related enzyme distinctively enhanced in resistant RCCs. Elevated intracellular glutathione levels add to resistance against doxorubicin, cisplatin, carboplatin or oxaliplatin [62]. In LRP mechanism, there is overexpression of the so-called lung resistance protein (LRP) or major vault protein. Vaults are cytoplasmic organelles that comprise a number of protein components, possibly in association with RNA. The octagonal symmetry of this organelle together with its ability to open out into a flower-like structure have suggested that its cellular function is to regulate the movement of molecules between the nucleus and cytoplasm, providing a basis for a potential drug resistance mechanism [63].

To overcome chemoresistance in kidney cancer, several MDR1-Pgp modulators have been used with the aim of reducing MDR [51, 64]. Agents such as medroxyprogesterone acetate, tamoxifen, cyclosporine and verapamil can reverse the MDR-mechanism to a certain degree, but do not enhance the response rates to cytotoxic drugs in mRCC [36]. There are two main approaches to overcoming transport MDR [65]. The first is to co-administer a drug that inhibits the action of the transporter [66] while the second is to design or utilise anticancer drugs whose activity is not significantly altered by the presence of transporters [60]. A variant of this approach is to co-administer a second drug that increases the cellular uptake of the anticancer drug: this has been examined in the case of paclitaxel through the administration of releasable octaarginine transporters [67].

Drugs reversing transport-mediated MDR are often referred to as first, second and third generation inhibitors. First generation inhibitors include verapamil, cyclosporine A, tamoxifen and calmodulin antagonists but their use involved comparatively high doses and consequent unacceptable side effects because of interaction with other cellular targets. Second generation inhibitors are generally more dose-potent and include dexverapamil, valspodar and biricodar. One of the potential problems is that the drugs inhibit cytochrome P450 activity in altered pharmacokinetics of the anticancer drugs with which they were co-administered. Third generation inhibitors are designed to overcome these disadvantages and include the drugs tariquidar, zosuquidar and laniquidar [55].

Resistance to Apoptosis

Another mechanism of resistance is the development of resistance to therapy-induced apoptosis. There are many potential mechanisms whereby tumour stem cells acquire changes that increase resistance to apoptosis [55, 68]. So far, two major apoptosis signalling pathways have been described: The extrinsic and the intrinsic apoptosis pathway [69, 70]. In both pathways, the initiator-caspase, caspase-8 plays an important role for transducing the death signal to more downstream death effectors. In the extrinsic apoptosis pathway binding of the death ligands to their corresponding receptors - including CD95, TRAIL-DR4 or TRAIL-DR5 - results in formation of the death inducing signalling complex (DISC) [71]. In the intrinsic pathway, caspase-8 cleavage is due to DNA-damage derived p53 activation which, on one hand results in transcriptional induction of death receptors including DR5 and CD95 and, on the other hand, in activation of Caspase-2, which, in turn can initiate sequential cleavage of caspase-8 [72].

Examples include inactivating mutations of the gene for p53 protein, activating mutations of the gene for PI3K, loss of expression of PTEN (a phosphatase controlling PI3K activity) and activating mutations of the genes for the RAS/RAF pathway. Modulation of these pathways affects the balance of activity of the bcl-2 family of proteins [73], which in turn control transition to apoptosis by modulating the stability of the outer mitochondrial membrane. Thus, a change in balance of bcl-2 family members can lead to a so-called permeability transition [74] where the outer mitochondrial membrane is disrupted, and proteins that are normally stored in the space between the inner and outer mitochondrial membranes are released into the cytoplasm. Induced overexpression of bcl-2 itself can also provide a mechanism of apoptosis resistance [75].

Strategies to overcome resistance to apoptosis have been studied in clinical trials and agents are being developed. Two broad strategies are involved here: first uses a drug that promotes apoptosis in combination with a cytotoxic agent to overcome an MDR, and the second uses a single agent to induce apoptosis without the need for combination therapy [55]. An example is obatoclax interferes with bcl-2 family-mediated resistance and restores sensitivity to several new anticancer drugs [76].

Hyperproliferation

Tumour growth is thought to be driven by a small population of self-renewing tumour cells [55], the so-called tumour stem cells, rather than the cells that comprised the majority of the tumour population. The tumour stem cell model, which has had increasing general acceptance, implies that the resistance properties of the tumour stem cell population will dictate overall response to therapy [55]. Stem cells appear to express multiple transport proteins of ABC family that exclude toxins and mutagens [77]. In addition, stem cells express pathways such as nuclear factor kappa B (NF-κB) and bcl-2 that protect them from the induction of apoptosis [78].

Recent Advances in Overcoming Chemotherapy Resistance

With the understanding of MDR and previous knowledge gained from conventional chemotherapy, there is renewed interest in chemotherapy and its combination with immunotherapy and targeted therapy. Three phase II trials have been performed testing capecitabine as oral monotherapy in patients with mRCC, all reporting a highly favorable tolerability profile, without significant major toxicity, suggesting a certain effectiveness of capecitabine after the failure of immunotherapy in this population. [79-81] Single-agent capecitabine has also been used in a particular population that included patients with non-clear-cell mRCC, reaching a good enrollment of individuals most of whom had papillary RCC, intermediate prognosis and had not been treated earlier. In this selected population, the overall response rate (RR) was 26%, also including complete responses (CRs), with a good median OS of 18.3 months [81]. Considering that no standard agent or combination regimen is established as an effective treatment for patients with advanced non-clear-cell RCC, in particular for those with a good or an intermediate prognosis, these findings with single-agent capecitabine represent important evidence, worthy of further investigation. Capecitabine, with more in-depth studies on selected patients with non-clear-cell RCC, could represent an effective alternative in the subset of good/intermediate-risk patient populations.

Another oral fluoropyrimidine has been explored for its activity on mRCC. In 2010, Naito et al. published the results of a phase II multicenter trial with S-1, a formulation combining tegafur (FT), 5-chloro-2,4-dihydroxypyridine, and potassium oxonate at a molar ratio of 1: 0.4: 1, in a study population of Japanese patients [82]. Considering the limitation of racial homogeneity, they reported the good tolerability profile and the effectiveness of this drug for mRCC, with an excellent response rate (RR) of 24.4%. Again, it is noteworthy that four of six patients who received sorafenib or sunitinib as previous therapy showed a partial response to chemotherapy, suggesting that patients whose disease has become resistant to targeted therapy may respond to S-1 [82].

Another study by Huang et al. explored the activity of ixabepilone, a novel microtubule-targeting agent analog to epothilone B, in patients affected by mRCC [83]. The study reported the good tolerability profile of ixabepilone, with low toxicity; the results in terms of response rates were more encouraging than those of the trials presented above, with an objective RR of 12.6%, including partial response (PR) and complete response (CR) [83].

In regards to combination chemotherapy, the most promising results as yet has been from the use of gemcitabine and capecitabine, an oral precursor of 5-flurouracil (5-FU). Multiple trials showed encouraging median overall survival (OS) and evidence of a certain activity of the regimen, with an RR of 11%. However, there were high rate of treatment discontinuation caused by the problematic toxicity observed in the study population, including Grade 3 or Grade 4 neutropenia in 45% of patients and high rates of minor toxicities, defined as persistent and unacceptable by a large percentage of treated patients and their physicians. With the dose reduction, reported a marked decrease in toxicity, without compromising the outcome in terms of results. Despite the pitfalls of comparisons across nonrandomized trials, particularly considering the heterogeneity of a disease such as mRCC, we can observe that the treatment with gemcitabine and capecitabine confirms quite good RRs and high survival rates in all published phase II studies, suggesting a certain activity on mRCC and encouraging further evaluations in selected patients after the necessary dose adjustments [84-87].

Chemotherapy has also been recently shown to be useful in the treatment of metastatic non clear cell RCCs. In 2009, Bylow et al. [88] published the results of a small phase II trial of carboplatin and paclitaxel in non-clear-cell RCC. With the assumption of the absence of standard care for patients with papillary mRCC, they included 16 patients with papillary histology and one patient with collecting duct RCC in the study. This last patient was unique because of a complete response of disease, with no better response other than stable disease in the rest of the treated population; the trial was closed after interim analysis showed minimal activity of the regimen in the study population. The authors concluded that the use of carboplatin and paclitaxel in patients with collecting duct tumors appears to warrant further investigation, whereas for the papillary histology, they suggested focusing efforts on the use of targeted therapies in future studies.

Sarcomatoid differentiation in mRCC tumours represent a difficult subset to treat as they are often characterized by rapid tumour growth and clinical deterioration with lack of response to cytokine treatment thus very poor prognosis. The regimen of doxorubicine and gemcitabine has been tested in patients with sarcomatoid features in various trials with promising results [89, 90]. Evidence provided by these studies has finally endorsed the approval of the chemotherapeutic regimen with doxorubicin and gemcitabine as an option included by guidelines for first-line therapy of renal cell cancer for patients with relapsed or medically unresectable stage IV disease with sarcomatoid histology [91].

Combination chemoimmunotherapy works by the synergistic premise that modulation of immune system by cytokine therapy can induce better response to cytotoxic drugs. Various chemotherapy agents such as gemcitabine, 5-FU were combined with IL-2 and IFN-α and modest results were obtained. One randomized prospective trial established the improved long-term therapeutic efficacy of IL-2 plus IFN-α based outpatient chemoimmunotherapies in comparison with IFN-α/ vinblastine on a large controlled multicenter basis; and also showed that the addition of 13-cis-retinoic acid does not confer considerable benefit to the present chemoimmunotherapy regimen [92]. A phase II trial was conducted by Sunela and colleagues [93] on 26 patients to evaluate the efficacy, tolerability, and safety of capecitabine and pegylated IFN-α combination. The overall RR was 27%. These data were confirmed by Padrik et al. [94] in a phase II study that tested the combination of capecitabine and IFN-α as a first-line treatment; the overall RR was 24%, with a median survival time of 248 days, suggesting the need for randomized trials to confirm the efficacy of adding capecitabine to IFN-α.

A retrospective study was carried out in mRCC patients treated with chemotherapy alone (gemcitabine and 5-FU) or chemotherapy plus low-dose IL-2 and IFN-α [95]. Overall time to progression (TTP) was 3.2 months and the median overall survival was 9.2 months; although not statistically significant, the response and disease control were better in pretreated patients, with a favorable trend for time to progression and OS, suggesting that previous immunotherapy treatment may increase the tumor cells' sensitivity to subsequent chemotherapy. The authors concluded that both chemotherapy and chemoimmunotherapy showed modest but definite activity and a chemotherapy-based regimen should be offered to patients with progressive mRCC [95].

Combination of chemotherapy with antiangiogenic targeted agents has also been extensively studied. Jonasch and colleagues showed combination of gemcitabine plus capecitabine with bevacizumab (anti-VEGF monoclonal antibody) provided potential efficacy and acceptable tolerability, in particular, in patients with intermediate and poor prognosis mRCC [96]. A recent study also investigated the role of sorafenib, a multikinase inhibitor, in mRCC in association with gemcitabine combined with metronomic capecitabine. The authors obtained a PFS of 12 months and a median OS of 25.8 months, with an objective RR of 50% and a disease control rate of 92%; these results support the hypothesis that chemo-switch (maximum tolerated dose plus metronomic) chemotherapy plus the inhibition of VEGF and platelet-derived growth factor have synergistic activity with manageable adverse events [97]. There are also several ongoing studies which include combination of mTOR inhibitor (everolimus) with cyclophosphamide (available at: http://www.clinicaltrial.gov, NCT01462214) and combination of sunitinib with gemcitabine (available at: http://www.clinicaltrial.gov, NCT00556049).

Future clinical trials of chemotherapy and combination with other agents together with further experimental insights into the molecular pathways will provide further hope for achieving better clinical outcomes for patients with mRCC.

Immunotherapy

RCC is a highly immunogenic tumour. Until the introduction of targeted therapy a few years ago, immunotherapy with IL-2 or IFN-α had been the mainstay of treatment for mRCC [98]. High-dose IL-2 was approved by the U.S. Food and Drug Administration for front-line treatment of advanced RCC in 1992 following publication of the results of seven phase II studies that had enrolled 255 patients affected by stage IV RCC [99]. The overall RR was 14% (90% CI, 10%–19%) with 5% complete responses and 9% partial responses; with median overall survival (OS) was 16.3 months. However, the treatment was associated with severe adverse events. Young and fit patients who tolerated the regime fared better with high dose IL-2. A dose reduction of IL-2 combined with IFN-α combination therapy was studied in a few studies [100-103]. The frequency and severity of side effects were reduced and the RR appeared somewhat similar to high dose IL-2.

IFN-α alone has been less extensively studied in advanced RCC. Several phase II studies have shown only modest antitumor activity with a response rate not exceeding 15% [104]. Moreover, although more favorable than that of IL-2, the toxicity profile of IFN-α can affect patients' quality of life [105].

Thus with the reasonable responses to immunotherapy in the past coupled with the inevitable failure with long term targeted agents, there is renewed interest in further development and use of immunotherapeutics. Various novel immunotherapeutics approaches have been studied in clinical trials and preclinical stages. These include dendritic cell based immunotherapy, gene modified tumour vaccine therapy, peptide based therapy, nonmyeloablative stem cell transplantation and regulatory T cells (treg cells). Phase I/II trials of vaccination with allogeneic dendritic cell/tumour fusions in patients with mRCC have demonstrated immunological and clinical responses in some patients [106, 107].

T-cell modulating agents (e. g. antibodies against programmed death 1 and cytotoxic T lymphocyte-associated antigen-4, or soluble lymphocyte activation gene-3) and dendritic cell-activating toll-like receptor agonists have also shown encouraging evidence of efficacy in early-phase clinical trials [108, 109]. These early studies suggest that immunotherapy may continue to be an effective approach for patients with mRCC. As such, a number of other strategies are currently under investigation, including adoptive cell transfer (ACT) with T cells modified to target proteins expressed by renal tumours such as MAGE-A3/12, DR4 and TRAIL, and ACT with autologous natural killer cells [110]. To realise the full benefit for patients, it is likely that immunotherapy will need to be combined with targeted agents or other agents. Novel therapies used in combination or sequentially have the potential to improve outcomes in mRCC, and results from ongoing/planned trials will shape future therapy.

Conclusion

Treatment of mRCC has come a long way from the humble beginnings of conventional monochemotherapy and radiotherapy that were largely ineffective against this disease, to the comforting limited but effective immunotherapy and now in the era of molecular targeted therapy which has provided effective clinical outcomes albeit inevitably not sustained responses or cure. However, these are exciting times as mentioned above, with numerous new therapeutic approaches involving chemotherapy, immunotherapy and targeted therapy being evaluated and constantly improved. Novel agents either working singly or in combination with the above therapeutics regimens targeting alternative pathways are also being developed with ongoing clinical trials. Efforts are also underway in developing predictive biomarkers via research to overcome some of the challenges of clinical efficacy and further advance the care of RCC patients. It is hoped that in the future, individualised, specific and effective therapy can be applied to patients with mRCC based on their unique tumour characteristics. Ultimate goal in the treatment of mRCC will always be patient centred with improved clinical responses, lesser toxicities and better quality of life.

References

[1] Davis C. J. Jr., Mostofi F. K., (1995). Sesterhenn IA. Renal medullary carcinoma. The seventh sickle cell nephropathy. *The American Journal of Surgical Pathology*. 1, 1-11.

[2] Cheville J. C., Lohse C. M., Zincke H., Weaver A. L., Leibovich B. C., Frank I. et al., (2004). Sarcomatoid renal cell carcinoma: an examination of underlying histologic subtype and an analysis of associations with patient outcome. *The American Journal of Surgical Pathology*. 28, 435-41.

[3] Farrow G. M., Harrison E. G. Jr., Utz D. C., ReMine W. H., (1968). Sarcomas and sarcomatoid and mixed malignant tumors of the kidney in adults. *I. Cancer*. 22, 545-50.

[4] Motzer R. J., Bacik J., Mariani T., Russo P., Mazumdar M., Reuter V., (2002). Treatment outcome and survival associated with metastatic renal cell carcinoma of non-clear-cell histology. *Journal of Clinical Oncology*. 20, 2376-81.

[5] Lee J. E., Hunter D. J., Spiegelman D., Adami H. O., Bernstein L., van den Brandt P. A. et al., (2007). Intakes of coffee, tea, milk, soda and juice and renal cell cancer in a pooled analysis of 13 prospective studies. *International Journal of Cancer*. 121, 2246-53.

[6] Rashidkhani B., Lindblad P., Wolk A., (2005). Fruits, vegetables and risk of renal cell carcinoma: a prospective study of Swedish women. *International Journal of Cancer*. 113, 451-5.

[7] McCredie M., Pommer W., McLaughlin J. K., Stewart J. H., Lindblad P., Mandel J. S. et al., (1995). International renal-cell cancer study. II. Analgesics. *International Journal of Cancer*. 60, 345-9.

[8] Parkin D. M., Bray F., Ferlay J., Pisani P., (2005). Global cancer statistics, 2002. *CA: a Cancer Journal for Clinicians*. 55, 74-108.

[9] Uzzo R. G., Novick A. C., (2001). Nephron sparing surgery for renal tumors: indications, techniques and outcomes. *The Journal of Urology*. 166, 6-18.

[10] Frank I., Blute M. L., Cheville J. C., Lohse C. M., Weaver A. L., Zincke H., (2003). Solid renal tumors: an analysis of pathological features related to tumor size. *The Journal of Urology*. 170, 2217-20.

[11] Remzi M., Ozsoy M., Klingler H. C., Susani M., Waldert M., Seitz C. et al., (2006). Are small renal tumorsn harmless? Analysis of histopathological features according to tumors 4 cm or less in diameter. *The Journal of Urology*. 176, 896-9.

[12] Chawla S. N., Crispen P. L., Hanlon A. L., Greenberg R. E., Chen D. Y., Uzzo R. G., (2006). The natural history of observed enhancing renal masses: meta-analysis and review of the world literature. *The Journal of Urology*. 175, 425-31.

[13] van Poppel H., Becker F., Cadeddu J. A., Gill I. S., Janetschek G., Jewett M. A. et al., (2011). Treatment of localised renal cell carcinoma. *European Urology*. 60, 662-72.

[14] Flanigan R. C., Mickisch G., Sylvester R., Tangen C., van Poppel H., Crawford E. D., (2004). Cytoreductive nephrectomy in patients with

metastatic renal cancer: a combined analysis. *The Journal of Urology*. 171, 1071-6.

[15] Flanigan R. C., Salmon S. E., Blumenstein B. A., Bearman S. I., Roy V., McGrath P. C. et al., (2001). Nephrectomy followed by interferon alfa-2b compared with interferon alfa-2b alone for metastatic renal-cell cancer. *The New England Journal of Medicine*. 345, 1655-9.

[16] Mickisch G. H., Garin A., van Poppel H. de Prijck L., Sylvester R., European Organisation for R. et al., (2001). Radical nephrectomy plus interferon-alfa-based immunotherapy compared with interferon alfa alone in metastatic renal-cell carcinoma: a randomised trial. *Lancet*. 358, 966-70.

[17] Rini B. I., Campbell S. C., (2007). The evolving role of surgery for advanced renal cell carcinoma in the era of molecular targeted therapy. *The Journal of Urology*. 177, 1978-84.

[18] Murthy S. C., Kim K., Rice T. W., Rajeswaran J., Bukowski R., de Camp M. M. et al., (2005). Can we predict long-term survival after pulmonary metastasectomy for renal cell carcinoma? *The Annals of Thoracic Surgery*. 79, 996-1003.

[19] Pfannschmidt J., Hoffmann H., Muley T., Krysa S., Trainer C,, Dienemann H., (2002). Prognostic factors for survival after pulmonary resection of metastatic renal cell carcinoma. *The Annals of Thoracic Surgery*. 74, 1653-7.

[20] Rini B. I., Campbell S. C., Escudier B., (2009). Renal cell carcinoma. *Lancet*. 373, 1119-32.

[21] Rosenberg S. A., Lotze M. T., Muul L. M., Chang A. E., Avis FP, Leitman S, et al., (1987). A progress report on the treatment of 157 patients with advanced cancer using lymphokine-activated killer cells and interleukin-2 or high-dose interleukin-2 alone. *The New England Journal of Medicine*. 316, 889-97.

[22] Leibovich B. C., Han K. R., Bui M. H., Pantuck A. J., Dorey F. J., Figlin R. A. et al., (2003). Scoring algorithm to predict survival after nephrectomy and immunotherapy in patients with metastatic renal cell carcinoma: a stratification tool for prospective clinical trials. *Cancer*. 98, 2566-75.

[23] Gupta K., Miller J. D., Li J. Z., Russell M. W., Charbonneau C., (2008). Epidemiologic and socioeconomic burden of metastatic renal cell carcinoma (mRCC): a literature review. *Cancer Treatment Reviews*. 34, 193-205.

[24] Escudier B., Goupil M. G., Massard C., Fizazi K., (2009). Sequential therapy in renal cell carcinoma. *Cancer*. 115, 2321-6.

[25] Bergers G., Hanahan D., (2008). Modes of resistance to anti-angiogenic therapy. *Nature Reviews Cancer*. 8, 592-603.

[26] Withers H. R., Mason K. A., Thames H. D. Jr., (1986). Late radiation response of kidney assayed by tubule-cell survival. *The British Journal of Radiology*. 59, 587-95.

[27] Kjaer M., Frederiksen P. L., Engelholm S. A., (1987). Postoperative radiotherapy in stage II and III renal adenocarcinoma. A randomized trial by the Copenhagen Renal Cancer Study Group. *International Journal of Radiation Oncology, Biology, Physics*. 13, 665-72.

[28] Finney R. The value of radiotherapy in the treatment of hypernephroma - a clinical trial., (1973). *British Journal of Urology*. 45, 258-69.

[29] Papac R. J., Ross S. A., Levy A., (1977). Renal cell carcinoma: analysis of 31 cases with assessment of endocrine therapy. *The American Journal of the Medical Sciences*. 274, 281-90.

[30] Pizzocaro G., di Fronzo G., Cappelletti V., Piva L., Salvioni R., Ronchi E. et al., (1983). Hormone treatment and sex steroid receptors in metastatic renal cell carcinoma: report of a multicentric prospective study. *Tumori*. 69, 215-20.

[31] Medical Research Council Renal Cancer Collaborators., (1999). Interferon-alpha and survival in metastatic renal carcinoma: early results of a randomised controlled trial. *Lancet*. 353, 14-7.

[32] Fossa S. D., Droz J. P., Pavone-Macaluso M. M., Debruyne F. J., Vermeylen K., Sylvester R., (1992) Vinblastine in metastatic renal cell carcinoma: EORTC phase II trial 30882. The EORTC Genitourinary Group. *European Journal of Cancer*. 28A, 878-80.

[33] Pyrhonen S., Salminen E., Ruutu M., Lehtonen T., Nurmi M., Tammela T. et al., (1999). Prospective randomized trial of interferon alfa-2a plus vinblastine versus vinblastine alone in patients with advanced renal cell cancer. *Journal of Clinical Oncology*. 17, 2859-67.

[34] Hrushesky W. J., von Roemeling R., Lanning R. M., Rabatin J. T., (1990). Circadian-shaped infusions of floxuridine for progressive metastatic renal cell carcinoma. *Journal of Clinical Oncology*. 8, 1504-13.

[35] Yagoda A, Abi-Rached B., Petrylak D., (1995). Chemotherapy for advanced renal-cell carcinoma: 1983-1993. *Seminars in Oncology*. 22, 42-60.

[36] Lilleby W., Fossa S. D., (2005). Chemotherapy in metastatic renal cell cancer. *World Journal of Urology*. 23, 175-79.
[37] Yagoda A., Petrylak D., Thompson S., (1993). Cytotoxic chemotherapy for advanced renal cell carcinoma. *The Urologic Clinics of North America*. 20, 303-21.
[38] Amato R. J., (2000). Chemotherapy for renal cell carcinoma. *Seminars in Oncology*. 27, 177-86.
[39] Carbonaro M., Escuin D., O'Brate A., Thadani-Mulero M., Giannakakou P., (2012). Microtubules regulate hypoxia-inducible factor-1alpha protein trafficking and activity: implications for taxane therapy. *The Journal of Biological Chemistry*. 287, 11859-69.
[40] Pu Y. S., Huang C. Y., Chen J. Y., Kang W. Y., Lin Y. C., Shiu Y. S. et al., (2012). Down-regulation of PKCzeta in renal cell carcinoma and its clinicopathological implications. *Journal of Biomedical Science*. 19, 39.
[41] Zhu H., Wang Z., Xu Q., Zhang Y., Zhai Y., Bai J. et al., (2012). Inhibition of STAT1 sensitizes renal cell carcinoma cells to radiotherapy and chemotherapy. *Cancer Biology & Therapy*. 13, 401-7.
[42] Vasko R., Mueller G. A., von Jaschke A. K., Asif A. R., Dihazi H., (2011). Impact of cisplatin administration on protein expression levels in renal cell carcinoma: a proteomic analysis. *European Journal of Pharmacology*. 670, 50-7.
[43] Doberstein K., Wieland A., Lee S. B., Blaheta R. A., Wedel S., Moch H. et al., (2011). L1-CAM expression in ccRCC correlates with shorter patients survival times and confers chemoresistance in renal cell carcinoma cells. *Carcinogenesis*. 32, 262-70.
[44] Walsh N., Larkin A., Kennedy S., Connolly L., Ballot J., Ooi W. et al., (2009). Expression of multidrug resistance markers ABCB1 (MDR-1/P-gp) and ABCC1 (MRP-1) in renal cell carcinoma. *BMC Urology*. 9,6.
[45] Roberts A. M., Watson I. R., Evans A. J., Foster D. A., Irwin M. S., Ohh M., (2009). Suppression of hypoxia-inducible factor 2alpha restores p53 activity via Hdm2 and reverses chemoresistance of renal carcinoma cells. *Cancer Research*. 69, 9056-64.
[46] Sato H., Senba H., Virgona N., Fukumoto K., Ishida T., Hagiwara H. et al., (2007). Connexin 32 potentiates vinblastine-induced cytotoxicity in renal cell carcinoma cells. *Molecular Carcinogenesis*. 46, 215-24.
[47] Kausch I., Jiang H., Thode B., Doehn C., Kruger S., Jocham D., (2005). Inhibition of bcl-2 enhances the efficacy of chemotherapy in renal cell carcinoma. *European Urology*. 47, 703-9.

[48] Oudard S., Levalois C., Andrieu J. M., Bougaran J., Validire P., Thiounn N. et al., (2002). Expression of genes involved in chemoresistance, proliferation and apoptosis in clinical samples of renal cell carcinoma and correlation with clinical outcome. *Anticancer Research*. 22, 121-8.

[49] Zellweger T., Miyake H., July L. V., Akbari M., Kiyama S., Gleave M. E., (2001). Chemosensitization of human renal cell cancer using antisense oligonucleotides targeting the antiapoptotic gene clusterin. *Neoplasia*. 3, 360-7.

[50] Kim W. J., Kakehi Y., Kinoshita H., Arao S., Fukumoto M., Yoshida O., (1996). Expression patterns of multidrug-resistance (MDR1), multidrug resistance-associated protein (MRP), glutathione-S-transferase-pi (GST-pi) and DNA topoisomerase II (Topo II) genes in renal cell carcinomas and normal kidney. *The Journal of Urology*. 156, 506-11.

[51] Mickisch G. H., Noordzij M. A., vd Gaast A., Gebreamlack P., Kohrmann K. U., Mogler-Drautz E. et al., (1995). Dexverapamil to modulate vinblastine resistance in metastatic renal cell carcinoma. *Journal of Cancer Research and Clinical Oncology*. 121, 11-6.

[52] Motzer R. J., Lyn P., Fischer P., Lianes P., Ngo R. L., Cordon-Cardo C., et al., (1995). Phase I/II trial of dexverapamil plus vinblastine for patients with advanced renal cell carcinoma. *Journal of Clinical Oncology*. 13, 1958-65.

[53] Volm M., Kastel M., Mattern J., Efferth T., (1993). Expression of resistance factors (P-glycoprotein, glutathione S-transferase-pi, and topoisomerase II) and their interrelationship to proto-oncogene products in renal cell carcinomas. *Cancer*. 71, 3981-7.

[54] Mickisch G. H., (1994). Chemoresistance of renal cell carcinoma: 1986-1994. *World Journal of Urology*. 12, 214-23.

[55] Baguley B. C., (2010). Multiple drug resistance mechanisms in cancer. *Molecular Biotechnology*. 46, 308-16.

[56] Juliano R. L., Ling V., (1976). A surface glycoprotein modulating drug permeability in Chinese hamster ovary cell mutants. *Biochimica et Biophysica Acta*. 455, 152-62.

[57] Ford J. M., Yang J. M., Hait W. N., (1996). P-glycoprotein-mediated multidrug resistance: experimental and clinical strategies for its reversal. *Cancer Treatment and Research*. 87, 3-38.

[58] Ling V., (1997). Multidrug resistance: molecular mechanisms and clinical relevance. *Cancer Chemotherapy and Pharmacology*. 40, S3-8.

[59] Gillet J. P., Efferth T., Remacle J., (2007). Chemotherapy-induced resistance by ATP-binding cassette transporter genes. *Biochimica et Biophysica Acta*. 1775, 237-62.

[60] Baguley B. C., (2002). Novel strategies for overcoming multidrug resistance in cancer. *Bio Drugs: Clinical Immunotherapeutics, Biopharmaceuticals and Gene Therapy*. 16, 97-103.

[61] Anderson M. E., (1998). Glutathione: an overview of biosynthesis and modulation. *Chemico-Biological Interactions*. 111-112, 1-14.

[62] Mickisch G., Bier H., Bergler W., (1999). P-170 glycoprotein, glutathione and associated enzymes in relation to chemoresistance of primary human renal cell carcinomas. *Urologia Internationalis*. 45, 170-6.

[63] Chugani D. C., Rome L. H., Kedersha N. L., (1993). Evidence that vault ribonucleoprotein particles localize to the nuclear pore complex. *J Cell Sci*. 106, 23-9

[64] Braybrooke J. P., Vallis K. A., Houlbrook S., Rockett H., Ellmen J., Anttila M. et al., (2000). Evaluation of toremifene for reversal of multidrug resistance in renal cell cancer patients treated with vinblastine. *Cancer Chemotherapy and Pharmacology*. 46, 27-34.

[65] Ozben T., (2006). Mechanisms and strategies to overcome multiple drug resistance in cancer. *FEBS letters*. 580, 2903-9.

[66] Szakacs G., Paterson J. K., Ludwig J. A., Booth-Genthe C., Gottesman M. M., (2006). Targeting multidrug resistance in cancer. *Nature Reviews Drug Discovery*. 5, 219-34.

[67] Dubikovskaya E. A., Thorne S. H., Pillow T. H., Contag C. H., Wender P. A., (2008). Overcoming multidrug resistance of small-molecule therapeutics through conjugation with releasable octaarginine transporters. *Proceedings of the National Academy of Sciences of the United States of America*. 105, 12128-33.

[68] Hanahan D., Weinberg R. A., (2000). The hallmarks of cancer. *Cell*. 100, 57-70.

[69] Gerharz C. D., Ramp U., Dejosez M. et al., (1999). Resistance to CD95 (APO-1/Fas)-mediated apoptosis in human renal cell carcinomas: an important factor for evasion from negative growth control. *Lab Invest*. 79, 1521–1534.

[70] Ramp U., Dejosez M., Mahotka C. et al., (2000). Deficient activation of CD95 (APO-1/Fas)-mediated apoptosis: a potential factor of multidrug resistance in human renal cell carcinoma. *Br J Cancer*. 82, 1851–1859.

[71] Wang S., El-Deiry W. S., (2003). TRAIL and apoptosis induction by TNF-family death receptors. *Oncogene*. 22, 8628–8633.

[72] Lin C. F., Chen C. L., Chang W. T. et al., (2004). Sequential caspase-2 and caspase-8 activation upstream of mitochondria during ceramide and etoposide-induced apoptosis. *J Biol Chem*. 279, 40755–40761.

[73] Danial N. N., (2007). BCL-2 family proteins: critical checkpoints of apoptotic cell death. *Clinical Cancer Research*.13, 7254-63.

[74] Forte M., Bernardi P., (2006). The permeability transition and BCL-2 family proteins in apoptosis: co-conspirators or independent agents? *Cell Death and Differentiation*. 13, 1287-90.

[75] Osford S. M., Dallman C. L., Johnson P. W., Ganesan A., Packham G., (2004). Current strategies to target the anti-apoptotic Bcl-2 protein in cancer cells. *Current Medicinal Chemistry*. 11, 1031-9.

[76] Nguyen M., Marcellus R. C., Roulston A., Watson M., Serfass L., Murthy Madiraju S. R. et al., (2007). Small molecule obatoclax (GX15-070) antagonizes MCL-1 and overcomes MCL-1-mediated resistance to apoptosis. *Proceedings of the National Academy of Sciences of the United States of America*. 104, 19512-7.

[77] Huls M., Russel F. G., Masereeuw R., (2009).The role of ATP binding cassette transporters in tissue defense and organ regeneration. *The Journal of Pharmacology and Experimental Therapeutics*. 328, 3-9.

[78] Turco M. C., Romano M. F., Petrella A., Bisogni R., Tassone P., Venuta S. (2004). NF-kappaB/Rel-mediated regulation of apoptosis in hematologic malignancies and normal hematopoietic progenitors. *Leukemia*. 18, 11-7.

[79] Wenzel C., Locker G. J., Bartsch R., Pluschnig U., Mader R., Hussian D. et al., (2003). Capecitabine monotherapy and in combination with immunotherapy in the treatment of metastatic renal cell carcinoma. *Anti-cancer Drugs*. 14, 779-84.

[80] Petrioli R., Paolelli L., Francini E., Marsili S., Pascucci A., Sciandivasci A. et al., (2007). Capecitabine as third-line treatment in patients with metastatic renal cell carcinoma after failing immunotherapy. *Anti-cancer Drugs*. 18, 817-20.

[81] Tsimafeyeu I., Demidov L., Kharkevich G., Petenko N., Galchenko V., Sinelnikov I. et al., (2012). Phase II, multicenter, uncontrolled trial of single-agent capecitabine in patients with non-clear cell metastatic renal cell carcinoma. *American Journal of Clinical Oncology*. 35, 251-4.

[82] Naito S., Eto M., Shinohara N., Tomita Y., Fujisawa M., Namiki M. et al., (2010). Multicenter phase II trial of S-1 in patients with cytokine-

refractory metastatic renal cell carcinoma. *Journal of Clinical Oncology*. 28, 5022-9.

[83] Huang H., Menefee M., Edgerly M., Zhuang S., Kotz H., Poruchynsky M. et al., (2010). A phase II clinical trial of ixabepilone (Ixempra; BMS-247550; NSC 710428), an epothilone B analog, in patients with metastatic renal cell carcinoma. *Clinical Cancer Research*. 16, 1634-41.

[84] Waters J. S., Moss C., Pyle L., James M., Hackett S., A'Hern R. et al., (2004). Phase II clinical trial of capecitabine and gemcitabine chemotherapy in patients with metastatic renal carcinoma. *British Journal of Cancer*. 91, 1763-8.

[85] Stadler W. M., Halabi S., Rini B., Ernstoff M. S., Davila E., Picus J. et al., (2006). A phase II study of gemcitabine and capecitabine in metastatic renal cancer: a report of Cancer and Leukemia Group B protocol 90008. *Cancer*. 107, 1273-9.

[86] Tannir N. M., Thall P. F., Ng C. S., Wang X., Wooten L., Siefker-Radtke A. et al., (2008). A phase II trial of gemcitabine plus capecitabine for metastatic renal cell cancer previously treated with immunotherapy and targeted agents. *The Journal of Urology*. 180, 867-72.

[87] van Veldhuizen P. J., Hussey M., Lara P. N., Jr., Mack P. C., Gandour-Edwards R., Clark J. I. et al., (2009). A phase II study of gemcitabine and capecitabine in patients with advanced renal cell cancer: Southwest Oncology Group Study S0312. *American Journal of Clinical Oncology*. 32, 453-9.

[88] Bylow K. A., Atkins M. B., Posadas E. M., Stadler W. M., McDermott D. F., (2009). Phase II trial of carboplatin and paclitaxel in papillary renal cell carcinoma. *Clinical Genitourinary Cancer*. 7, 39-42.

[89] Nanus D. M., Garino A., Milowsky M. I., Larkin M., Dutcher J. P., (2004). Active chemotherapy for sarcomatoid and rapidly progressing renal cell carcinoma. *Cancer*. 101, 1545-51.

[90] Haas N. B., Lin X., Manola J., Pins M., Liu G., McDermott D. et al., (2012). A phase II trial of doxorubicin and gemcitabine in renal cell carcinoma with sarcomatoid features: ECOG 8802. *Medical Oncology*. 29, 761-7.

[91] Motzer R. J., Agarwal N., Beard C., Bhayani S., Bolger G. B., Buyyounouski M. K., (2012). NCCN Clinical Practice Guidelines in Oncology. *Kidney Cancer*. 1, 8-22.

[92] Atzpodien J., Kirchner H., Rebmann U., Soder M., Gertenbach U., Siebels M. et al., (2006). Interleukin-2/interferon-alpha2a/13-retinoic

acid-based chemoimmunotherapy in advanced renal cell carcinoma: results of a prospectively randomised trial of the German Cooperative Renal Carcinoma Chemoimmunotherapy Group (DGCIN). *British Journal of Cancer*. 95, 463-9.

[93] Sunela K. L., Koskinen S., Kellokumpu-Lehtinen P. L., (2010). A phase-II study of combination of pegylated interferon alfa-2a and capecitabine in locally advanced or metastatic renal cell cancer. *Cancer Chemotherapy and Pharmacology*. 66, 59-67.

[94] Padrik P., Leppik K., Arak A., (2004). Combination therapy with capecitabine and interferon alfa-2A in patients with advanced renal cell carcinoma: a phase II study. *Urologic Oncology*. 22, 387-92.

[95] Buti S., Brighenti M., Bongiovanni C., Buzio C., Chiesa M. D., Alberici F. et al., (2007). Role of chemotherapy with gemcitabine plus 5-fluorouracil and chemoimmunotherapy in metastatic renal cell cancer (mRCC). *Journal of Immunotherapy*. 30, 780-6.

[96] Jonasch E., Lal L. S., Atkinson B. J., Byfield S. D., Miller L. A., Pagliaro L. C. et al., (2011).Treatment of metastatic renal carcinoma patients with the combination of gemcitabine, capecitabine and bevacizumab at a tertiary cancer centre. *BJU International*. 107, 741-7.

[97] Bellmunt J., Trigo J. M., Calvo E., Carles J., Perez-Gracia J. L., Rubio J. et al., (2010). Activity of a multitargeted chemo-switch regimen (sorafenib, gemcitabine, and metronomic capecitabine) in metastatic renal-cell carcinoma: a phase 2 study (SOGUG-02-06). *The Lancet Oncology*. 11, 350-7.

[98] Itsumi M., Tatsugami K., (2010). Immunotherapy for renal cell carcinoma. *Clinical & Developmental Immunology*. 2010, 284581.

[99] Fyfe G., Fisher R. I., Rosenberg S. A., Sznol M., Parkinson D. R., Louie A. C., (1995). Results of treatment of 255 patients with metastatic renal cell carcinoma who received high-dose recombinant interleukin-2 therapy. *Journal of Clinical Oncology*. 13, 688-96.

[100] Dutcher J. P., Atkins M., Fisher R., Weiss G., Margolin K., Aronson F. et al., (1997). Interleukin-2-based therapy for metastatic renal cell cancer: the Cytokine Working Group experience, 1989-1997. *The Cancer Journal from Scientific American*. 3, S73-8.

[101] Dutcher J. P., Fisher R. I., Weiss G., Aronson F., Margolin K., Louie A., et al. (1997). Outpatient subcutaneous interleukin-2 and interferon-alpha for metastatic renal cell cancer: five-year follow-up of the Cytokine Working Group Study. *The Cancer Journal from Scientific American*. 3, 157-62.

[102] Dutcher J. P., Logan T., Gordon M., Sosman J., Weiss G., Margolin K. et al., (2000). Phase II trial of interleukin 2, interferon alpha, and 5-fluorouracil in metastatic renal cell cancer: a cytokine working group study. *Clinical Cancer Research*. 6, 3442-50.

[103] Negrier S., Caty A., Lesimple T., Douillard J. Y., Escudier B., Rossi J. F. et al., (2000). Treatment of patients with metastatic renal carcinoma with a combination of subcutaneous interleukin-2 and interferon alfa with or without fluorouracil. Groupe Francais d'Immunotherapie, Federation Nationale des Centres de Lutte Contre le Cancer. *Journal of Clinical Oncology*. 18, 4009-15.

[104] Atkins M. B., Regan M., McDermott D., (2004). Update on the role of interleukin 2 and other cytokines in the treatment of patients with stage IV renal carcinoma. *Clinical Cancer Research*. 10, 6342S-6S.

[105] Basso M., Cassano A., Barone C., (2010). A survey of therapy for advanced renal cell carcinoma. *Urol Oncol*. 28, 121-33.

[106] Therapeutics A., (2011). New phase 2 data showing Arcelis immunotherapy AGS-003 in combination with sunitinib improves progression free survival in patients with advanced renal cell carcinoma. www.argostherapeutics.com/pdfs/news_release_posterepre- sentation ASCO-final.pdf2011.

[107] Figlin R. A., Nicollete C. A., Amin A., (2011). Monitoring T-cell responses in a phase IIstudy of AGS-003, an autologous dnedritic cell-based therapy in patients with newly diagnosed advanced stage renal cell carcinoma in combination with sunitinib. *Journal of Clinical Oncology*. 29, 2532.

[108] Chambers C. A., Kuhns M. S., Egen J. G., Allison J. P., (2001). CTLA-4-mediated inhibition in regulation of T cell responses: mechanisms and manipulation in tumor immunotherapy. *Annual Review of Immunology*. 19, 565-94.

[109] Keir M. E., Butte M. J., Freeman G. J., Sharpe A. H., (2008). PD-1 and its ligands in tolerance and immunity. *Annual Review of Immunology*. 26, 677-704.

[110] Escudier B., (2012). Emerging immunotherapies for renal cell carcinoma. *Annals of Oncology*. 23, 35-40.

In: Advances in Drug Resistance Research ISBN: 978-1-63117-131-4
Editor: Christudas Morais

Chapter 8

Resistance of Renal Cell Carcinoma to Targeted Therapy

Retnagowri Rajandram [*1, 2, 5], ***Teng Aik Ong*** [1] ***and Marniza Saad*** [3, 4]

[1] Department of Surgery, Faculty of Medicine, University of Malaya, Kuala Lumpur, Malaysia
[2] Centre for Kidney Disease Research, University of Queensland,Brisbane, Australia
[3] Clinical Oncology Unit, University Malaya Medical Centre, Kuala Lumpur, Malaysia
[4] Faculty of Medicine, University of Malaya, Kuala Lumpur, Malaysia
[5] University of Malaya Cancer Research Institute, University of Malaya, Kuala Lumpur, Malaysia

Abstract

Targeted therapy has replaced immunotherapy as the standard of care for metastatic renal cell carcinoma (RCC). Currently available targeted agents include multi- tyrosine kinase inhibitors (axitinib, sunitinib, sorafenib and pazopanib), mammalian target of rapamycin (mTOR) kinase inhibitors (temsirolimus and everolimus) and bevacizumab, a

* Author for Correspondence: retnagowri@gmail.com. This work was supported by Fundamental Research Grant Scheme, Malaysia; ID: FRGS FP012-2013B.

humanized monoclonal antibody against vascular endothelial growth factor (VEGF). Despite the beneficial clinical outcomes, resistance to therapy is emerging as a new challenge. Resistance to therapy can be either intrinsic or extrinsic (acquired). About 30% of patients have intrinsic resistant and almost all patients who respond initially will develop acquired resistance within 12 months of treatment. In this chapter, we summarize the current challenges of drug resistance in the effective treatment of metastatic RCC with particular emphasis on targeted therapies.

Keywords: Renal cell carcinoma, resistance, targeted therapy, multi-tyrosine kinase, mTOR

Introduction

Renal cell carcinoma (RCC), thought to arise from the epithelial cells of the renal tubules [1], are a heterogeneous group of diseases. They are highly metastatic, and account for about 3% of all adult malignancies [2, 3]. Clear cell carcinoma is the predominant subtype (70-80%), followed by papillary (10-15%), chromophobe (5%) and collecting duct (<1%) carcinomas [1, 4]. Metastatic RCC is highly resistant to conventional radio and immunotherapies. The field of RCC study has undergone a revolution in the past decade, largely because of our understanding of the role of the von-Hippel Lindau (VHL) gene in RCC biology. The VHL gene mutations are the most important risk factors for the development of RCC. A functional VHL degrades hypoxia inducible factor-1 alpha (HIF-1α). In the absence of a functional VHL, either through mutations or hyper-methylation, HIF-1α is stabilized, leading to the transcriptional activation of over 300 genes, especially pro-angiogenic factors such as vascular endothelial growth factor (VEGF), its tyrosine kinase receptors (VEGF-R1-3) and platelet-derived growth factor (PDGF) (Figure 1) [5, 6].

VEGF binds to VEGF-R1 and VEGF-R2, and promotes angiogenesis through endothelial cell proliferation, migration and vascular permeability [7]. Elucidation of these molecular pathways has led to the development of VEGF and multi-tyrosine kinase inhibitors as summarized in Figure 2 and Table 1.

Mammalian Target of Rapamycin (MTOR) Inhibitors

Mammalian target of rapamycin (mTOR) is a serine/threonine protein kinase that regulates cell growth, proliferation, motility and survival [5]. It is composed of two molecular complexes: mTORC1 and mTORC2 [30]. mTORC1 can be activated by many factors including VEGFR, PDGFR, EGFR and IGFR through the PI3K/Akt pathway [31].

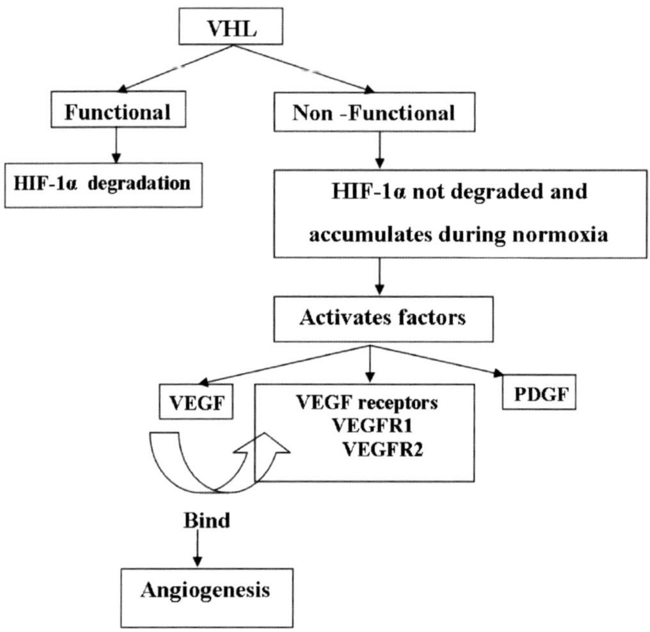

Figure 1. Schema of the role of VHL in angiogenesis of RCC. A non-functional VHL gene leads to the stabilization of HIF-1α and subsequent activation of angiogenesis [7].

Activated mTORC1 regulates cyclin D, m-Myc and other proteins involved in cell proliferation through the disassociation of 4E binding protein-1 (4E-BP1) and eukaryotic initiation factor-4 subunit E (EIF-4E) [32, 33]. mTORC2, through protein kinase Cα, regulates cell morphology and adhesion [8, 34] (Figure 3). mTOR activity is enhanced in RCC [35-37]. The two major mTOR inhibitors in clinical practice are temsirolimus and everolimus. Their mode of action is summarized in Figure 3 and Table 2 [36].

Resistance to Targeted Therapy

Despite the availability of the novel targeted therapeutics, and the promising clinical outcomes, nearly all patients with metastases will develop resistance to treatment.

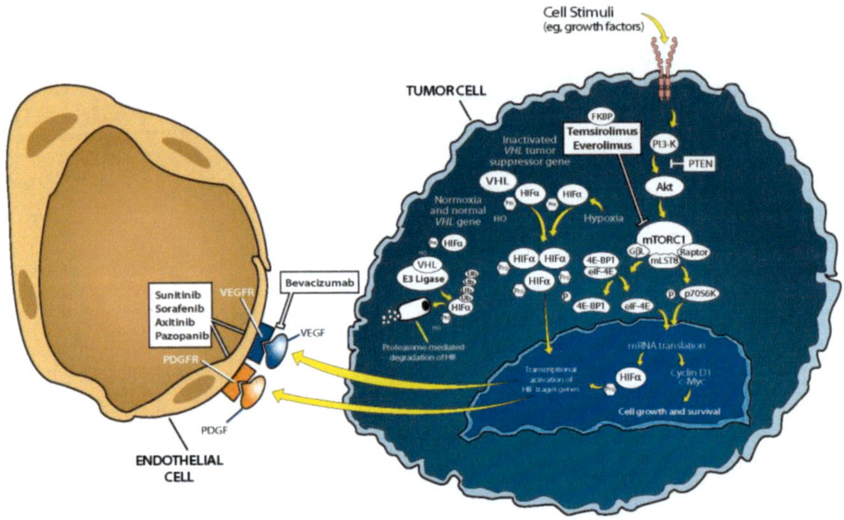

Figure 2. An overview of the VHL-HIF-VEGF pathway in RCC and the mode of action of targeted therapy. A functional *VHL gene* targets hypoxia-inducible factor (HIF)-α for proteolysis. When the *VHL* gene is inactivated, either through mutations, hyper-methylations or loss of heterozygosity, HIF is stabilised, activated and translocated to the nucleus, where it binds to HIF-responsive elements leading to the transcription of many hypoxia-inducible genes, including VEGF, mTOR and platelet-derived growth factor (PDGF). The binding sites of the targeted therapies on VEGF, mTOR and TKI pathways are emphasized. *FKBP, FK binding protein; PI3K, phosphoinositide 3-kinase; AKT, protein kinase B; mTORC1/2, mammalian target of rapamycin complex 1 or 2; mLST8, mammalian lethal with SEC13 protein 8; 4E-BP1, 4E binding protein-1; eIF-4E, eukaryotic initiation factor-4 subunit E; VEGFR, vascular endothelial growth factor receptor; PDGFR, platelet-derived growth factor receptor; Pro, proline; P, phosphorous; Ub, Ubiquitin; FGF, fibroblast growth factor; IL-8, interleukin-8; PTEN, phosphatase and tensin homologue; P70S6K, P70S6 kinase, TKI, tyrosine kinase inhibitor.* Modified from (8).

Approximately 30% of patients are intrinsically resistant to therapy [42] and almost all patients who initially respond to therapy will eventually develop extrinsic or acquired resistance. In intrinsic or primary resistance, tumors do not respond to targeted therapy from the beginning of the treatment. Extrinsic resistance is the result of adaptive mechanisms to the action of angiogenesis inhibitors leading to the re-emergence of tumor angiogenesis [5, 43].

Table 1. Summary of currently available VEGF inhibitors and TKI for the treatment of metastatic RCC

Drug	Mechanism	Outcome
Vascular endothelial growth factor (VEGF) monoclonal antibody		
Bevacizumab (Avastin®, Genentech Inc.)	Binds and neutralizes all biologically active isoforms of VEGF [2, 9, 10]	Predominantly used in combination with interferon-alpha (IFN-α); median overall survival 18.3-23.3months; overall response rate, 25.5% [11-13]
Multi-tyrosine kinase inhibitors		
Sunitinib (SUTENT®, Pfizer Inc.)	Inhibits PDGFR-α and β, c-KIT, FLT-3, VEGFR1-3, CSF-1R and neurotropic factor receptor [14-16]	Standard first-line of therapy; median overall survival, 26.4 months; objective response rate, 31-47% [11, 17, 18]
Sorafenib (Nexavar®, Bayer HealthCare/Onyx Pharmaceuticals)	Inhibits VEGFR 1-3,PDGFRα & β and Raf kinase, RET [19]	First or second line of therapy; overall survival 12.5-17.8 months; response rate 40%; stable disease 80% [11, 20, 21, 22]
Pazopanib (Votrient®, GlaxoSmithKline)	Inhibits VEGFR 1-3, PDGFR α & β and c-KIT [23, 24]	Objective response rate 30-31%; progression free survival 9.2-13 months [11, 24, 25]
Axitinib (Pfizer Inc.)	Inhibits VEGFRs 1 and 2, PDGFRβ and c-KIT [26, 27]	Overall response rate 44.2%; median overall survival 20·1-29.9 months; [11, 28, 29]

While the mechanisms of intrinsic resistance are largely elusive, the understanding of the extrinsic or acquired resistance is rapidly expanding. In a nutshell, the acquired resistance to targeted therapy can be summarized under four categories: activated alternative angiogenic pathways, inadequate target inhibition, up-regulation of HIF, and faulty mTOR pathway as illustrated in Figure 4 [7, 8, 42].

Alternative Pro-Angiogenic Pathways in Drug Resistance

One of the mechanisms of resistance to targeted therapy is the activation of VEGF-independent alternate angiogenic pathways. The emerging consensus is that these alternate angiogenic pathways activate a variety of pro-angiogenic factors, which would compensate for the inhibited VEGF signalling and promote angiogenesis [5, 42].

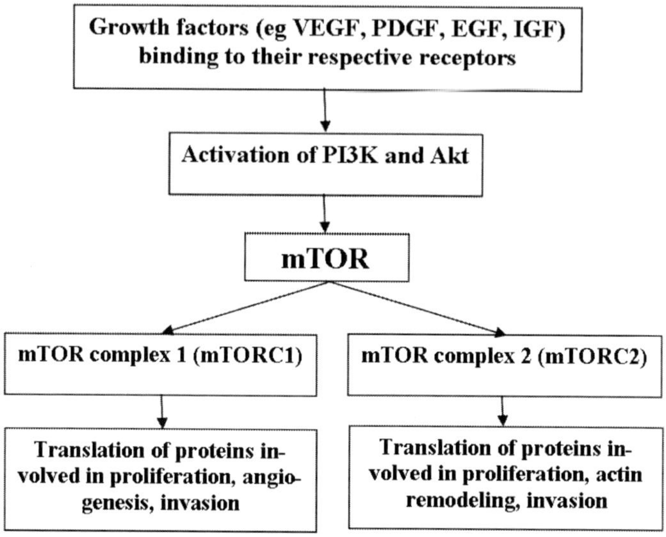

Figure 3. Overview of the role of mTOR in RCC progression [7]. *PI3K, phosphoinositide 3-kinase; AKT, protein kinase B; mTORC1/2, mammalian target of rapamycin complex 1 or 2; VEGF, vascular endothelial growth factor; PDGF, platelet-derived growth factor; IGF, Insulin-like growth factor; EGF, Epidermal growth factor.*

For example, the proposed mechanism of sunitinib resistance includes the activation or up-regulation of FGF-s, ephrins and angiopoietins, and for sorafenib, the recruitment of pro-angiogenic bone marrow-derived cells and monocytes to the tumor site [5, 42, 43]. The recruitment of pericytes that help to maintain vessels permeable and functional, and prevent endothelial cells from being affected by anti-angiogenic therapies, is the proposed mechanisms of resistance to pazopanib [44]. For bevacizumab, the increased potential of tumor cells to invade without the need of neovascularization is thought to be the mechanism [7, 43].

It is well-known that interleukin-8 (IL-8) is a potent pro-angiogenic factor and a prognostic factor for RCC. Emerging data show that IL-8 is also a key player in the development of resistance to sunitinib.

Table 2. mTOR inhibitors in clinical practice

Drug	Mechanism	Outcome
Temsirolimus (Torisel®, Pfizer Inc.)	Inhibits *VHL*/HIF/VEGF and PI3K/AKT/mTOR pathways [32, 38] [5, 39].	Second line of treatment after sunitinib [40, 41]; overall survival10.9 months; median progression-free survival 3.8-5.5 months; objective response rate 8.6%; stable disease 32.1% [11, 22, 35]
Everolimus (Afinitor®, Novartis Pharmaceuticals)	Inhibits mTOR serine-threonine kinase [37]	Second line of treatment after sunitinib or sorafenib; median progression free survival 4-4.9 months; median overall survival 14.8months; stable disease 66.8% [11, 36, 37]

In a xenograft model of RCC, increased IL-8 secretion was associated with reactivation of tumor angiogenesis and subsequent resistance to sunitinib [36, 45]. Administration of IL-8 neutralizing antibody re-sensitized the tumors to sunitinib. Furthermore, elevated IL-8 expression was found in RCC patients who did not respond to sunitinib [36, 45].

Angiopoietin-2 (Ang-2) and sphingosine kinase are potent pro-angiogenic agents. It is emerging that they also play crucial roles in conferring resistance to sunitinib. Ang-2 and SIP are decreased at the initiation of sunitinib treatment. However, with the development of resistance, their expression and activation are significantly increased [42]. Neutralizing antibodies against sphingosine kinase have been shown to reverse resistance in animal models of RCC [42]. Down-regulation of angiostatic factors is another mechanism of resistance to TKIs. Treatment with sunitinib and sorafenib decreases the expression of several IFN-γ inducible molecules including the angiostatic chemokines CXCL 10 and CXCL 11 [42, 46, 47]. Furthermore, recruitment of bone marrow-derived cells, especially CD11b + GR1 + myeloid cells, to the tumour site, enables the development of resistance to sunitinib [42]. In other instances invasion of tumour cells into normal tissue and the recruitment by these invaded tumour cells of normal tissue vasculature protect them from anti-angiogenic therapy [46-48].

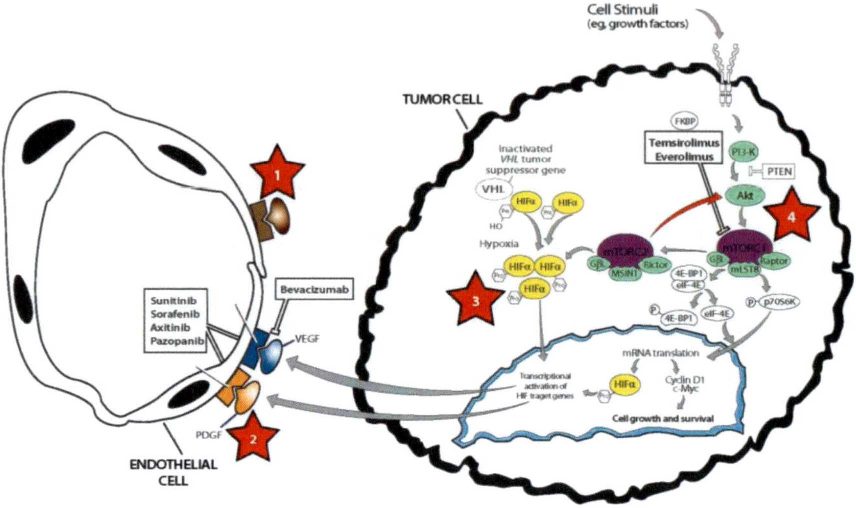

Figure 4. Mechanisms of resistance to targeted therapy. Resistance to targeted therapy can be summarised under four broad categories: (1) up-regulation of alternative angiogenic pathways (e.g. FGF, PDGF & IL8); (2) ineffective target inhibition due to reduced drug levels and/or enhanced receptor signaling; (3) up-regulation of HIF due to sustained VEGF blockade; and (4) up-regulation of mTORC2 in response to sustained mTORC1 inhibition, largely mediated by increased P13K and AKT activity. Modified from [8].

Inadequate Target Inhibition and Resistance to Therapy

Although research into this aspect of drug resistance is still in its infancy, there is emerging data that inadequate target inhibition could be a player in resistance to axitinib, sunitinib and sorafenib [49-51]. Inadequate target inhibition can be either due to enhanced receptor signalling or reduced intracellular drug levels (Figure 4). Over time, physiological changes can lead to reduced plasma concentrations of the drugs that in turn lead to resistance through inadequate inhibition of the VEGFR signalling. These data, although support the concept of physiological resistance, fail to identify dose-escalation as the best clinical strategy for overcoming resistance.

Therapy-Mediated VEGF Up-Regulation in Drug Resistance

VEGFR inhibition in clear cell RCC patients leads to a significant increase in serum VEGF levels within the first few weeks of treatment as seen with bevacizumab. However it has been shown that the amount of available unbound bevacizumab is sufficient to adsorb this excess VEGF [52]. It has been hypothesised that this increase reflects effective VEGFR blockade and that an intracellular or intercellular feedback loop leads to greater HIF activity and more VEGF production. If this increase reflects the degree to which VEGFR are inhibited, as opposed to a macroscopic effect on tumour blood vessel architecture leading to increased tumor hypoxia and HIF activation, then one might expect greater increases in VEGF would associate with improved clinical outcome [53, 54]. However, this does not appear to be the case. The emerging consensus regarding the significant rise in VEGF levels following VEGFR inhibition is that tumor progression might in time be mediated by overcoming incomplete receptor inhibition or stimulation of lower affinity VEGFR. Although experimental evidence may be lacking, animal models of tumor angiogenesis (not in RCC) show that VEGF or VEGFR inhibition leads to increased production of PDGF and FGF by tumours. PDGF up-regulation may be addressed by the cross reactivity to PDGFRβ inherent with sorafenib and sunitinib but pro-angiogenic growth factors including basic bFGF, transforming growth factor β (TGFβ), hepatocyte growth factor (HGF) Ang, and ephrins may mediate tumor escape in the face of VEGF and VEGFR inhibition [9, 54, 55].

Faulty Mammalian Target of Rapamycin (MTOR) Pathway in Drug Resistance

mTOR plays a critical role in tumour angiogenesis [32, 56-59]. Temsirolimus, exerts its inhibitory effects on both the tumor and endothelial cells [35]. The mechanisms of resistance to mTOR inhibition may be quite distinct compared to that observed with VEGF-targeted therapy [32, 60]. It has been proposed that acquired resistance is the result of activation of feedback loops that promotes cell survival through the activation of mTORC2, IGF and extracellular signal-regulated kinase/mitogen-activated protein kinase (ERK/MAPK) signaling pathway [43, 61]. The rapamycin analogs inhibit only one of the two signaling complexes of which mTOR is a part. TORC1 is inhibited by temsirolimus and other rapamycin analog mTOR inhibitors, whereas TORC2 is not [38]. As a result, part of the downstream mTOR activation is unopposed. It has been demonstrated in preclinical studies that mTOR inhibition with rapamycin analogs results in feedback up-regulation of the PI3K pathway, assessed by activation of Akt, which is more proximal in the PI3K pathway than mTOR. This is analogous to VEGF up-regulation in the setting of VEGF receptor blockade. Because Akt can activate the TORC2 complex, which is not inhibited in rapamycin analogs, it is possible that the up-regulation of this pathway compensates for TORC1 inhibition in tumors that are refractory to temsirolimus [42, 43, 60, 62]. Other proposed mechanisms of resistance to mTOR are redundant signaling pathways including KRAS or BRAF mutations and loss of PTEN [5, 42].

Advances in Overcoming Resistance to Targeted Therapy

The approaches that have been employed to overcome resistance to targeted therapy are summarized in Table 3. In a nutshell, the available evidence suggests that the use of a second TKI after the failure of the first could 'reset' the tumor microenvironment and overcome resistance [43]. Apart from the approaches described in Table 3, there is emerging evidence that a third line of treatment may restore the sensitivity to the initial treatment [5-7, 63-65]. That is, re-challenging with VEGF-TKI as a third line of treatment after the failures of VEGF-TKI as a first line and mTOR inhibitors as a second line. [7]. Ferrari and team compared the administration of mTOR inhibitors everolimus or temsirolimus as a third line therapy, and illustrated them to be promising treatment options [66]. Di Lorenzo et al. showed that sorafenib could be considered as a third line of treatment for metastatic RCC after the failure on sunitinib and mTOR inhibitor, however, with adverse events such as hand-foot syndrome, anaemia, fatigue, diarrhoea and neutropenia [63].

Future Directions

Currently, patients with metastatic RCC can obtain benefit from multiple lines of targeted therapy. Resistance to TKI and mTOR inhibitors seem to be at least partially reversible. Re-challenging with the inhibitors from the same group in subsequent lines of therapy may be a therapeutic option if toxicity does not limit it. Tailoring treatment to a particular patient is of utmost importance [5, 6, 64].

Table 3. Current approaches to overcome RCC resistance to targeted therapies

Approach	Description	References
Alternating dose	Scheduling 4 weeks on drug and 2 weeks off drug (e.g. sunitinib); re-challenging the same drug after a discontinuation period (e.g. sorafenib)	[36, 42]
Combined TKI and immunotherapy	Sunitinib and sorafenib with or without IFN-α	[67, 68]
New agents	Dovitinib alone or in combination with VEGF-TKI/mTOR inhibitors; Tivozanib	[69, 70]
Combination therapy		
– Two TKIs together	Combination of temsirolimus and sunitinib	[39, 42, 43]
– mTOR inhibitor after first line TKI	Sunitinib followed by everolimus	[35, 64, 68, 71,72]
– TKIs after first line anti VEGF	Sunitinib or sorafenib after bevacizumab	[5, 43]
– Second line VEGF TKI after first line VEGF-TKI	Sorafenib after sunitinib	[5-7, 43, 64, 73]

Below are some possible interventions that could improve treatment outcome for metastatic RCCs.

Fourth-Line Therapy Regimens

Even though no clinical guidelines exist for a fourth-line targeted therapy, some reports suggest that patients may gain clinical benefit of sequential targeted agents with different mechanisms of action. Up to 48 months of progression-free survival was achieved in metastatic RCC patients treated with four lines of targeted therapies (sunitinib, everolimus, sorafenib, and temsirolimus), advocating use of the sunitinib, everolimus, sorafenib and temsirolimus for better treatment outcome and overcoming resistance [7, 51, 73].

New Agents

Novel agents that modulate c-MET and Ang/Tie-2 may be effective in overcoming drug resistance. c-MET is a significant player in papillary RCC [74, 75] and c-MET inhibitors such as tivantinib and cabozantinib hold potential as either first or second line therapy [76-79]. Ang/Tie 2 signaling axis is a well-known promoter of angiogenesis. Metastatic RCC is positively associated with circulating Ang-2, making it an interesting therapeutic target [80]. For example, the Ang-2 inhibitors AMG386, CVX060 and CVX241 have been shown to be effective in pre-clinical models of RCC (81-83). The PI3K pathway is related with poor prognosis and serine/threonine Akt kinase is a critical player downstream from PI3K and crucial for cell survival. BKM-120 is a pan-class I PI3K inhibitor, and has undergone phase I trial in combination with bevacizumab (84). Moreover the Akt inhibitor MK2206 is also in phase II clinical trial [85].

Conclusion

Despite the immense advancement, resistance to targeted therapy is emerging as a major hurdle for the treatment of metastatic RCC. Defining the mechanisms and pathways of resistance to therapy will help develop methods to overcome therapy resistance. Many issues remain unanswered and open in this emerging field. Further research will shed more light into the mechanisms of drug resistance, and enable the development of better therapeutics for the treatment of metastatic RCC.

References

[1] Curti B.D., (2004) Renal cell carcinoma. *JAMA,*292:(1), 97-100.

[2] Amato R.J., (2005) Renal cell carcinoma: review of novel single-agent therapeutics and combination regimens. *Ann Oncol,*16:(1), 7-15.

[3] Gupta K., Miller J.D., Li J.Z., Russell M.W., Charbonneau C., (2008) Epidemiologic and socioeconomic burden of metastatic renal cell carcinoma (mRCC): a literature review. *Cancer Treat Rev,*34:(3), 193-205.

[4] Morais C., Gobe G., Johnson D.W., Healy H., (2011) The emerging role of nuclear factor kappa B in renal cell carcinoma. *Int J Biochem Cell Biol,*43:(11), 1537-49.

[5] Gonzalez Larriba J.L., Espinosa E., Garcia Carbonero I., Garcia-Donas J., Lopez M., Meana A., Puente J., Bellmunt J., (2012) Sequential therapy in metastatic renal cell carcinoma: pre-clinical and clinical rationale for selecting a second- or subsequent-line therapy with a different mechanism of action. *Cancer Metastasis Rev,*31 Suppl 1 S11-7.

[6] Porta C., Szczylik C., Escudier B., (2012) Combination or sequencing strategies to improve the outcome of metastatic renal cell carcinoma patients: a critical review. *Crit Rev Oncol Hematol,*82:(3), 323-37.

[7] Oudard S., Elaidi R.T., (2012) Sequential therapy with targeted agents in patients with advanced renal cell carcinoma: optimizing patient benefit. *Cancer Treat Rev,*38:(8), 981-7.

[8] Rini B.I., Atkins M.B., (2009) Resistance to targeted therapy in renal-cell carcinoma. *Lancet Oncol,*10:(10), 992-1000.

[9] Hegde P.S., Jubb A.M., Chen D., Li N.F., Meng Y.G., Bernaards C., Elliott R., Scherer S.J., Chen D.S., (2013) Predictive impact of circulating vascular endothelial growth factor in four phase III trials evaluating bevacizumab. *Clin Cancer Res,*19:(4), 929-37.

[10] Presta L.G., Chen H., O'Connor S.J., Chisholm V., Meng Y.G., Krummen L., Winkler M., Ferrara N., (1997) Humanization of an anti-vascular endothelial growth factor monoclonal antibody for the therapy of solid tumors and other disorders. *Cancer Res,*57:(20), 4593-9.

[11] Administration U.S.F.a.D. FDA Approved Drug Products. 2013.

[12] Escudier B., Bellmunt J., Negrier S., Bajetta E., Melichar B., Bracarda S., Ravaud A., Golding S., Jethwa S., Sneller V., (2010) Phase III trial of bevacizumab plus interferon alfa-2a in patients with metastatic renal cell carcinoma (AVOREN): final analysis of overall survival. *J Clin Oncol,*28:(13), 2144-50.

[13] Rini B.I., Halabi S., Rosenberg J.E., Stadler W.M., Vaena D.A., Archer L., Atkins J.N., Picus J., Czaykowski P., Dutcher J., Small E.J., (2010) Phase III trial of bevacizumab plus interferon alfa versus interferon alfa monotherapy in patients with metastatic renal cell carcinoma: final results of CALGB 90206. *J Clin Oncol,*28:(13), 2137-43.

[14] Gale N.W., Yancopoulos G.D., (1999) Growth factors acting via endothelial cell-specific receptor tyrosine kinases: VEGFs, angiopoietins, and ephrins in vascular development. *Genes Dev,*13:(9), 1055-66.

[15] Mendel D.B., Laird A.D., Xin X., Louie S.G., Christensen J.G., Li G., Schreck R.E., Abrams T.J., Ngai T.J., Lee L.B., Murray L.J., Carver J., Chan E., Moss K.G., Haznedar J.O., Sukbuntherng J., Blake R.A., Sun L., Tang C., Miller T., Shirazian S., McMahon G., Cherrington J.M., (2003) In vivo antitumor activity of SU11248, a novel tyrosine kinase inhibitor targeting vascular endothelial growth factor and platelet-derived growth factor receptors: determination of a pharmacokinetic/pharmacodynamic relationship. *Clin Cancer Res,*9:(1), 327-37.

[16] Rajagopalan S., Mohler E., 3rd, Lederman R.J., Saucedo J., Mendelsohn F.O., Olin J., Blebea J., Goldman C., Trachtenberg J.D., Pressler M., Rasmussen H., Annex B.H., Hirsch A.T., (2003) Regional Angiogenesis with Vascular Endothelial Growth Factor (VEGF) in peripheral arterial disease: Design of the RAVE trial. *Am Heart J,*145:(6), 1114-8.

[17] Motzer R.J., Hutson T.E., Tomczak P., Michaelson M.D., Bukowski R.M., Oudard S., Negrier S., Szczylik C., Pili R., Bjarnason G.A., Garcia-del-Muro X., Sosman J.A., Solska E., Wilding G., Thompson J.A., Kim S.T., Chen I., Huang X., Figlin R.A., (2009) Overall survival and updated results for sunitinib compared with interferon alfa in patients with metastatic renal cell carcinoma. *J Clin Oncol,*27:(22), 3584-90.

[18] Motzer R.J., Hutson T.E., Tomczak P., Michaelson M.D., Bukowski R.M., Rixe O., Oudard S., Negrier S., Szczylik C., Kim S.T., Chen I., Bycott P.W., Baum C.M., Figlin R.A., (2007) Sunitinib versus interferon alfa in metastatic renal-cell carcinoma. *N Engl J Med,*356:(2), 115-24.

[19] Flaherty K.T., (2007) Sorafenib: delivering a targeted drug to the right targets. *Expert Rev Anticancer Ther,*7:(5), 617-26.

[20] Escudier B., Eisen T., Stadler W.M., Szczylik C., Oudard S., Staehler M., Negrier S., Chevreau C., Desai A.A., Rolland F., Demkow T., Hutson T.E., Gore M., Anderson S., Hofilena G., Shan M., Pena C.,

Lathia C., Bukowski R.M., (2009) Sorafenib for treatment of renal cell carcinoma: Final efficacy and safety results of the phase III treatment approaches in renal cancer global evaluation trial. *J Clin Oncol,*27:(20), 3312-8.

[21] Stadler W.M., Figlin R.A., McDermott D.F., Dutcher J.P., Knox J.J., Miller W.H., Jr., Hainsworth J.D., Henderson C.A., George J.R., Hajdenberg J., Kindwall-Keller T.L., Ernstoff M.S., Drabkin H.A., Curti B.D., Chu L., Ryan C.W., Hotte S.J., Xia C., Cupit L., Bukowski R.M., (2010) Safety and efficacy results of the advanced renal cell carcinoma sorafenib expanded access program in North America. *Cancer,*116:(5), 1272-80.

[22] Agency E.M. Science Medicine Health 2013. Available from: http://www.ema.europa.eu/ema/.

[23] Hutson T.E., Bukowski R.M., Cowey C.L., Figlin R., Escudier B., Sternberg C.N., (2011) Sequential use of targeted agents in the treatment of renal cell carcinoma. *Critical Reviews in Oncology Hematology,*77:(1), 49-63.

[24] Hutson T.E., Davis I.D., Machiels J.P., De Souza P.L., Rottey S., Hong B.F., Epstein R.J., Baker K.L., McCann L., Crofts T., Pandite L., Figlin R.A., (2010) Efficacy and safety of pazopanib in patients with metastatic renal cell carcinoma. *J Clin Oncol,*28:(3), 475-80.

[25] Sternberg C.N., Davis I.D., Mardiak J., Szczylik C., Lee E., Wagstaff J., Barrios C.H., Salman P., Gladkov O.A., Kavina A., Zarba J.J., Chen M., McCann L., Pandite L., Roychowdhury D.F., Hawkins R.E., (2010) Pazopanib in locally advanced or metastatic renal cell carcinoma: results of a randomized phase III trial. *J Clin Oncol,*28:(6), 1061-8.

[26] Escudier B., Gore M., (2011) Axitinib for the management of metastatic renal cell carcinoma. *Drugs R D,*11:(2), 113-26.

[27] Kessler E.R., Bowles D.W., Flaig T.W., Lam E.T., Jimeno A., (2012) Axitinib, a new therapeutic option in renal cell carcinoma. *Drugs Today (Barc),*48:(10), 633-44.

[28] Motzer R.J., Escudier B., Tomczak P., Hutson T.E., Michaelson M.D., Negrier S., Oudard S., Gore M.E., Tarazi J., Hariharan S., Chen C., Rosbrook B., Kim S., Rini B.I., (2013) Axitinib versus sorafenib as second-line treatment for advanced renal cell carcinoma: overall survival analysis and updated results from a randomised phase 3 trial. *Lancet Oncol,*14:(6), 552-62.

[29] Rini B.I., de La Motte Rouge T., Harzstark A.L., Michaelson M.D., Liu G., Grunwald V., Ingrosso A., Tortorici M.A., Bycott P., Kim S., Bloom

J., Motzer R.J., (2013) Five-year survival in patients with cytokine-refractory metastatic renal cell carcinoma treated with axitinib. *Clin Genitourin Cancer,*11:(2), 107-14.

[30] Wullschleger S., Loewith R., Hall M.N., (2006) TOR signaling in growth and metabolism. *Cell,*124:(3), 471-84.

[31] Gossage L., Eisen T., (2010) Targeting multiple kinase pathways: a change in paradigm. *Clin Cancer Res,*16:(7), 1973-8.

[32] Land S.C., Tee A.R., (2007) Hypoxia-inducible factor 1alpha is regulated by the mammalian target of rapamycin (mTOR) via an mTOR signaling motif. *J Biol Chem,*282:(28), 20534-43.

[33] Mazzoletti M., Bortolin F., Brunelli L., Pastorelli R., Di Giandomenico S., Erba E., Ubezio P., Broggini M., (2011) Combination of PI3K/mTOR inhibitors: antitumor activity and molecular correlates. *Cancer Res,*71:(13), 4573-84.

[34] Banumathy G., Cairns P., (2010) Signaling pathways in renal cell carcinoma. *Cancer Biol Ther,*10:(7), 658-64.

[35] Hudes G., Carducci M., Tomczak P., Dutcher J., Figlin R., Kapoor A., Staroslawska E., Sosman J., McDermott D., Bodrogi I., Kovacevic Z., Lesovoy V., Schmidt-Wolf I.G., Barbarash O., Gokmen E., O'Toole T., Lustgarten S., Moore L., Motzer R.J., (2007) Temsirolimus, interferon alfa, or both for advanced renal-cell carcinoma. *N Engl J Med,*356:(22), 2271-81.

[36] Motzer R.J., Escudier B., Oudard S., Hutson T.E., Porta C., Bracarda S., Grunwald V., Thompson J.A., Figlin R.A., Hollaender N., Kay A., Ravaud A., (2010) Phase 3 trial of everolimus for metastatic renal cell carcinoma : final results and analysis of prognostic factors. *Cancer,*116:(18), 4256-65.

[37] Motzer R.J., Escudier B., Oudard S., Hutson T.E., Porta C., Bracarda S., Grunwald V., Thompson J.A., Figlin R.A., Hollaender N., Urbanowitz G., Berg W.J., Kay A., Lebwohl D., Ravaud A., (2008) Efficacy of everolimus in advanced renal cell carcinoma: a double-blind, randomised, placebo-controlled phase III trial. *Lancet,*372:(9637), 449-56.

[38] Flaherty K.T., Puzanov I., (2010) Building on a foundation of VEGF and mTOR targeted agents in renal cell carcinoma. *Biochem Pharmacol,*80:(5), 638-46.

[39] Bellmunt J., (2007) Current treatment in advanced renal cell carcinoma (RCC): Impact of targeted therapies in the management of RCC. *European Urology Supplements,*6:(7), 484-91.

[40] Gerullis H., Bergmann L., Maute L., Ecke T.H., Eimer C., Bagner J.W., Otto T., (2010) Feasibility of sequential use of sunitinib and temsirolimus in advanced renal cell carcinoma. *Med Oncol,*27:(2), 373-8.

[41] Grundbichler M., Mlineritsch B., Ressler S., Moik M., Kappacher A., Rosenlechner S., Greil R., (2011) Efficacy of temsirolimus after previous treatment with sunitinib, sorafenib or everolimus in advanced renal cell cancer. *Oncology,*80:(1-2), 34-41.

[42] Ravaud A., Gross-Goupil M., (2012) Overcoming resistance to tyrosine kinase inhibitors in renal cell carcinoma. *Cancer Treat Rev,*38:(8), 996-1003.

[43] Rini B.I., (2010) New strategies in kidney cancer: therapeutic advances through understanding the molecular basis of response and resistance. *Clin Cancer Res,*16:(5), 1348-54.

[44] Larriba J.L.G, Espinosa E, Carbonero I.C., García-Donas J, López M, Meana A, Puente J, J B., (2012) Sequential therapy in metastatic renal cell carcinoma: pre-clinical and clinical rationale for selecting a second- or subsequent-line therapy with a different mechanism of action. *Cancer and Metastasis Reviews,*31:(1), 11-7.

[45] Huang D., Ding Y., Zhou M., Rini B.I., Petillo D., Qian C.N., Kahnoski R., Futreal P.A., Furge K.A., Teh B.T., (2010) Interleukin-8 mediates resistance to antiangiogenic agent sunitinib in renal cell carcinoma. *Cancer Res,*70:(3), 1063-71.

[46] Cowey C.L., Hutson T.E., (2010) Molecularly targeted agents for renal cell carcinoma: the next generation. *Clin Adv Hematol Oncol,*8:(5), 357-60, 61-4.

[47] Figlin R.A., Kaufmann I., Brechbiel J., (2013) Targeting PI3K and mTORC2 in metastatic renal cell carcinoma: new strategies for overcoming resistance to VEGFR and mTORC1 inhibitors. *Int J Cancer,*133:(4), 788-96.

[48] Khattak M., Larkin J., (2013) Sequential therapy with targeted agents in metastatic renal cell carcinoma: beyond second-line and overcoming drug resistance. *World J Urol.*

[49] Gross-Goupil M., Massard C., Ravaud A., (2012) Targeted therapies in metastatic renal cell carcinoma: overview of the past year. *Curr Urol Rep,*13:(1), 16-23.

[50] Lombardi G., Zustovich F., Donach M., Dalla Palma M., Nicoletto O., Pastorelli D., (2012) An update on targeted therapy in metastatic renal cell carcinoma. *Urol Oncol,*30:(3), 240-6.

[51] Afonso F.J., Anido U., Fernandez-Calvo O., Vazquez-Estevez S., Leon L., Lazaro M., Ramos M., Anton-Aparicio L., (2013) Comprehensive overview of the efficacy and safety of sorafenib in advanced or metastatic renal cell carcinoma after a first tyrosine kinase inhibitor. *Clin Transl Oncol,*15:(6), 425-33.

[52] Gordon M.S., Margolin K., Talpaz M., Sledge G.W., Jr., Holmgren E., Benjamin R., Stalter S., Shak S., Adelman D., (2001) Phase I safety and pharmacokinetic study of recombinant human anti-vascular endothelial growth factor in patients with advanced cancer. *J Clin Oncol,*19:(3), 843-50.

[53] Bose D., Meric-Bernstam F., Hofstetter W., Reardon D.A., Flaherty K.T., Ellis L.M., (2010) Vascular endothelial growth factor targeted therapy in the perioperative setting: implications for patient care. *Lancet Oncol,*11:(4), 373-82.

[54] Rini B.I., Flaherty K., (2008) Clinical effect and future considerations for molecularly-targeted therapy in renal cell carcinoma. *Urol Oncol,*26:(5), 543-9.

[55] Gore M.E., Larkin J.M., (2011) Challenges and opportunities for converting renal cell carcinoma into a chronic disease with targeted therapies. *Br J Cancer,*104:(3), 399-406.

[56] Thomas G.V., Tran C., Mellinghoff I.K., Welsbie D.S., Chan E., Fueger B., Czernin J., Sawyers C.L., (2006) Hypoxia-inducible factor determines sensitivity to inhibitors of mTOR in kidney cancer. *Nat Med,*12:(1), 122-7.

[57] Wilhelm S.M., Adnane L., Newell P., Villanueva A., Llovet J.M., Lynch M., (2008) Preclinical overview of sorafenib, a multikinase inhibitor that targets both Raf and VEGF and PDGF receptor tyrosine kinase signaling. *Molecular cancer therapeutics,*7:(10), 3129-40.

[58] Hamada K., Sasaki T., Koni P.A., Natsui M., Kishimoto H., Sasaki J., Yajima N., Horie Y., Hasegawa G., Naito M., Miyazaki J., Suda T., Itoh H., Nakao K., Mak T.W., Nakano T., Suzuki A., (2005) The PTEN/PI3K pathway governs normal vascular development and tumor angiogenesis. *Genes Dev,*19:(17), 2054-65.

[59] Riesterer O., Zingg D., Hummerjohann J., Bodis S., Pruschy M., (2004) Degradation of PKB/Akt protein by inhibition of the VEGF receptor/mTOR pathway in endothelial cells. *Oncogene,*23:(26), 4624-35.

[60] Inoki K., Guan K.L., (2006) Complexity of the TOR signaling network. *Trends Cell Biol,*16:(4), 206-12.

[61] Fisher R., Larkin J., Swanton C., (2011) Delivering preventive, predictive and personalised cancer medicine for renal cell carcinoma: the challenge of tumour heterogeneity. *EPMA J*,3:(1), 1.

[62] Inoki K., Ouyang H., Zhu T., Lindvall C., Wang Y., Zhang X., Yang Q., Bennett C., Harada Y., Stankunas K., Wang C.Y., He X., MacDougald O.A., You M., Williams B.O., Guan K.L., (2006) TSC2 integrates Wnt and energy signals via a coordinated phosphorylation by AMPK and GSK3 to regulate cell growth. *Cell,*126:(5), 955-68.

[63] Di Lorenzo G., Casciano R., Malangone E., Buonerba C., Sherman S., Willet J., Wang X., Liu Z., De Placido S., (2011) An adjusted indirect comparison of everolimus and sorafenib therapy in sunitinib-refractory metastatic renal cell carcinoma patients using repeated matched samples. *Expert Opin Pharmacother,*12:(10), 1491-7.

[64] Larkin J., Swanton C., Pickering L., (2011) Optimizing treatment of metastatic renal cell carcinoma by changing mechanism of action. *Expert Rev Anticancer Ther,*11:(4), 639-49.

[65] Valcamonico F., Ferrari V., Amoroso V., Rangoni G., Simoncini E., Marpicati P., Vassalli L., Grisanti S., Marini G., (2009) Long-lasting successful cerebral response with sorafenib in advanced renal cell carcinoma. *J Neurooncol,*91:(1), 47-50.

[66] Ferrari V.D., Fogazz G.I., Valcamonico F., Amoroso V., Procopio G., Nonnis D., Vassalli P., Marpicati S., Grisanti E., Simoncini, (2010) III-IV line of target therapy in advanced renal cell carcinoma (RCC). *Journal of Clinical Oncology,*28 (Suppl), e15148.

[67] Boris R.S., Benhammou J., Merino M., Pinto P.A., Linehan W.M., Bratslavsky G., (2011) The impact of germline BHD mutation on histological concordance and clinical treatment of patients with bilateral renal masses and known unilateral oncocytoma. *J Urol,*185:(6), 2050-5.

[68] Escudier B., Roigas J., Gillessen S., Harmenberg U., Srinivas S., Mulder S.F., Fountzilas G., Peschel C., Flodgren P., Maneval E.C., Chen I., Vogelzang N.J., (2009) Phase II study of sunitinib administered in a continuous once-daily dosing regimen in patients with cytokine-refractory metastatic renal cell carcinoma. *J Clin Oncol,*27:(25), 4068-75.

[69] Angevin E., Lopez-Martin J.A., Lin C.C., Gschwend J.E., Harzstark A., Castellano D., Soria J.C., Sen P., Chang J., Shi M., Kay A., Escudier B., (2013) Phase I study of dovitinib (TKI258), an oral FGFR, VEGFR, and PDGFR inhibitor, in advanced or metastatic renal cell carcinoma. *Clin Cancer Res,*19:(5), 1257-68.

[70] Hepgur M., Sadeghi S., Dorff T.B., Quinn D.I., (2013) Tivozanib in the treatment of renal cell carcinoma. *Biologics,*7 139-48.

[71] Barrios C.H., Hernandez-Barajas D., Brown M.P., Lee S.H., Fein L., Liu J.H., Hariharan S., Martell B.A., Yuan J., Bello A., Wang Z., Mundayat R., Rha S.Y., (2012) Phase II trial of continuous once-daily dosing of sunitinib as first-line treatment in patients with metastatic renal cell carcinoma. *Cancer,*118:(5), 1252-9.

[72] Calvo E., Escudier B., Motzer R.J., Oudard S., Hutson T.E., Porta C., Bracarda S., Grunwald V., Thompson J.A., Ravaud A., Kim D., Panneerselvam A., Anak O., Figlin R.A., (2012) Everolimus in metastatic renal cell carcinoma: Subgroup analysis of patients with 1 or 2 previous vascular endothelial growth factor receptor-tyrosine kinase inhibitor therapies enrolled in the phase III RECORD-1 study. *Eur J Cancer,*48:(3), 333-9.

[73] Dutcher J.P., Mourad W.F., Ennis R.D., (2012) Integrating innovative therapeutic strategies into the management of renal cell carcinoma. *Oncology (Williston Park),*26:(6), 526-30, 32, 34.

[74] Jeffers M., Schmidt L., Nakaigawa N., Webb C.P., Weirich G., Kishida T., Zbar B., Vande Woude G.F., (1997) Activating mutations for the met tyrosine kinase receptor in human cancer. *Proc Natl Acad Sci U S A,*94:(21), 11445-50.

[75] Schmidt L., Duh F.M., Chen F., Kishida T., Glenn G., Choyke P., Scherer S.W., Zhuang Z., Lubensky I., Dean M., Allikmets R., Chidambaram A., Bergerheim U.R., Feltis J.T., Casadevall C., Zamarron A., Bernues M., Richard S., Lips C.J., Walther M.M., Tsui L.C., Geil L., Orcutt M.L., Stackhouse T., Lipan J., Slife L., Brauch H., Decker J., Niehans G., Hughson M.D., Moch H., Storkel S., Lerman M.I., Linehan W.M., Zbar B., (1997) Germline and somatic mutations in the tyrosine kinase domain of the MET proto-oncogene in papillary renal carcinomas. *Nat Genet,*16:(1), 68-73.

[76] Nagi F.M., Omar A.A., Mostafa M.G., Mohammed E.A., Abd-Elwahed Hussein M.R., (2011) The expression pattern of Von Hippel-Lindau tumor suppressor protein, MET proto-oncogene, and TFE3 transcription factor oncoprotein in renal cell carcinoma in Upper Egypt. *Ultrastruct Pathol,*35:(2), 79-86.

[77] Schoffski P., Garcia J.A., Stadler W.M., Gil T., Jonasch E., Tagawa S.T., Smitt M., Yang X., Oliner K.S., Anderson A., Zhu M., Kabbinavar F., (2011) A phase II study of the efficacy and safety of AMG 102 in patients with metastatic renal cell carcinoma. *BJU Int,*108:(5), 679-86.

[78] Sharma N., Adjei A.A., (2011) In the clinic: ongoing clinical trials evaluating c-MET-inhibiting drugs. *Ther Adv Med Oncol,*3:(1 Suppl), S37-50.

[79] Yee D., (2011) Receptor kinase inhibitors target NSCLC: two antibodies and a small-molecule MET inhibitor. *BioDrugs,*25:(4), 271-3.

[80] Currie M.J., Gunningham S.P., Turner K., Han C., Scott P.A., Robinson B.A., Chong W., Harris A.L., Fox S.B., (2002) Expression of the angiopoietins and their receptor Tie2 in human renal clear cell carcinomas; regulation by the von Hippel-Lindau gene and hypoxia. *The Journal of pathology,*198:(4), 502-10.

[81] Pal S.K., Williams S., Josephson D.Y., Carmichael C., Vogelzang N.J., Quinn D.I., (2012) Novel therapies for metastatic renal cell carcinoma; efforts to expand beyond the VEGF/mTOR signaling paradigm. *Molecular cancer therapeutics,*11:(3), 526-37.

[82] Buhimschi C.S., Bhandari V., Dulay A.T., Thung S., Razeq S.S., Rosenberg V., Han C.S., Ali U.A., Zambrano E., Zhao G., Funai E.F., Buhimschi I.A., (2010) Amniotic fluid angiopoietin-1, angiopoietin-2, and soluble receptor tunica interna endothelial cell kinase-2 levels and regulation in normal pregnancy and intraamniotic inflammation-induced preterm birth. *J Clin Endocrinol Metab,*95:(7), 3428-36.

[83] Gordon M.S., Sweeney C.S., Mendelson D.S., Eckhardt S.G., Anderson A., Beaupre D.M., Branstetter D., Burgess T.L., Coxon A., Deng H., Kaplan-Lefko P., Leitch I.M., Oliner K.S., Yan L., Zhu M., Gore L., (2010) Safety, pharmacokinetics, and pharmacodynamics of AMG 102, a fully human hepatocyte growth factor-neutralizing monoclonal antibody, in a first-in-human study of patients with advanced solid tumors. *Clin Cancer Res,*16:(2), 699-710.

[84] Martini M., Ciraolo E., Gulluni F., Hirsch E., (2013) Targeting PI3K in Cancer: Any Good News? *Front Oncol,*3 108.

[85] Elfiky A.A., Sonpavde G., (2012) Novel molecular targets for the therapy of renal cell carcinoma. *Discov Med,*13:(73), 461-71.

In: Advances in Drug Resistance Research
Editor: Christudas Morais
ISBN: 978-1-63117-131-4

Chapter 9

Molecular Mechanisms of Sunitinib Resistance in Renal Cell Carcinoma

Turibius Simon[1], Glenda C. Gobe[2], Chung-Shu Wu[1], Fu-Hsiang Ko[1] and Christudas Morais[2]*

[1]Graduation Program for Nanotechnology, Department of Materials Science and Engineering, National Chiao Tung University, Hsinchu, Taiwan

[2] Centre for Kidney Disease Research, School of Medicine, The University of Queensland at Translational Research Institute, Brisbane, Queensland, Australia

Abstract

Renal cell carcinoma (RCC) is a treatment resistant cancer. The identification of the link between the von Hippel Lindau (VHL) gene and the vascular endothelial growth factor (VEGF) pathway has led to development of the multi-tyrosine kinase inhibitor sunitinib. The introduction of sunitinib in clinical practice for the treatment of metastatic RCC has significantly increased the overall survival of patients. However resistance to sunitinib is emerging as a challenge. About 30% of patients

* Author of correspondence, c.morais@uq.edu.au.

are intrinsically resistant to sunitinib and almost all patients who show initial response to sunitinib develop extrinsic (acquired) resistance after a median of 6–15 months. While the molecular mechanisms of sunitinib resistance are multifactorial, the emerging consensus is that, sustained VEGF/VEGF receptor (VEGFR) inhibition by sunitinib 'resets' the tumor microenvironment leading to the development of VEGF/VEGFR-independent alternate angiogenic pathways. This chapter summarises the advances in understanding of the molecular mechanisms of sunitinib resistance in RCC.

Keywords: Renal cell carcinoma, sunitinib, vascular endothelial growth factor, resistance

Introduction

Renal cell carcinoma (RCC), which is adenocarcinoma of the renal tubular epithelium, is a heterogeneous group of disease with an ever growing number of subtypes [1-3]. RCC accounts for about 3% of all adult neoplasms and its incidence has been increasing at a rate of 2-3% since 1999. The increase may be due, in part, to the increase in use of diagnostic imaging techniques, but there also seems to be an actual increase in incidence of RCC [3, 4]. Clear cell RCC is the most common subtype accounting for 70-80 % of renal neoplasms, followed by papillary (10-15%), chromophobe (5%) and collecting duct (<1%) RCC [5, 6]. Radical or partial nephrectomy remains the mainstay of treatment for localised RCC. However, RCC is a highly metastatic disease, with about a third of patients diagnosed with metastatic disease, and another third of patients who undergo surgical resection for localised RCC having recurrence [7]. RCC is also a treatment resistant cancer. Prior to 2005, patients with metastatic or locally invasive RCC received immunotherapies such as interferon-alpha (IFNα) and interleukin-2 (IL-2), with an objective response rate of 15 to 20% [8, 9]. Since then the understanding of the link between the von Hippel-Lindau (VHL) gene and the vascular endothelial factor (VEGF) pathway has led to the development of many targeted therapies, which has revolutionised the treatment of metastatic RCC [10].

The major risk factor for the development of RCC, especially clear cell RCC, is the inactivation of the VHL gene. In the majority of clear cell RCC, the VHL gene is frequently deleted, mutated, or epigenetically silenced, leading to the stabilisation and constitutive activation of the transcription factor, hypoxia-inducible factor 1α (HIF-1α), which would be otherwise degraded by the pVHL, a product of the functional VHL [9, 11, 12]. HIF-1α is translocated to the nucleus, where it binds to hypoxia responsive elements of the DNA and induces the transcription of a variety of pro-angiogenic factors including VEGF and platelet-derived growth factor (PDGF) [13, 14]. They bind to their respective tyrosine kinase receptors, for example VEGFR1, VEGFR2 and VEGFR3 for VEGF and PDGFR-α and PDGFR-β for PDGF, and promote tumor angiogenesis. The dependency of RCC on VEGF-mediated angiogenesis has led to the development of many agents that directly target the VEGF pathway [12, 14]. These include the anti-VEGF antibody bevacizumab and the multi-tyrosine kinase inhibitors [TKIs] sunitinib, sorafenib and pazopanib [3, 15, 16], of which, sunitinib is the focus of this chapter.

Sunitinib inhibits the tyrosine kinase activity of VEGF receptors (VEGFR-1, VEGFR-2, and VEGFR-3), PDGF receptors (PDGFR-α and PDGFR-β), fms-related tyrosine kinase 3 (FLT3), stem cell growth factor receptor KIT, and REarranged during Transfection (RET) [17, 18]. Sunitinib has replaced immunotherapy as the standard of care for first-line therapy of metastatic RCC. Compared with IFNα treatment, sunitinib doubles progression-free survival of patients with metastatic RCC [10, 19, 20]. Apart from its anti-angiogenic activities, sunitinib has been reported to have direct anti-proliferative and apoptotic effects on tumor cells [21].

About 70% of patients show initial positive response to sunitinib treatment [4]. However, durable responses are rare, and acquired resistance to treatment develops in almost all of them after a median of 6–15 months [3, 4, 22, 23]. The remaining 30% of patients are intrinsically resistant to sunitinib treatment [4, 22, 23]. The mechanisms of sunitinib resistance are varied and multifactorial. This chapter summarises the advances in understanding of the molecular mechanisms of sunitinib resistance in RCC.

Sphingosine Kinase-1

Sphingolipids are important lipid signaling molecules that regulate diverse cellular processes. One of the bioactive sphingolipid metabolites, sphingosine 1-phosphate (S1P), plays a critical role in tumor growth, survival, angiogenesis and drug resistance [24-27]. The formation of S1P from the shingolipid sphingosine is catalysed by sphingosine kinases (SKs). Two SKs exist in humans, SK1 and SK2, of which SK1 has been extensively studied. SK1 is elevated in many human cancers and contributes to carcinogenesis, chemotherapeutic resistance and poor patient outcome [28, 29]. The expression and activation of SK1 is enhanced in sunitinib-resistant 786-O and A498 RCC cell lines. SK1 inhibition re-sensitises these cells to sunitinib, and delays the development of resistance [26]. Furthermore, sunitinib-resistant cells have a higher S1P, and S1P inhibitors delay the development of sunitinib resistance in tumor bearing mice [26, 30].

At least two mechanisms have been suggested to play a role in SKI-mediated resistance to sunitinib, activation of ERK, and the inhibition of ATP-binding cassette (ABC) drug transporter family. It has been reported that ERK and AKT are downstream effectors of SK1-S1P pathway and that the phosphorylation and activation of these two molecules are associated with resistance to tyrosine kinase inhibitors in many cancers [25, 31-33]. In contrast, only ERK not AKT, is activated in sunitinib-resistant RCC cell lines, which is abrogated by SKI inhibition (26). The ABC transporter family includes multidrug resistance-associated protein 1, ABCC1, ABCA1, and breast cancer resistance protein (ABCG2). Sunitinib blocks the function of the ABC transporters [34, 35]. It has been suggested that continuous blockade of ABC transporters by sunitinib inhibits the export of S1P from cells leading to AKT activation and subsequent drug resistance. Given that AKT is not activated in response to sunitinib in RCC [26], it is not clear if this mechanism is applicable to RCC.

p53, HDM2 and HDMX

Inactivation of the tumor suppressor gene p53 plays a central role in oncogenesis and tumor angiogenesis. While nearly half of all human tumors inactivate p53 through gene mutation or deletion, the remaining half, including RCC, have intact wild type p53 but their transcriptional activity is inhibited [36-40]. For example, kidney cancer-related POK transcription factor [KR-POK] is over expressed in RCC [41]. KR-POK, along with its co-repressors NCoR and BCoR interacts with p53, resulting in reduced histone H3 and H4 acetylation at the promoter region of certain p53-dependent genes, for example, $p21^{waf1}$/CDKN1A. As a result, despite the integrity of p53, its ability to inhibit angiogenesis is inhibited [36, 41].

HDM2 and HDMX are well-documented transcriptional inhibitors of p53, and their overexpression has been linked to tumor aggression and drug resistance [42-47]. Both HDM2 and HDMX bind to the same site of p53, however, the mechanism by which they inhibit the p53 transcription activity is different. Upon binding to p53, HDM2 acts as a ubiquitin ligase to degrade p53 [42, 48]. In contrast, HDMX lacks ubiquitin ligase activity and, therefore, blocks p53 activity without promoting degradation [42, 49]. In RCC xenograft models, sunitinib activates p53, however, its anti-angiogenic activity is short-lived because of the up-regulation of HDM2 and HDMX. There is an inverse correlation between the expression of these two proteins and the development of resistance to sunitinib. HDM2 is initially induced by sunitinib [42]. As resistance develops, its activity is decreased. In contrast, HDMX is constitutively expressed in RCC, decreases with the initiation of sunitinib treatment, and reappears as resistance develops. Compounds that block the interaction of HDM2 or HDMX with p53, for example MI-319, restore p53 transcriptional activity, delay the development of sunitinib resistance, and inhibit angiogenesis [42].

The transcriptional activation of p53 by MI-319 and the subsequent inhibition of angiogenesis is mediated through the suppression of the sunitinib-induced $CD11b^{+}/Gr\text{-}1^{+}$ myeloid-derived suppressor cells (MDSC) influx into the tumor [36]. MDSC are a heterogeneous group of myeloid-derived cells that down-regulate anti-tumor immunity and help tumors evade immune-mediated destruction [50-52]. The influx of MDSC into the tumor is largely mediated by chemokines, especially SDF-1 [36, 53, 54]. Thus sunitinib-induced MDSC and SDF-1 appear to be the key players in conferring resistance to RCC.

Cycloxygenase-2

Cycloxygenase-2 (COX-2) is the key enzyme of the cycloxygenase pathway that produces prostaglandin E and arachidonic acid [55, 56]. COX-2 expression correlates with poor prognosis of RCC [57-60] and inhibition of COX-2 attenuates tumor progression and angiogenesis in pre-clinical models of RCC [61-63]. Since sunitinib reduces tumor perfusion and angiogenesis, sunitinib-treated tumors exhibit enhanced hypoxia [55, 64]. In due course, this leads to further enhancement of the hypoxia-dependent angiogenic pathway, restoration of angiogenesis and acquired sunitinib-resistance [55]. Hypoxia is also an inducer of COX-2. In RCC xenograft models, sunitinib resistance is accompanied by an increase in COX-2 expression, especially in areas of tumor hypoxia. Combining sunitinib and celecoxib, a COX-2 inhibitor, enhances anti-tumor efficacy and delays disease progression [55]. However, this synergistic effect was not the result of decreased perfusion or angiogenesis, but yet to be discovered mechanisms.

Akt and p44/42 MAPK Signalling Pathways

Several studies have shown the involvement of signal transduction pathways in the acquisition of drug resistance [65-67]. A comparison between ACHN parental RCC and sunitinib-resistant sublines of ACHN showed no significant difference in the baseline expression of phosphorylated Akt and p44/42 mitogen-activated protein kinase (MAPK). However, after sunitinib treatment, Akt and p44/42 MAPK were significantly inactivated in the parental cell line when compared with the resistant sublines (65). Treatment of resistant cell lines with LY294002, a selective inhibitor of phosphoinositol 3′-kinase (PI3K) in conjunction with sunitinib resulted in a level of growth inhibition similar to that in ACHN parent cell lines. However no such effect was observed in response to co-treatment with U0126, a MAPK inhibitor, suggesting the involvement of Akt, and not MAPK, in the induction of resistance to sunitinib (65). Furthermore, sunitinib treatment markedly inhibited the expression of several tyrosine kinases including phosphorylated bone marrow X kinase (BMX), hematopoietic cell kinase (HCK), megakaryocyte-associated tyrosine kinase (MATK), RET, thirty-eight-negative kinase 1 (TNK1) and resting lymphocyte kinase (RLK) in the parental ACHN cells when compared to the sunitinib-resistant ACHN cells [65]. Interestingly, no significant differences in VEGFR and PDGFR families were observed between ACHN sublines in response to sunitinib [65]. Whilst further confirmation is required, these findings question the concept of angiogenesis inhibition as a mechanism of development of sunitinib resistance [65, 68-70].

Micro RNA

The micro RNA miR-141 is part of the miR-200 family with a pivotal role in tumor biology [71-74]. The miR-200 family suppresses epithelial mesenchymal transition [EMT] in tumors and in normal renal epithelium [75-78]. miR-141 inhibits the activity of ZEB1 and 2, which are implicated in EMT, tumor metastasis, angiogenesis induction and chemotherapy resistance [79]. The expression of miR-141 is decreased in RCC when compared to adjacent normal renal cortex and is an indicator of sunitinib resistance in RCC [71, 75-77]. Patients with unfavourable response to sunitinib, defined as progression-free survival less than 6 months, had significantly lower miR-141 than those with favourable response, defined as progression-free survival more than one year. Furthermore, ZEB2 expression was significantly increased in patients with lower miR-141 or the poor responders with lower miR -141 [71].

EMMPRIN

Extracellular matrix metalloproteinase inducer [EMMPRIN] is a cell-surface glycoprotein [80-82] implicated in tumor progression [83-85]. Apart from its direct pro-proliferative effects on cancer cells, EMMPRIN stimulates the peri-tumoral fibroblasts to secrete matrix metalloproteinases, which in turn degrades extracellular matrix proteins and promote angiogenesis and tumor progression [86, 87]. EMMPRIN expression is increased in RCC and correlates with proliferation, angiogenesis, tumor aggression and poor prognosis of RCC [88]. Elevated EMMPRIN levels have been recorded in patients who were resistant to sunitinib, and also in sunitinib-resistant 786-0 RCC cell lines [80]. EMMPRIN-mediated sunitinib resistance is thought to be the result of hyaluronan-mediated activation of the ErbB2 signaling pathway [89, 90].

PTEN AKT/mTOR

Another mechanism of sunitinib resistance is the constitutive activation of the phosphoinositide 3-kinase (PI3K)/Akt/mTOR pathway [69]. The PI3K/Akt/mTOR signalling pathway regulates many cellular events, including cell cycle, proliferation, angiogenesis and tumor initiation and progression [69, 91]. PTEN is a negative regulator of PI3K/Akt/mTOR, and under normal conditions acts as a tumor suppressor by inhibiting PI3K/Akt/mTOR - mediated cell survival signalling pathway. Inactivation of PTEN, either by mutation or deletion, leads to the activation of PI3K/Akt/mTOR and subsequent tumor progression [69, 91]. In 786-0 RCC cell lines, PTEN expression inversely correlates with sunitinib resistance and restoration of PTEN in PTEN-negative tumor cells markedly increased tumor sensitivity to sunitinib and suppressed the production of pro-tumoric cytokines such as IL-6 and IL-8 [18, 69, 92]. Furthermore, inhibition of PI3K/Akt/mTOR signaling in PTEN negative cells with GDC-0980, GSK690693, and temsirolimus led to the restoration of sensitivity to sunitinib [69]. These results indicate that lack of PTEN expression may contribute to intrinsic sunitinib resistance, and that the activity of the PI3K/Akt/mTOR pathway may be a marker of response to treatment. Co-administration of sunitinib with PI3K/Akt/mTOR inhibitors may represent a rational treatment strategy for patients with resistant RCC.

PRKX

The serine threonine kinase, protein kinase x-linked (PRKX), is involved in renal development, epithelial cell migration, uretic bud branching and glomerular formation [93, 94]. In A498 RCC cell lines, over expression of PRKX leads to sunitinib resistance and its inhibition re-sensitizes the cells to sunitinib. While the mechanism of PRKX-mediated resistance to sunitinib is not clear, the up-regulation of microphthalmia-associated transcription factor (MITF) has been implicated [95, 96]. Aberrant expression of MITF has been reported in papillary renal cell carcinoma [93, 97, 98].

Lysosomal Sequestration

One of the classical mechanisms of drug resistance is enhanced drug efflux leading to decreased intracellular concentration [99, 100]. Contrary to this well-known mechanism, in the sunitinib-resistant 786-0 RCC cell line, the intracellular concentration of sunitinib is increased up to a thousand fold when compared with the parental cell lines. Sunitinib is preferentially sequestered in acidic lysosomes, and inhibition of lysosomal function with specific inhibitors reduced the lysosomal sequestration of Sunitinib [99]. Furthermore, the lysosomal capacity, and the expression of the major lysosome-associated membrane proteins (LAMP) 1 and LAMP-2 [101] are significantly increased in sunitinib-resistant 786-O cells [99]. However, the phosphorylation status of ERK 1/2 and Akt (see above for the role of Akt in drug resistance) is similar, suggesting the lack of bio-availability because of lysosomal sequestration. Sunitinib is hydrophobic (logP = 5.2) and therefore easily crosses the plasma membrane. Sunitinib is also a weak base (pKa = 8.95) [99, 102]. This means at pH below 9, sunitinib will be increasingly protonated and, thereby, lose its ability to cross membranes. At a pH of 5, all sunitinib will be protonated, and therefore, upon entering an acidic lysosome, sunitinib becomes protonated and cannot cross membranes anymore [99]. Thus, despite higher intracellular concentration of sunitinib in resistant cells, reduced cytoplasmic availability provides a novel mechanism of resistance to sunitinib.

Angiostatic Signaling

Down-regulation of tumor-derived IFN-γ is another mechanism of sunitinib-resistance [64]. IFN-γ signalling produces three angiostatic chemokines CXCL9, CXCL10 and CXCL11 [64, 103]. In a murine model of RCC, sunitinib resistance coincided with a significant reduction of IFN-γ and its receptor IFN-γR. This was accompanied by further reduction in IFN-γ-regulated chemokines, especially the angiostatic CXCL9 [64]. Co-treatment of RCC xenofrafts with sunitinib and CXCL9 significantly delayed the development of resistance largely the result of significant reduction in tumor microvascular density [64].

IL-8

Interleukin-8 is a well-known pro-angiogenic chemokine [104], and its up-regulation is an emerging mechanism of extrinsic and intrinsic resistance to sunitinib [18]. In a murine xenograft model of RCC, acquired sunitinib resistance was associated with a significant increase in plasma levels of IL-8, tumor growth and tumor micro vascular density, and neutralization of IL-8 re-sensitized tumors to sunitinib and inhibited angiogenesis [18]. Over-expression of IL-8 in response to treatment is not uncommon in RCC [105]. IL-8 also appears to play a role in intrinsic resistance to sunitinib. As mentioned earlier, about 30% of the patients are intrinsically resistant to sunitinib [4, 22]. A comparison of IL-8 expression in RCC before and after sunitinib treatment showed that tumors from patients who progressed while on sunitinib treatment had a significantly higher IL-8 expression than tumors from patients who did not progress on sunitinib treatment [18]. Thus IL-8 status may be a useful biomarker to predict sunitinib resistance.

RLIP76

Glutathione is a ubiquitous sulfhydryl tripeptide that protects cells from electrophilic oxidants generated by endo and xenobiotics. Glutathione S-transferases play a major role in this detoxification process by catalyzing the reaction of electrophilic compounds with the sulfhydryl group of glutathione [106, 107].The resulting glutathione S-electrophilic conjugates (GS-E) are transported out of cells and thus the cells are protected from electrophilic or oxidative stress. The ral-interacting protein (RLIP76) is the prominent transporter of nearly 80% of the GS-E and protects cells from apoptosis [106, 107]. Blocking RLIP76-mediated transport of GS-E results in the accumulation of endogenous electrophiles, and apoptosis of cells [106, 107]. RLIP76 belongs to the Ras family, and is activated in many cancers, including RCC [106, 107]. Sunitinib is a substrate for transport by RLIP76, and administration of RLIP76 antisense, siRNA or anti-RLIP76 IgG to nude mice leads to nearly complete and sustained regression of RCC xenograft models [107].

Epithelial Mesenchymal Transition

Based on a case report, the *de novo* onset of EMT is suggested to be one of the mechanisms of drug resistance [9]. In a patient with conventional clear cell RCC on sunitinib treatment, acquired resistance was associated with EMT. When cells from these tumors were implanted into mice, the cells reverted to epithelial-like morphology and regained response to sunitinib. Treatment-associated tumor hypoxia is one of the drivers of EMT [9]. The authors observed an increased expression of HIF-1α staining in the skin metastasis as compared with the nephrectomy sample that resolved in the xenografts. Based on these findings the authors suggested that EMT, mediated by HIF-α is a potential mechanism for sunitinib resistance in RCC [9].

Genetic Polymorphisms

Genetic polymorphisms also play a role in resistance to sunitinib. Retrospective and prospective analysis of patients treated with sunitinib showed that worse sunitinib response and shorter progression-free survival were associated with *CYP3A5* rs776746, VEGFR2 rs1870377, VEGFR3 rs307826 (T494A), rs307821 (R1324L) and rs448012, PDGFRA rs1800812, IL-8 rs4073, PXR rs3814055 and ABCB1 rs2032582 and rs1128503 [108-111]. There is considerable inter-ethnic difference in the allelic frequency of these single nucleotide polymorphisms (SNP). For example, the allele frequency of VEGFR3 rs307826 in the Caucasian population is 10%, and is either absent or at a very low frequency in Asians and Africans [108, 112]. The *CYP3A5*1* rs776746 has 6, 28 and 83% allele frequency in Caucasians, Asians and Africans, respectively [108, 113]. These suggest that considerable inter-ethnic differences in response to sunitinib could be expected [108].

Conclusion

Resistance to therapy, either intrinsic or extrinsic, continues to be one of the major challenges in the effective treatment of metastatic RCC. While there have been advances in our understanding of the mechanisms of extrinsic resistance to sunitinib, the molecular mechanisms of intrinsic resistance still remain elusive. The possible mechanisms of intrinsic resistance could include stage of progression, genetic make-up, subtype, and microenvironment of RCC. Much research is required in this largely unexplored area of intrinsic resistance. In contrast, as discussed in this chapter, a greater understanding has developed of the molecular mechanisms of extrinsic resistance. However, most of these data have been generated using selected cell lines and their clinical relevance needs to be independently verified. Despite this, the available information has led to an emerging consensus that these mechanisms converge to a final common pathway that 'resets' the tumor microenvironment leading to the development of a VEGF/VEGFR-independent alternate angiogenic pathway through the up-regulation of angiogenic factors other than VEGF [3, 114]. For example, up-regulation of IL-8 or down-regulation IFN-γ, as discussed above [18, 64], may circumvent the anti-angiogenic effects of sunitinib, and functionally compensate for the VEGF/VEGFR-mediated inhibition of angiogenesis. To overcome such resistance, sequential and combination therapies with other anti-angiogenic agents or mTOR inhibitors has been tested, with promising results [3, 114]. Furthermore, it is also emerging that the resistance is transient and that after a short treatment interruption, sensitivity to sunitinib can be restored by subsequent rechallenge [9, 115, 116]. These advances will lead to the development of better treatment modalities to overcome sunitinib resistance in the days to come.

References

[1] Eble J, Sauter G, Epstein J, Sesterhenn I. (2001). Pathology and genetics. Tumors of the urinary system and male genital organs. Lyon, IARC Press.

[2] Lopez-Beltran A, Scarpelli M, Montironi R, Kirkali Z. (2006). (2004) WHO classification of the renal tumors of the adults. *Eur. Urol.* 49,798-805.

[3] Santos N, Wenger JB, Havre P, Liu Y, Dagan R, et al. (2011). Combination therapy for renal cell cancer, what are possible options? *Oncology (Williston Park)* 81,220-9.

[4] Porta C, Sabbatini R, Procopio G, Paglino C, Galligioni E, Ortega C. (2012). Primary resistance to tyrosine kinase inhibitors in patients with advanced renal cell carcinoma, state-of-the-science. *Expert Rev. Anticancer Ther.* 12,1571-7.

[5] Curti BD. (2004). Renal cell carcinoma. *Jama* 292,97-100.

[6] Morais C, Gobe G, Johnson DW, Healy H. (2011). The emerging role of nuclear factor kappa B in renal cell carcinoma. *Int. J. Biochem. Cell. Biol.* 43,1537-49.

[7] Society AC. (2011). Cancer facts and figures (2011). Atlanta. American Cancer Society. .

[8] Rini BI, Campbell SC, Escudier B. (2009). Renal cell carcinoma. *Lancet* 373,1119-32.

[9] Hammers HJ, Verheul HM, Salumbides B, Sharma R, Rudek M, et al. (2010). Reversible epithelial to mesenchymal transition and acquired resistance to sunitinib in patients with renal cell carcinoma, evidence from a xenograft study. *Mol. Cancer. The.r* 9,1525-35.

[10] Motzer RJ, Hutson TE, Tomczak P, Michaelson MD, Bukowski RM, et al. (2009). Overall survival and updated results for sunitinib compared with interferon alfa in patients with metastatic renal cell carcinoma. *J. Clin. Oncol.* 27,3584-90.

[11] Maxwell PH, Wiesener MS, Chang GW, Clifford SC, Vaux EC, et al. 1999. The tumor suppressor protein VHL targets hypoxia-inducible factors for oxygen-dependent proteolysis. *Nature* 399,271-5.

[12] Morais C, Johnson DW, Gobe GC. (2011). The VHL-HIF signaling in renal cell carcinoma, Promises and pitfalls. In *Emerging Research and Treatments in Renal Cell Carcinoma*, ed. R Amato,57-82. Croatia, InTech Publishers. Number of 57-82 pp..

[13] Forsythe JA, Jiang BH, Iyer NV, Agani F, Leung SW, et al. 1996. Activation of vascular endothelial growth factor gene transcription by hypoxia-inducible factor 1. *Mol. Cell. Biol.* 16,4604-13.

[14] Baldewijns MM, van VIJ, Vermeulen PB, Soetekouw PM, van EM, de BAP. (2010). VHL and HIF signalling in renal cell carcinogenesis. *J. Pathol.* 221,125-38.

[15] Hutson TE. (2011). Targeted therapies for the treatment of metastatic renal cell carcinoma, clinical evidence. *Oncologist* 16 Suppl 2,14-22.

[16] Powles T, Chowdhury S, Jones R, Mantle M, Nathan P, et al. (2011). Sunitinib and other targeted therapies for renal cell carcinoma. *Br. J. Cancer* 104,741-5.

[17] Faivre S, Demetri G, Sargent W, Raymond E. (2007). Molecular basis for sunitinib efficacy and future clinical development. *Nat. Rev. Drug Discov.* 6,734-45.

[18] Huang D, Ding Y, Zhou M, Rini BI, Petillo D, et al. (2010). Interleukin-8 mediates resistance to antiangiogenic agent sunitinib in renal cell carcinoma. *Cancer Res.* 70,1063-71.

[19] Reddy K. (2006). Phase III study of sunitinib malate (SU11248) versus interferon-alpha as first-line treatment in patients with metastatic renal cell carcinoma. *Clin. Genitourin. Cancer* 5,23-5.

[20] Motzer RJ, Hutson TE, Tomczak P, Michaelson MD, Bukowski RM, et al. (2007). Sunitinib versus interferon alfa in metastatic renal-cell carcinoma. *N. Engl. J. Med.* 356,115-24.

[21] Huang D, Ding Y, Li Y, Luo WM, Zhang ZF, et al. (2010). Sunitinib acts primarily on tumor endothelium rather than tumor cells to inhibit the growth of renal cell carcinoma. *Cancer Res.* 70,1053-62.

[22] Heng DY, Mackenzie MJ, Vaishampayan UN, Bjarnason GA, Knox JJ, et al. (2012). Primary anti-vascular endothelial growth factor (VEGF)-refractory metastatic renal cell carcinoma, clinical characteristics, risk factors, and subsequent therapy. *Ann. Oncol.* 23,1549-55.

[23] Busch J, Seidel C, Weikert S, Wolff I, Kempkensteffen C, et al. (2011). Intrinsic resistance to tyrosine kinase inhibitors is associated with poor clinical outcome in metastatic renal cell carcinoma. *BMC Cancer* 11,295.

[24] Song L, Xiong H, Li J, Liao W, Wang L, et al. (2011). Sphingosine kinase-1 enhances resistance to apoptosis through activation of PI3K/Akt/NF-kappaB pathway in human non-small cell lung cancer. *Clin. Cancer Re.s* 17,1839-49.

[25] Pyne NJ, Pyne S. (2010). Sphingosine 1-phosphate and cancer. *Nat Rev Cancer* 10,489-503.

[26] Gao H, Deng L. (2013). Sphingosine Kinase-1 Activation Causes Acquired Resistance Against Sunitinib in Renal Cell Carcinoma Cells. *Cell. Biochem. Biophys* . Epub ahead of print.

[27] Cuvillier O, Ader I, Bouquerel P, Brizuela L, Malavaud B, et al. (2010). Activation of sphingosine kinase-1 in cancer, implications for therapeutic targeting. *Curr Mol Pharmacol* 3,53-65.

[28] Billich A, Bornancin F, Mechtcheriakova D, Natt F, Huesken D, Baumruker T. (2005). Basal and induced sphingosine kinase 1 activity in A549 carcinoma cells, function in cell survival and IL-1beta and TNF-alpha induced production of inflammatory mediators. *Cell Signal.* 17,1203-17.

[29] Taha TA, Argraves KM, Obeid LM. (2004). Sphingosine-1-phosphate receptors, receptor specificity versus functional redundancy. *Biochim. Biophys. Acta* 1682,48-55.

[30] Bhatt RS, Zhang L, Bullock A, Moreno K, Signoretti S, et al. (2010). Sphingosine-1-phosphate (S1P) as a novel target in renal cancer (RCC). In *AACR 101st Annual Meeting (2010)* .

[31] Kuroda K, Horiguchi A, Sumitomo M, Asano T, Ito K, et al. (2009). Activated Akt prevents antitumor activity of gefitinib in renal cancer cells. *Urology* 74,209-15.

[32] Li H, Schmid-Bindert G, Wang D, Zhao Y, Yang X, et al. (2011). Blocking the PI3K/AKT and MEK/ERK signaling pathways can overcome gefitinib-resistance in non-small cell lung cancer cell lines. *Adv. Med. Sci.* 56,275-84.

[33] Pchejetski D, Bohler T, Stebbing J, Waxman J. (2011). Therapeutic potential of targeting sphingosine kinase 1 in prostate cancer. *Nat. Rev. Urol.* 8,569-678.

[34] Hu S, Chen Z, Franke R, Orwick S, Zhao M, et al. (2009). Interaction of the multikinase inhibitors sorafenib and sunitinib with solute carriers and ATP-binding cassette transporters. *Clin. Cancer Res* 15,6062-9.

[35] Shukla S, Robey RW, Bates SE, Ambudkar SV. (2009). Sunitinib (Sutent, SU11248), a small-molecule receptor tyrosine kinase inhibitor, blocks function of the ATP-binding cassette (ABC) transporters P-glycoprotein (ABCB1) and ABCG2. *Drug. Metab. Dispos.* 37,359-65.

[36] Panka DJ, Liu Q, Geissler AK, Mier JW. (2013). Effects of HDM2 antagonism on sunitinib resistance, p53 activation, SDF-1 induction, and

tumor infiltration by CD11b+/Gr-1+ myeloid derived suppressor cells. *Mol. Cancer* 12,17.

[37] Szymanska K, Moore LE, Rothman N, Chow WH, Waldman F, et al. (2010). TP53, EGFR, and KRAS mutations in relation to VHL inactivation and lifestyle risk factors in renal-cell carcinoma from central and eastern Europe. *Cancer Lett.* 293,92-8.

[38] Gurova KV, Hill JE, Razorenova OV, Chumakov PM, Gudkov AV. (2004). p53 pathway in renal cell carcinoma is repressed by a dominant mechanism. *Cancer Res.* 64,1951-8.

[39] Gurova KV, Hill JE, Guo C, Prokvolit A, Burdelya LG, et al. (2005). Small molecules that reactivate p53 in renal cell carcinoma reveal a NF-kappaB-dependent mechanism of p53 suppression in tumors. *Proc. Natl. Acad. Sci. U S A* 102,17448-53.

[40] An J, Rettig MB. (2005). Mechanism of von Hippel-Lindau protein-mediated suppression of nuclear factor kappa B activity. *Mol. Cell. Biol.* 25,7546-56.

[41] Jeon BN, Kim MK, Choi WI, Koh DI, Hong SY, et al. (2012). KR-POK interacts with p53 and represses its ability to activate transcription of p21WAF1/CDKN1A. *Cancer Res* 72,1137-48.

[42] Hayashi R, Wang D, Hara T, Iera JA, Durell SR, Appella DH. (2009). N-acylpolyamine inhibitors of HDM2 and HDMX binding to p53. *Bioorg. Med. Chem.* 17,7884-93.

[43] Vogelstein B, Lane D, Levine AJ. 2000. Surfing the p53 network. *Nature* 408,307-10.

[44] Han X, Garcia-Manero G, McDonnell TJ, Lozano G, Medeiros LJ, et al. (2007). HDM4 (HDMX) is widely expressed in adult pre-B acute lymphoblastic leukemia and is a potential therapeutic target. *Mod. Pathol.* 20,54-62.

[45] Ramos YF, Stad R, Attema J, Peltenburg LT, van dEAJ, Jochemsen AG. (2001). Aberrant expression of HDMX proteins in tumor cells correlates with wild-type p53. *Cancer Res* 61,1839-42.

[46] Wade M, Wong ET, Tang M, Stommel JM, Wahl GM. (2006). Hdmx modulates the outcome of p53 activation in human tumor cells. *J. Biol. Chem.* 281,33036-44.

[47] Stad R, Ramos YF, Little N, Grivell S, Attema J, et al. 2000. Hdmx stabilizes Mdm2 and p53. *J. Biol. Chem.* 275,28039-44.

[48] Momand J, Wu HH, Dasgupta G. 2000. MDM2--master regulator of the p53 tumor suppressor protein. *Gene* 242,15-29.

[49] Marine JC, Dyer MA, Jochemsen AG. (2007). MDMX, from bench to bedside. *J. Cell. Sci* .120,371-8.

[50] Yang L, Huang J, Ren X, Gorska AE, Chytil A, et al. (2008). Abrogation of TGF beta signaling in mammary carcinomas recruits Gr-1+CD11b+ myeloid cells that promote metastasis. *Cancer Cell* 13,23-35.

[51] Shojaei F, Wu X, Malik AK, Zhong C, Baldwin ME, et al. (2007). Tumor refractoriness to anti-VEGF treatment is mediated by CD11b+Gr1+ myeloid cells. *Nat. Biotechnol.* 25,911-20.

[52] Yang L, DeBusk LM, Fukuda K, Fingleton B, Green-Jarvis B, et al. (2004). Expansion of myeloid immune suppressor Gr+CD11b+ cells in tumor-bearing host directly promotes tumor angiogenesis. *Cancer Cell* 6,409-21.

[53] Moskovits N, Kalinkovich A, Bar J, Lapidot T, Oren M. (2006). p53 Attenuates cancer cell migration and invasion through repression of SDF-1/CXCL12 expression in stromal fibroblasts. *Cancer Res.* 66,10671-6.

[54] Addadi Y, Moskovits N, Granot D, Lozano G, Carmi Y, et al. (2010). p53 status in stromal fibroblasts modulates tumor growth in an SDF1-dependent manner. *Cancer Res.* 70,9650-8.

[55] Wang X, Zhang L, O'Neill A, Bahamon B, Alsop DC, et al. (2013). Cox-2 inhibition enhances the activity of sunitinib in human renal cell carcinoma xenografts. *Br. J. Cancer.* 108,319-26.

[56] Ghosh N, Chaki R, Mandal V, Mandal SC. (2010). COX-2 as a target for cancer chemotherapy. *Pharmacol. Rep.* 62,233-44.

[57] Miyata Y, Koga S, Kanda S, Nishikido M, Hayashi T, Kanetake H. (2003). Expression of cyclooxygenase-2 in renal cell carcinoma, correlation with tumor cell proliferation, apoptosis, angiogenesis, expression of matrix metalloproteinase-2, and survival. *Clin. Cancer Res.* 9,1741-9.

[58] Tuna B, Yorukoglu K, Gurel D, Mungan U, Kirkali Z. (2004). Significance of COX-2 expression in human renal cell carcinoma. *Urology* 64,1116-20.

[59] Sozen S, Gurocak S, Erdem O, Acar C, Kordan Y, et al. (2008). Cyclooxygenase-2 expression, does it have a probable role in tumorigenesis mechanisms of renal cell carcinoma? *Int. Urol. Nephrol.* 40,295-301.

[60] Kankuri-Tammilehto MK, Soderstrom KO, Pelliniemi TT, Vahlberg T, Pyrhonen SO, Salminen EK. (2010). Prognostic evaluation of COX-2 expression in renal cell carcinoma. *Anticancer Res.* 30,3023-30.

[61] Chen Q, Shinohara N, Abe T, Harabayashi T, Nonomura K. (2004). Impact of cyclooxygenase-2 gene expression on tumor invasiveness in a human renal cell carcinoma cell line. *J. Urol.* 172,2153-7.

[62] Chen Q, Shinohara N, Abe T, Watanabe T, Nonomura K, Koyanagi T. (2004). Significance of COX-2 expression in human renal cell carcinoma cell lines. *Int. J. Cancer* 108,825-32.

[63] Sato N, Mizutani Y, Li YN, Fujiwara J, Ishida H, et al. (2010). Enhancement of the sensitivity of renal cell carcinoma cells to fas-mediated cytotoxicity and apoptosis by the selective cyclooxygenase-2 inhibitor JTE-522. *Urol. Int.* 84,362-8.

[64] Bhatt RS, Wang X, Zhang L, Collins MP, Signoretti S, et al. (2010). Renal cancer resistance to antiangiogenic therapy is delayed by restoration of angiostatic signaling. *Mol. Cancer. Ther.* 9,2793-802.

[65] Sakai I, Miyake H, Fujisawa M. (2013). Acquired resistance to sunitinib in human renal cell carcinoma cells is mediated by constitutive activation of signal transduction pathways associated with tumor cell proliferation. *BJU Int.* 112,E211-20.

[66] Okabe T, Okamoto I, Tsukioka S, Uchida J, Hatashita E, et al. (2009). Addition of S-1 to the epidermal growth factor receptor inhibitor gefitinib overcomes gefitinib resistance in non-small cell lung cancer cell lines with MET amplification. *Clin. Cancer Res.* 15,907-13.

[67] Di NF, Arena S, Tabernero J, Grosso S, Molinari F, et al. (2010). Deregulation of the PI3K and KRAS signaling pathways in human cancer cells determines their response to everolimus. *J. Clin. Invest.* 120,2858-66.

[68] Serova M, de GA, Tijeras-Raballand A, Dos SC, Riveiro ME, et al. (2013). Benchmarking effects of mTOR, PI3K, and dual PI3K/mTOR inhibitors in hepatocellular and renal cell carcinoma models developing resistance to sunitinib and sorafenib. *Cancer Chemother. Pharmacol.* 71,1297-307.

[69] Makhov PB, Golovine K, Kutikov A, Teper E, Canter DJ, et al. (2012). Modulation of Akt/mTOR signaling overcomes sunitinib resistance in renal and prostate cancer cells. *Mol. Cancer Ther.* 11,1510-7.

[70] Figlin RA, Kaufmann I, Brechbiel J. (2013). Targeting PI3K and mTORC2 in metastatic renal cell carcinoma, new strategies for overcoming resistance to VEGFR and mTORC1 inhibitors. *Int. J. Cancer* 133,788-96.

[71] Berkers J, Govaere O, Wolter P, Beuselinck B, Schoffski P, et al. (2013). A possible role for microRNA-141 down-regulation in sunitinib

resistant metastatic clear cell renal cell carcinoma through induction of epithelial-to-mesenchymal transition and hypoxia resistance. *J. Urol.* 189,1930-8.

[72] Gregory PA, Bert AG, Paterson EL, Barry SC, Tsykin A, et al. (2008). The miR-200 family and miR-205 regulate epithelial to mesenchymal transition by targeting ZEB1 and SIP1. *Nat. Cell Biol.* 10,593-601.

[73] Brabletz S, Brabletz T. (2010). The ZEB/miR-200 feedback loop--a motor of cellular plasticity in development and cancer? *EMBO Rep.* 11,670-7.

[74] Mateescu B, Batista L, Cardon M, Gruosso T, de FY, et al. (2011). miR-141 and miR-200a act on ovarian tumorigenesis by controlling oxidative stress response. *Nat. Med.* 17,1627-35.

[75] Juan D, Alexe G, Antes T, Liu H, Madabhushi A, et al. (2010). Identification of a microRNA panel for clear-cell kidney cancer. *Urology* 75,835-41.

[76] Nakada C, Matsuura K, Tsukamoto Y, Tanigawa M, Yoshimoto T, et al. (2008). Genome-wide microRNA expression profiling in renal cell carcinoma, significant down-regulation of miR-141 and miR-200c. *J. Pathol.* 216,418-27.

[77] Slaby O, Jancovicova J, Lakomy R, Svoboda M, Poprach A, et al. (2010). Expression of miRNA-106b in conventional renal cell carcinoma is a potential marker for prediction of early metastasis after nephrectomy. *J. Exp. Clin. Cancer Res.* 29,90.

[78] Xiong M, Jiang L, Zhou Y, Qiu W, Fang L, et al. (2012). The miR-200 family regulates TGF-beta1-induced renal tubular epithelial to mesenchymal transition through Smad pathway by targeting ZEB1 and ZEB2 expression. *Am J Physiol Renal Physiol* 302, F369-79.

[79] Gerlinger M, Rowan AJ, Horswell S, Larkin J, Endesfelder D, et al. (2012). Intratumor heterogeneity and branched evolution revealed by multiregion sequencing. *N. Engl. J. Med* . 366,883-92.

[80] Sato M, Nakai Y, Nakata W, Yoshida T, Hatano K, et al. (2013). EMMPRIN promotes angiogenesis, proliferation, invasion and resistance to sunitinib in renal cell carcinoma, and its level predicts patient outcome. *PLoS One* 8,e74313.

[81] Biswas C, Zhang Y, DeCastro R, Guo H, Nakamura T, et al. 1995. The human tumor cell-derived collagenase stimulatory factor (renamed EMMPRIN) is a member of the immunoglobulin superfamily. *Cancer Res.* 55,434-9.

[82] Guo H, Majmudar G, Jensen TC, Biswas C, Toole BP, Gordon MK. 1998. Characterization of the gene for human EMMPRIN, a tumor cell surface inducer of matrix metalloproteinases. *Gene* 220,99-108.

[83] Gabison EE, Hoang-Xuan T, Mauviel A, Menashi S. (2005). EMMPRIN/CD147, an MMP modulator in cancer, development and tissue repair. *Biochimie* 87,361-8.

[84] Zhu P, Ding J, Zhou J, Dong WJ, Fan CM, Chen ZN. (2005). Expression of CD147 on monocytes/macrophages in rheumatoid arthritis, its potential role in monocyte accumulation and matrix metalloproteinase production. *Arthritis. Res. Ther.* 7,R1023-33.

[85] Nabeshima K, Iwasaki H, Koga K, Hojo H, Suzumiya J, Kikuchi M. (2006). Emmprin (basigin/CD147), matrix metalloproteinase modulator and multifunctional cell recognition molecule that plays a critical role in cancer progression. *Pathol. Int.* 56,359-67.

[86] Kanekura T, Chen X, Kanzaki T. (2002). Basigin (CD147) is expressed on melanoma cells and induces tumor cell invasion by stimulating production of matrix metalloproteinases by fibroblasts. *Int. J. Cancer* 99,520-8.

[87] Tang Y, Nakada MT, Kesavan P, McCabe F, Millar H, et al. (2005). Extracellular matrix metalloproteinase inducer stimulates tumor angiogenesis by elevating vascular endothelial cell growth factor and matrix metalloproteinases. *Cancer Res.* 65,3193-9.

[88] Liang YX, He HC, Han ZD, Bi XC, Dai QS, et al. (2009). CD147 and VEGF expression in advanced renal cell carcinoma and their prognostic value. *Cancer Invest.* 27,788-93.

[89] Misra S, Ghatak S, Zoltan-Jones A, Toole BP. (2003). Regulation of multidrug resistance in cancer cells by hyaluronan. *J. Biol. Chem.* 278,25285-8.

[90] Marieb EA, Zoltan-Jones A, Li R, Misra S, Ghatak S, et al. (2004). Emmprin promotes anchorage-independent growth in human mammary carcinoma cells by stimulating hyaluronan production. *Cancer Res.* 64,1229-32.

[91] Ciuffreda L, Di SC, Incani UC, Milella M. (2010). The mTOR pathway, a new target in cancer therapy. *Curr. Cancer Drug Targets* 10,484-95.

[92] Zhu AX, Meyerhardt JA, Blaszkowsky LS, Kambadakone AR, Muzikansky A, et al. (2010). Efficacy and safety of gemcitabine, oxaliplatin, and bevacizumab in advanced biliary-tract cancers and correlation of changes in 18-fluorodeoxyglucose PET with clinical outcome, a phase 2 study. *Lancet Oncol.* 11,48-54.

[93] Bender C, Ullrich A. (2012). PRKX, TTBK2 and RSK4 expression causes Sunitinib resistance in kidney carcinoma- and melanoma-cell lines. *Int. J. Cancer* 131,E45-55.

[94] Li X, Hyink DP, Polgar K, Gusella GL, Wilson PD, Burrow CR. (2005). Protein kinase X activates ureteric bud branching morphogenesis in developing mouse metanephric kidney. *J Am Soc Nephrol* 16,3543-52.

[95] Di PG, Stacey SN. 1998. Adeno-associated virus Rep78 protein interacts with protein kinase A and its homolog PRKX and inhibits CREB-dependent transcriptional activation. *J. Virol.* 72,7916-25.

[96] Saha B, Singh SK, Sarkar C, Bera R, Ratha J, et al. (2006). Activation of the Mitf promoter by lipid-stimulated activation of p38-stress signalling to CREB. *Pigment Cell Res.* 19,595-605.

[97] Davis IJ, Hsi BL, Arroyo JD, Vargas SO, Yeh YA, et al. (2003). Cloning of an Alpha-TFEB fusion in renal tumors harboring the t(6,11)(p21,q13) chromosome translocation. *Proc. Natl. Acad. Sci. U S A* 100,6051-6.

[98] Argani P, Antonescu CR, Illei PB, Lui MY, Timmons CF, et al. (2001). Primary renal neoplasms with the ASPL-TFE3 gene fusion of alveolar soft part sarcoma, a distinctive tumor entity previously included among renal cell carcinomas of children and adolescents. *Am. J. Pathol.* 159,179-92.

[99] Gotink KJ, Broxterman HJ, Labots M, de HRR, Dekker H, et al. (2011). Lysosomal sequestration of sunitinib, a novel mechanism of drug resistance. *Clin. Cancer Res.* 17,7337-46.

[100] Broxterman HJ, Gotink KJ, Verheul HM. (2009). Understanding the causes of multidrug resistance in cancer, a comparison of doxorubicin and sunitinib. *Drug Resist. Updat.* 12,114-26.

[101] Saftig P, Klumperman J. (2009). Lysosome biogenesis and lysosomal membrane proteins, trafficking meets function. *Nat. Rev. Mol. Cell Biol.* 10,623-35.

[102] Goodman VL, Rock EP, Dagher R, Ramchandani RP, Abraham S, et al. (2007). Approval summary, sunitinib for the treatment of imatinib refractory or intolerant gastrointestinal stromal tumors and advanced renal cell carcinoma. *Clin. Cancer Res.* 13,1367-73.

[103] Strieter RM, Burdick MD, Mestas J, Gomperts B, Keane MP, Belperio JA. (2006). Cancer CXC chemokine networks and tumor angiogenesis. *Eur. J. Cancer* 42,768-78.

[104] Brat DJ, Bellail AC, Van MEG. (2005). The role of interleukin-8 and its receptors in gliomagenesis and tumoral angiogenesis. *Neuro. Oncol.* 7,122-33.

[105] Morais C, Gobe G, Johnson DW, Healy H. (2009). Anti-angiogenic actions of pyrrolidine dithiocarbamate, a nuclear factor kappa B inhibitor. *Angiogenesis* 12,365-79.

[106] Singhal SS, Sehrawat A, Mehta A, Sahu M, Awasthi S. (2009). Functional reconstitution of RLIP76 catalyzing ATP-dependent transport of glutathione-conjugates. *Int. J. Oncol.* 34,191-9.

[107] Singhal SS, Sehrawat A, Sahu M, Singhal P, Vatsyayan R, et al. (2010). Rlip76 transports sunitinib and sorafenib and mediates drug resistance in kidney cancer. *Int. J. Cancer* 126,1327-38.

[108] Rodriguez-Antona C, Garcia-Donas J. (2012). Constitutional genetic variants as predictors of antiangiogenic therapy outcome in renal cell carcinoma. *Pharmacogenomics* 13,1621-33.

[109] van dVAA, Eechoute K, Gelderblom H, Gietema J, Guchelaar HJ, et al. (2011). Genetic polymorphisms associated with a prolonged progression-free survival in patients with metastatic renal cell cancer treated with sunitinib. *Clin. Cancer Res.* 17,620-9.

[110] Garcia-Donas J, Esteban E, Leandro-Garcia LJ, Castellano DE, del AAG, et al. (2011). Single nucleotide polymorphism associations with response and toxic effects in patients with advanced renal-cell carcinoma treated with first-line sunitinib, a multicentre, observational, prospective study. *Lancet Oncol.*12,1143-50.

[111] Beuselinck B, Karadimou A, Couchy G. (2012). A pharmacogenomic scoring system predicting median time to progression (mTTP) on sunitinib (SUN) as first-line treatment in patients (pts) with metastatic renal cell carcinoma (mRCC). Abstarct 359. *J. Clin. Oncol.* 30 (Suppl. 5).

[112] International HapMap Project. www.hapmap.org.

[113] The 1000 Genomes Project. www.1000genomes.org.

[114] Gonzalez LJL, Espinosa E, Garcia CI, Garcia-Donas J, Lopez M, et al. (2012). Sequential therapy in metastatic renal cell carcinoma, pre-clinical and clinical rationale for selecting a second- or subsequent-line therapy with a different mechanism of action. *Cancer Metastasis Rev.* 31 Suppl 1,S11-7.

[115] Ravaud A, Gross-Goupil M. (2012). Overcoming resistance to tyrosine kinase inhibitors in renal cell carcinoma. *Cancer Treat Rev.* 38,996-1003.

[116] 116. Zama IN, Hutson TE, Elson P, Cleary JM, Choueiri TK, et al. (2010). Sunitinib rechallenge in metastatic renal cell carcinoma patients. *Cancer* 116,5400-6.

About the Editor

Dr. Christudas Morais
Research Officer
Centre for Kidney Disease Research, School of Medicine
The University of Queensland Translational Research Institute
37 Kent Street
Brisbane, Queensland, Australia, 4102
Tel: +61 7 3443 8012
e-mail: c.morais@uq.edu.au

Index

A

B

C

D

E

H

K

L

M

N

Q

R

S

T

U

V

W

X

Y

Z